T'ai Chi Ch'uan
The Wellspring Source Book

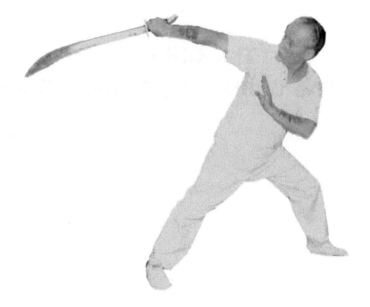

Grandmaster Symonds performing Taiji Dao

T'ai Chi Ch'uan
The Wellspring Source Book.

Written by Shih-Jo Myke Symonds©.
Way of Heaven & Earth™ Taoist School:
Wellspring 'Shadow Boxing' Style™.

Published by Life Force Books, Life Force Publishing.
This First Edition: December 2015.
Paperback: Royal / Laminated Cover / 12 pt text / Illustrated.

ISBN (10): 0-9542932-5-8
ISBN (13): 978-0-9542932-5-3

The titles of the other books in this series so far are (Size in brackets):
*Tai Chi Diet: food for life (Royal)
*Kung Fu – The Way of Heaven & Earth (Royal)
*Qigong & Baduanjin (Royal)
* Practical Philosophy of Tao, for teachers and individuals (Letter)

* [Still to come] K'ai Men – Taoist Yoga_____

Foreword.

Many westerners have heard of something that they call "Tai Chi", a misspelling that has come about by the media or press software being originally unable to add the apostrophe needed in "T'ai". T'ai Chi *Ch'uan*, as is should be, is much, much more than a lazy person's exercise form or slow dance exercise; as many ill-informed people thought it was at first.

The earliest style of T'ai Chi Ch'uan in the UK, as far as we know, was my Old Master's style, the Li Family Style (Li often written as "Lee" as westerners could not understand the pronunciation). Then followed a style based on Yang Style, but truly debased and treated as a "dance" with no meaning! Only when the Chinese Arts became very popular did Chen Style come along, plus a few modern Chinese "Competition style" Forms; again bastardised, but deliberately.

There are Five Major Styles of T'ai Chi Ch'uan recognised by China, Chen, Yang, Wu, Wu/Hao and Sun, but there are literally hundreds of other styles, many of which sadly never see the light of day, so to speak. Factually, some of the unknown styles may be more like the original Forms than some of the mainstream styles, mentioned above. It is the author's educated opinion that the original style, accredited to Ch'eung Sam-feng, was the '13 Methods' but was taught in a way that many newcomers could not quite comprehend, perhaps due to their training in more physical styles of Ch'uan-shu (Chinese Boxing styles). Personalisation followed to suit the recipient and their current style and/or way of doing things. This is very common in Martial Arts and one reason why there are so many styles. History of a factual nature only goes back as far as Chen Style, so much has been lost.

Of course, everyone who has invested time and energy into learning one style likes to think that what they do is "de rigour", the best or the only "real" style. The facts about the original style were never recorded or transmitted, so we do not know.

Jingquanshitaijiquan, or Wellspring Style, is one of the relatively new styles created last century (20th century) but is already causing a stir and gaining much interest. Even a few Chinese, trained in China, have commented on its practicality and that it has "meaning" and "practical applications" in the Form; unlike altered Competition Forms or "People's Tai Chi" from mainland China. In just under one year "you can feel your ch'i developing and flowing within the Form!" said one student "But I never felt any ch'i flow while training in the other style I used to do."

Whether someone chooses to do this style, that style or the other style, there is always something more to learn. Keep an open mind, open heart and open eyes and enjoy the life changing system of Taoist Health that we now know as T'ai Chi Ch'uan.

This subject is dear to me and one I describe as being "as wide as the oceans of Earth, and just like the oceans, most just see the surface but there is a depth and breadth beneath that awaits discovery!"

T'ai Chi Ch'uan is not just exercise; it includes subtle ways of developing the mind and spirit as well as helping stave off diseases and imbalances that can shorten life. Study, practice, learn and enjoy the many benefits.

Dedication and Thanks.

As usual, I thank my Old Taoist Arts Master C. Chee Soo, for his invitation to learn with him in his Teacher's Choi Kung Classes and his guidance and wisdom. Many thanks to my many other guides and mentors, in Kung Fu and Internal Arts, etcetera, making sure that the right information came to me in the best order.

Thanks to my senior student, Shih-Kung Terry Windsor, who has trained with me now for around 38+ years and for the help with my terrible English grammar.

To other senior and long term students, Lou Lloyd, Ian Draycott, Ian England, PJ Whiting and Lynda Lee for their encouragement and good questions: which I always like to hear; asking questions about detailed technique is a good sign of learning! My student's dedication and positive feedback has been a great signpost in my development of the Art.

Thanks also to my many Chinese friends, both in UK and world-wide. They have given me details of the history, current status of places or other important information and have also given me positive feedback regarding my progress with this book and encouragement to put the right information within it. Some have also warned me "do not give Tao away!" However, without certain information being available good students cannot progress. Only those who are dedicated will learn and discover the true secrets! So, with this in mind I have left out some key points which any genuine instructor should be able to teach and composed the book for the discerning students.

Finally, a heartfelt and belated thank you to my parents. When we are young we barely have time for our parents and later regret this. In later life I knew that my mother was proud of what I did and what I achieved. However, my father died when I was in my twenties and it was not until I was almost fifty that I realised that he had suspected at least what my path in life might be; it was my father who mysteriously kept the brass

Snake & Crane aside; found many years after his death. He must have known something, but never said and just showed me unswerving love and trust while he was alive. Being a man that loved Nature I am sure that he would appreciate T'ai Chi Ch'uan and the amazing Taoist Arts.

To you, dear reader, I leave the last message of gratitude. The Taoist Arts are the result of thousands of years of development by hundreds of thousands of dedicated people. The knowledge that I bring you has been brought to me to improve my life. In turn and in the true spirit of Taoism I pass on this knowledge and skills to you so that you may enhance your life, and hoping that in turn you will enhance the lives of at least ten others.

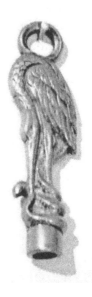

Contents

CONTENTS

Chapter Three

Chapter Four

Chapter Five

Chapter Six

Chapter Seven

Chapter Seven·One

Chapter Eight

WELLSPRING T'AI CHI CH'UAN:

Chapter Eleven

Chapter Twelve

Chapter Thirteen

Chapter Fourteen

AIR

A cloud drifts by on sea of air
Corn sways lazily growing fair
The Swallow glides down and by
All in a heated summer sky
Scent is carried to deer that scurry
Breeze ruffles hair when in a hurry
Pollen carried makes us tearful.
The hurricane comes to be so fearful
Sound of a tractor is carried afar, like
Spray and smoke and fumes from car
A man breathes deep in wooded way
Relaxed of mind in T'ai Chi Play.

Chapter One

Introduction to T'ai Chi Ch'uan

Chinese Boxing has been around for centuries. Circumstances such as World War 2 and contact with Japan lead to the discovery of Karate in Europe before we heard of Ch'uan-shu, Wushu or even "Kung Fu", which did not arrive here in UK until 1970-71. Some American troops were astounded by the discovery of both Japanese Ju Jitsu and Chinese Ch'uan-shu when they served around Japan and the South Pacific islands during that war. It must have come as quite a shock to those who were used to western boxing Oriental Arts for the very first time; or even the second!

In the mid to late 1960's Kung Fu hit America. Bruce Lee and a few others followed in the wake of Hong Kong Shaw Brothers movies which depicted fantastic fight scenes, the likes of which had never been seen by most western eyes before. Bruce Lee, who, like my Old Master had one Chinese parent and one western, suddenly showed the west what Chinese people could do and do very well indeed. In his early films he often depicted a racially abused Chinese person who was either fighting back against the Japanese or corrupt westerners. The Chinese movies on the other hand often showed the struggle of the ordinary Chinese person against the abusive Warlord or the Japanese invaders of the sino-asian wars. Many of these films depicted fights to the death, common place in old China but rarely seen in the West since olden days pistol duelling!

Young men, mainly, across America and UK, France, Germany and many other places with TV and cinema, decided that they would like to fight like Bruce Lee, Jackie Chan, Sammo Hung, Bolo, Carter Wong or David Carradine, etcetera. Most failed. The failure was not their fault but sadly a lack of understanding, a lack of technique and an absence of teachers. This spurred an almost tragic wave of imposters. Some men with a little knowledge of Karate or later

Taekwondo decided to don a Black Belt, one they had not earned, and call themselves "Master". A few of these are still around, selling black belt courses at a high price monetarily and sometimes at cost of injury or disillusion to the unwary customer, when many find out that what they have been shown does not work in real self-defence, or that their health or body has been damaged because of it.

All of this is pertinent to the introduction of the "mystical art of Tai Chi" as one scribe put it. I am not sure when it was first screened publicly, apart from a few brief encounters on those early "Chop Suey" movies, as they were unceremoniously nicknamed; often because of the visible wires and other props used. The first book on T'ai Chi Ch'uan in UK, as far as I know, was by an American author, Robert Smith, in coordination with a Chinese Teacher called Cheng, Man Ching. It was not only funny to see someone trying to learn these movements from a book but also quite sad that there were apparently no Chinese teachers of real knowledge over here to correct or help spread these wonderfully promising skills. But there were, as I later discovered when I was invited to Grandmaster C. Chee Soo's 'Teacher Training Classes' in Dunstable.

The problem existed then that many Chinese were going through very difficult times themselves, so had little time to worry about what was going on over in UK, Europe or in USA. Although later, when communications improved, many did make their homes in USA, UK and Europe to teach their beloved family treasures to keen students. Many more died and took their family secrets to the grave.

The situation has come about that China is now trying to renew its traditional Arts. Many traditional Arts and skills had been replaced with a modern programme of Wushu, a mix of Martial arts and Athletics without the traditional philosophy or folklore. This was aimed at promoting competition amongst men and women for "gold", not for self-defence. The traditional Chinese Arts were more often *less* "flowery" or show-off, but were far more practical both for fitness, self-defence and health. This is especially true of T'ai Chi Ch'uan which was developed by Taoist adepts specifically for those needs, not for demonstrations or competitions; Many Chinese people born thirty or so years ago knew nothing of the traditional skills or forms, as they had been banned, the newer Wushu being taught in schools in their place alongside various propaganda and brain-washing. Imagine their surprise when some of them discovered that the western world not only had "real Kung Fu" but that some of the teachers were western too. This induced another change in China and the authorities decided to call Wushu 'Kung Fu' instead, which has caused much confusion since.

Further to all of these changes and confusion many people in the western world thought at first that T'ai Chi Ch'uan was just another Martial Art, and not that it had great depth behind it in the form of the Philosophy of Tao. As you will see from reading this little book all the way through, it is an Art, it is wide, deep and very profound; although one does not have to study all aspects to enjoy the many benefits of health or even self-defence. However, even such "surface study" can have a profound effect on the practitioner's life and create changes in the way we live almost sub-consciously. The calmness of the movements, the rhythm, flow and necessary relaxation all has a good effect. Being built around the philosophy of TAO, with its Yin and Yang, expansion and contraction, action and reaction, etcetera, the movements are all designed to reproduce these elements within the human body and mind.

This book is aimed at the serious student of Jingquanshitaijiquan and is most useful when thinking about the various lessons learned in the classes. It is a reference point, guide and serves to provide more in-depth information than is possible in the average class. Considering that, the book's overall content may be useful to students of other styles, as long as they have a good teacher. The teacher is necessary to observe posture, progress, mistakes and even energy levels. It is not possible to learn T'ai Chi Ch'uan from a book; or even a video. Postures have to be correct, as do attitudes and awareness. It can take many years to learn on Form (set of movements) from beginning to end, then even more to do it properly. It may take many westerners longer than many Chinese, for example, because of the differences in lifestyle, body build, in-built attitude to physical tasks or posture. The mind has to be trained and the body changed in a sort of metamorphosis that gives the practitioner a new wave of life as a proverbial butterfly, rather than a slow and clumsy caterpillar. The joy of T'ai Chi Ch'uan is not confined to physical health and more fluid or adroit movements, it is also a source of great joy, feelings of well-being and mental calmness leading to observation and much more. It is a journey on a path – The Way – Tao.

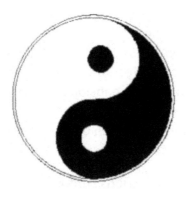

Spelling Notes.

Due to the fact that there have been changes introduced to the Chinese language last century, there are now two commonly used systems of language in use, the traditional or Mandarin, plus the new simplified and Pinyin.

In traditional Chinese the popular Taoist Boxing would have been written as 太極拳, meaning "Supreme Ultimate Fist"; fist can refer, as it does here, to any method of exercise based around self-defence applications whether Martial or Health and self-protection based. This was Romanized by Wade Giles as "T'ai Chi Ch'uan" in English; Anglicised pronunciation. Modern Chinese Simplified uses the same Chinese characters (太極拳) but is written in Pinyin as "Taijiquan", the three words being joined together. The actual pronunciation of this in English varies from person to person, but should sound something like "Tie-chee-chewann" or "Tei-jee-chewahn". This is influenced by different regional accents in China, such as Guangdong (Cantonese) or Peking (Mandarin), the equivalent in England to what they used to call "Queen's English" (well pronounced) or a "broad" Norfolk dialect, for example.

The exercises known as 氣功 in Traditional Chinese, or 气功 in Simplified Chinese is pronounced as "Chee gong "or "Chee kung", regardless. The Wade Giles is written as Ch'i Kung whilst the Modern Pinyin is written as Qigong, respectively.

There are far too many Chinese words or names used in this book to explain all here so both or just one may be used. The reader is urged to lean one pronunciation, either traditional or modern, and learn to use this for each reference. In T'ien Ti Tao or Tiandidao, we use mainly traditional but will use modern Pinyin if it helps in visual writing or web search facilities.

What most people call "Tai Chi" is just relaxing, slow exercise. T'ai Chi *Ch'uan* or *Taijiquan* is the full programme with many layers.

Most people in the western world who have never studied anything "eastern" could be forgiven for thinking that all Martial Arts are alike, or worse still, that they are all like the fight scenes that we see in elaborate films, with people swinging on wires, etcetera. Nothing could be further from the truth.

Styles and Categories.

There are "styles" which emanated from military training. These were mainly used to train guards or Special Forces, such as an Emperor's Elite Guard Unit, although infantrymen would also be trained in spear, staff, archery and other weapons too.

There are family styles too. These were often created by the need to protect themselves from marauding bandits, bad soldiers or just thieves. Family style depended on and was shaped by what the practitioner had learned before.

Other styles may have been influenced by many people over many years. This is certainly the case for what is generically called Shaolin Ch'uan nowadays. The original Shao-lin (Young Forest) Monastery in the Song-shan region was a retreat. Many people stayed there as either a resting place on their travels or literally to "retreat" from their normal lives. Amongst many notable characters that stayed there were travelling guards, ex-soldiers, transcontinental sight-seers and people such as the notorious Lo-han, a bandit of sorts. Even Lo-han contributed to a style of fighting at Shaolin and, somewhat surprising to many, a vegetarian dish now sometimes found in Chinese Takeaways! At various times people travelled between Shaolin, Wudang and other well-known centres for Chinese Boxing practitioners to meet up, stay and exchange ideas. Ch'eung Sam-feng stayed there and learned the original Five Animals style associated with Shaolin Ssu. Eventually the Shaolin Ssu became a place for Buddhists to gather, live and study, so developing a set of styles that suited their philosophy and way of life.

Wudangshan or Wu Tang Shan is another great place of repute. You will read more detailed descriptions of Wudang later on in this book, but suffice to say it was a famous centre for the study of Tao and Taoism, so gaining its own reputation for Taoist Kung Fu styles.

The word "style" separates one school from another. Each style may be influenced by need, previous learning, philosophy or belief and the desire to imitate animals, such as Crane, Snake, Tiger, Panther, Dog or Monkey, to name a few.

T'ai Chi Ch'uan is not a "martial" style. It is a style which is influenced by a philosophy, the philosophy of Tao, to be precise. Again, this subject is covered in greater depth later in this book. The history of Chinese Boxing for self-defence, the belief in imitating animals for keeping healthy tissues and internal organs, plus the desire to have and exercise which follows the Taoist principles all helped mould the style we call T'ai Chi Ch'uan. However, this was further influenced by personal preference or previous training and then re moulded into new styles; Chen, Yang, Wu, Li, Sun, etcetera.

There are so many styles of T'ai Chi Ch'uan in China alone that nobody has been able to count them all. Add to this the even larger number of schools or styles of Chinese Martial arts and we have a staggering picture of the diversity of Chinese Boxing. The Chinese Communist Government or CCG tried to alter this at one stage and replace all traditional styles with modern variants. This has not helped, and now added to the confusion!

The average person who gets involved with T'ai Chi Ch'uan usually does so because they wish to improve their health, learn to relax and rid their body of tensions or just try it out of curiosity. On finding that it is not that easy to learn, requiring great concentration and patience, many drop out. A few may like this and get a little deeper into the skills, enjoying a challenge and reaping more benefits. For those few there are other aspects that await them, exploration, discoveries and new skills to learn and master. That is where the beauty of T'ai Chi Ch'uan lays.

Note on Wellspring T'ai Chi Ch'uan:

Ching-chuan T'ai Chi Ch'uan (Jingquanshitaijiquan) serves as a introduction and compressed essential Form. It contains "pure" principles or forms; as perhaps intended by the "founder" of Taoist Internal Arts, Ch'eung Sam Feng (Cheng San-feng).

Please note: The early Mandarin Romanized - e.g. T'ai Chi Ch'uan - is shown at first but then later Romanized (Taijiquan) is shown in brackets and then used alternately throughout this book as it has become more common. This is simply because the newer, Romanization is said to represent the pronunciation more accurately; i.e. Taiji = "Tai-jee" or "Tai-chi". You can get used to both.

T'IEN TI TAO KUOSHU

T'ien Ti Tao was "officially" founded in 1975 by Shih-Jo Mike Symonds after many years of study and basic development. Then in mid-1985 tested over two years plus and then accepted by China (ICKF, R.o. China) as "Genuine traditional Chinese Arts" in 1987. After years of intense study, development and trial of traditional techniques the improvements and testing continue. Covering exercise to self-defence, T'ai Chi to healing therapies, the Arts include all aspects of daily life. T'IEN TI TAO has been proven in self-defence as a system with control built in. It is not necessary for a skilful person to cause "excess" damage to his/her attacker - though very positive results are required.

T'IEN TI TAO KUOSHU P'AI has been favourably featured in *COMBAT, FIGHTERS, FIGHTING ARTS INTERNATIONAL, FIGHTING

FOCUS and INSIDE KUNG-FU (USA), and latterly F.A.I., Martial Arts Illustrated, and Kung Fu International since around 1979 onwards.

Shih-fu Mike Symonds has been registered in R.o. China (Taiwan: ICKF) and P.R.o. China (Peking), England (BKPA & AMA) and was appointed East Anglian Representative for Kuoshu (Kung Fu) with both associations. He developed fighting skills when young and began training seriously in the mid-sixties. He studied popular Eastern philosophies and as many forms of Eastern Arts as were possible including Kempo, Yoga and Meditations Skills. In late 1974 he was invited by Grand-master C. Chee Soo to join Teacher's Training classes in T'ai Chi Ch'uan (Taijiquan), Ch'i Kung (Qigong), Taoist Yoga (K'ai Men), Defence & Healing Arts.

Kuoshu means, Kuo = China, Shu = Arts; historically taken as Traditional Chinese Arts which includes study of the "Five Excellences".

Now dear reader, now you can appreciate just what T'ai Chi Ch'uan is, read on and discovers some of the depth and breadth of the Art so that you too may appreciate and explore it more fully.

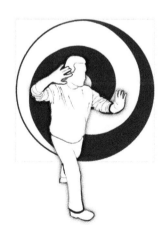

Chapter Two.
The Wealth of Taoist Arts

FINDING TAO

Follow The Way
And you will find home,
The path is wide,
The view complete.

Atop highest mountain
You'll sit alone,
But in the Market Place
Your friends you meet.

_____

Shih-fu Myke Symonds. c.1997.

The Wealth of Taoist Arts

There are few places in the world where there is a dedicated area, the size of Wales almost, that specialise in the practice and development of health and spiritually related skills. Wu Tang is such a place. There are no other countries in the world like China. The Chinese are a unique race of people whose collective spirit is likened to a Dragon. The inventions that have arisen from the Chinese cultural mind are phenomenal, not only that, most form the proverbial backbone of western society and its needs: e.g. banknotes, spectacles, gunpowder, irrigation methods, takeaway foods, speedometer, kites, fireworks and many, many more commonly accepted things.

Many people see China as a developing country, but this is not really accurate. It was developed, both culturally and technically, many hundreds of years ago when people in my home county of Norfolk were still running around with Wode on their faces, trying to look scary! Well, it certainly upset the Romans, but nobody else. It is said that the Chinese discovered the world, and mapped it, in 1421: a book by Gavin Menzies – 1421 The Year the Chinese Discovered the World.

In Chapter Six you will read how Dr Hua not only developed Acupuncture, but used it in a live heart swap over 700 years before Christ was born. Medicine and healing in China was far in advance of anything else in the world. Natural remedies were used in the main, but surgery was not unheard of.

The great Yellow Emperor decreed that he would help his people, and so he did. Not only did he introduce new ways of farming, irrigation and crop planting but also extolled the virtues of harmony, in marriage as well as in the country. He gathered information on Taoist practises, wisdom and humanitarian ways from all over China: an awesome task in those days with no air travel, phones or

Internet! Sexism was something that was virtually unknown. Men and women worked together to create a better society, an equal society. They looked up to their wise leader who had indeed set them free and helped them to enjoy life in a more natural way.

So, if China had all this then, what happened? What went wrong and why have there been so much conflict, death and destruction of the society which was so far advanced? The "revolution" was probably the main factor. When someone comes along with "new ideas" and declares that anyone with old ideals will be punished or killed, if they do not declare allegiance, then change can be bad. It is said that 36,000,000 people died during the 'Cultural Revolution' of Chairman Mao. Traditions were banned, as was folklore, history and any part of the old traditional culture. It is always a sad indictment of humans that the majority suffer because of the minority. The vast majority of Chinese people are intelligent, warm, friendly and try to live harmonious lives whilst not interfering with others.

Many people fled to Taiwan (Formosa) or other parts of the world to escape the death threats and "ghost squads" that came to take people from their homes in the middle of the night. Many stories came out of China about firing squads, vital organs being removed whilst sill conscious and before bleeding to death, and worse. Some of these innocent people were old, some young, male or female. It did not matter. The revolutionists forced change and what was left of Chinese Culture was about to be changed too.

Wudang Mountains was not immune. Temples and historic places of study were smashed, burned and destroyed. Anyone who resisted was also destroyed by the new army of the People's Republic of China (CPR). Change lasted for many decades, and now it is changing again. Industry and wealth are the goals now.

Some of the old cultural ways, only those deemed harmless but attractive to tourism or business, are allowed to resurface. This change, oddly enough, was brought about by the western demands for Chinese culture and this was really propagated in the west by the love of Chinese Martial Arts. Another irony as Bruce Lee was part American, but gave us all insight into something deep, mysterious and awe inspiring. This lead to the TV series called 'Kung Fu' starring David Carradine and ten many "Chop Suey" movies from Hong Kong. Here we are today with an insatiable thirst for all things Chinese, whether they be Martial arts or Mobile Phones!

China is re-emerging. The Phoenix rises from the ashes, again. The indomitable spirit of the greater Chinese people is once again leading the way. Many "traditional" Arts are re-emerging too, albeit slightly cautiously, like a tortoise slowly seeing if it is safe to stick its neck out.

The Wudang Mountains are now a thriving destination for tourists. Among those tourists are people wanting to stay there a while and learn something of the Taoist Arts. What is it that is so special about Tao, Taoism and the Taoist Arts?

You will see more in a later chapter that will help you to see just how special the place is, but let us look at the quintessential ingredient that makes Wudang what it is, health. Better health is something that everyone wants, at some stage, especially when they become ill! In Wudang Mountains live many people who study, practice and research health issues. This has happened in that area since before the first temple was built. With health comes the promise of longevity. Who in their right minds would not want to live a longer, healthier and therefore happier life?

It has not been uncommon to hear stories; many well documented, about old people who study Taoist ways living to 130, 150, 180 or more years. Their secrets are not really secrets at all. They lived in cleaner environments, ate natural herbs and drank pure spring water, worked all day and trained in special exercises, like Qigong and Taijiquan.

What is so special about Taijiquan and Qigong?

These exercises have not only been around for many hundreds of years, but have been developed by Doctors, Generals and others who are and were very well studied in these matters. A

Most Chinese systems are what you might call "specialist" subjects and nothing like common or garden fitness regimes found in the western hemisphere of the past two or three centuries. Most exercise system are very basic, "pump and grunt", as someone once called them. Weight lifting, running, aerobics and even most popular sports have very little scientific input, save for sport strategies. When talking about "scientific input" I mean in the development. Most Qigong (Energy Training) exercises are developed for medical reasons. Anyone familiar with the principles of Acupuncture will have heard of Qi (Ch'i – in old Pinyin Mandarin) and of how it is controlled using Acupuncture needles on certain points along the Meridians or "energy channels": like this one below, showing only the lower arm part of the Triple Burner energy channel.

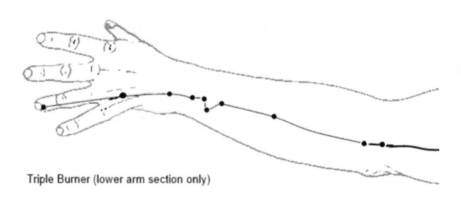

Triple Burner (lower arm section only)

In most Qigong exercises the energy channels are "tuned" by specific movements, combined with breathing, that will both open and regulate channels. There are many Medical Qigong exercises that are designed specifically to correct energy flow that has either become "blocked" or "out of control". There are many terms to describe various symptoms, like "weak" or "damp heat", etcetera that would only be understood by a well-trained Chinese Medical practitioner. They may treat with acupuncture to give immediate effect but also prescribe qigong exercises or even dietary and lifestyle changes for a long term effect. This is what we call TCM – Traditional Chinese Medicine. TCM recognises all factors in life and the diagnosis searches for the cause, not the symptoms. The cause is then treated by appropriate actions, somewhat like a reversal of the cause but using targeted methods. These methods have been proven over many hundreds of years.

Other types of qigong exercise include 'General Health Qigong'. These are also well developed. You can read about a popular exercise called "Baduanjin" in a book written specifically for the subject and part of this series. The book is called 'Qigong and Baduanjin" (by me), Mike Symonds, and can be found in any bookstore list or on-line using that search criteria. You will notice that it has the 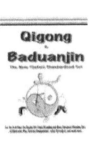 same coloured bars atop the cover pages, grey and gold. This is representative of the old Taoist adage "turning lead into gold" or otherwise "turning base metal into precious metal". This actually refers to the whole purpose of the Taoist Arts and Studies, to change yourself from a basic being into someone healthier, more enlightened and more spiritually in tune with the Universe or Tao.

General health qigong, performed on a regular basis, and accompanied by a cleaner diet, can change your life quite dramatically: as many past students have found to their delight. There are many different exercises know around China and the world, but the uniqueness of Baduanjin is that it a set of eight exercises, done eight times each, that combine to make a superb health routine and is tested by time and millions of people. The name in English is "Eight Strands of Silk Brocade". Chinese people traditionally used to wear fine silk brocade clothing for special occasions, this would make them feel good, feel special. So it is that Baduanjin also makes you feel special, hence the adopted nickname.

In much the same way as qigong exercises were developed for medical practice or general health reasons, Taijiquan was developed by Taoists who were seeking the right kind of exercise that was in harmony with their principles. The nature of Taoism is to study Tao, the Way of Nature: or as I call it "Life, The Universe and everything!" If one is trying to become more natural, then natural exercise is a good idea.

How Do We Define 'Natural Exercise'?
Good question. Oh you are on the ball! If you look at the animal kingdom, as many old Taoists did, you will see that they run, climb, swing, leap, stretch, massage, move with stealth or fast but relaxed. So it was deemed that they do not use weights, artificial equipment or anything else that is "unnatural". The species that we call Human is also animal. However, most human animals tend to stray off the path of naturalness. Just look at your diet, your clothing materials, your home and your environment and see how much is "natural".

Following the examples of many animals, the studiers concluded that a mixture of what they do should also be good for human animals to stay fit, healthier and even defend oneself. So the early exercises were devised. Further observation told them that these types of exercise were good to do, for not only did they work externally (muscle and sinew, etc.) but they also worked internally too. So history was made and Qigong started on a long upwards curve of development.

The same applied to Taoist Boxing Exercises. Animal antics were copied alongside more conventional human responses, like punching or tripping. None was more famous than the Shaolin Five

Animals Set: the original one which was "lost", not the one you may find today, made up to replace it. The original Set was learned by a gentleman with the family name of Ch'eung. As you will read later, he is said to have developed the first T'ai Chi Ch'uan Form that was "complete" in terms of essential elements that are now collectively known as "T'ai Chi Ch'uan" or "Taijiquan. The Well-spring Form uses some of these original tributes, like the coiling Snake or flapping Crane style movements. Over the centuries, since the first style of this type was developed, it has become the most popular form of exercise in the world, bar none. There must be good reason for this, of course. If I sang its praises in copious words, you might be forgiven for thinking that I was just trying to sell it to you. No, I have had more than my fair share of leading proverbial horses to water! You go out and find someone you know who practises Taijiquan on a regular, daily basis, and then ask them how it makes them feel.

University Studies.
Harvard University has been a leading light in recent years. There they have conducted experiments which are monitored to discover the health giving claims about Taijiquan. One article begins "Tai chi is often described as 'meditation in motion', but it might well be called "*medication* in motion." There is growing evidence that this mind-body practice, which originated in China ... has value in treating or preventing many health problems. And you can get started even if you aren't in top shape or the best of health."

Their studies go on to give sterling advice, like checking with your doctor if you have musculoskeletal problems, suffer from dizziness or balance problems, for example. No hesitation here in suggesting that any reader unsure of what he or she should do should visit their page and read the advice: http://www.health.harvard.edu/staying-healthy/the-health-benefits-of-tai-chi

Medical conditions that have been tested and said to be helped by doing this form of exercise are:
o Heart Condition

o Arthritis
o Breast Cancer
o Hypertension
o Stress and PTSD
o Stroke
o Sleep difficulty
o Parkinson's disease
o Low bone density and more.

It has also been stated that for healthy adults Taijiquan can help aspects of mental health such as concentration or attention, thinking, learning or retaining memory, perception and special awareness, to name a few. In learning we have to learn movements that may be unusual to most in everyday life. Then we have to retain that memory by concentration and practice. This process produces a deeper state of concentration than most people use in the normal course of everyday life or work.

The Letchworth Centre for Healthy Living in UK also states the positive benefits of practising Taijiquan on a regular basis. "Better physical and mental health statuses, lower blood pressure, less mood disturbance, more positive mood states than those who did not practice T'ai Chi' in a study of 80 community-dwelling Taiwanese aged 65-88, 40 of whom practiced T'ai Chi, and 40 of whom did not" to quote one of their research articles.

They use a quote from Georgia University who discovered that "Young people: significant improvement in general health, vitality, perceptions of mental health (in 'Effects of T'ai Chi exercise on physical and mental health of college students' , Department of Physical Therapy, Georgia State University, Atlanta, Georgia, 2004)," This is of as great importance as research on older people, especially in these modern days of poor diet, use of drugs, mental health issues and a lack of focus on personal development in many young people.

Stanford Prevention Research Centre, School of Medicine, Stanford University, Stanford, California, (2006) reported that "Psychosocial status, mood and stress of ethnic minority group: significant improvement in mood state, reduction in perceived stress, self-confidence, and in all measures of psychosocial status (in 'Change in perceived psychosocial status' following a 12-week T'ai Chi exercise programme." This is great news for anyone of an "ethnic minority" who considers himself or herself to be an outcast, not as worthy as others or just plain "brow beaten" as we call it in the West. Personally I would like to see more "mixed race" groups practising Taijiquan, feeling better about themselves, improving life and meeting new friends too. This could have an effect on the social separation that tends to go on far too much nowadays. If more people made an effort to say "Hello" to strangers, of any race, then the mood in the streets would change for the better.

PTSD is one of the conditions that would benefit from daily practice of Taijiquan. For those who do not understand what PTSD is, but may have heard much about it in the news, it is this. The human mind is as prone to injury as any part of the physical anatomy. Whereas physical "trauma" can occur with a sudden accident, the mind can be "injured" by a sudden shock. Many war veterans have experienced such things as they witnessed horrific sights that they were not trained to expect. Many close relatives are affected for life by the sudden and unexpected loss of a loved one, perhaps in a shooting or bombing. Other people may be traumatised by unexpected events in many other ways, such as being falsely accused or even arrested for something that they are not guilty of. Trauma is not something which "heals" easily or will "go away after a year or two". The mind is further disturbed by what are called "triggers". These triggers are sights, sounds, television programmes or even titles such as "Falsely Accused", "The Horrors of War" or "Psycho". Sounds, such as explosions, sirens or other sounds that represent the "event" are also triggers. Other factors may be sight related, such as uniforms, vehicles, fires or dead bodies.

The effects of trauma may never go away. Taijiquan can help by giving the victim something to concentrate on, a new focus. It will also give a feeling of wellbeing, calm and being centred. The longer, more traditional Forms would be of more help here. As the Forms are usually longer, taking longer to learn: so giving more to focus on. The traditional Forms usually have other aspects to learn as well, such as Taiji Staff or Taiji Sword, thus giving even more to occupy the mind as well as even more health giving effects.

The benefits of Taijiquan are many, yet there are still many people in the world who could be helped to overcome their problems by taking up this beautiful exercise form for the body, internal energies and the mind. An old friend of mine has a favourite saying, "Procrastination is the thief of time!" How true that is. Never put off something as important as health issues, no matter how small you may perceive them to be at the time. O out and join a reputable Taijiquan class and do it this week!

How Do I Find A Class?
The obvious first method of choice for most people nowadays is searching the World Wide Web or "Internet" as many call it. Use search terms that are local, but also look for the most important factors on their websites.

- Experience. An old Chinese saying goes "It takes ten years to make a teacher. Twenty to make a good one!" The reason for this is that Taijiquan is a complex subject and takes time to learn, so therefore longer to know well enough to teach.
- Qualifications. These are not de rigor in Chinese Arts, but it is traditional at least to issue a new Student-Instructor with a letter of introduction. Grade books going back to the acclaimed 'Master' or his school may be seen more in the West. Beware as there are many frauds out there claiming to teach "Tai Chi" of sorts.
- Websites. Many of the abovementioned fakes may have a website where they are stated as being a 'Master' or

'Grandmaster' of 'Tai Chi', etcetera. There may be no mention of lineage (who they learned from) or even a mention of someone unheard of that is also not "linked", so untraceable. You do not have to learn from an old Chinese Master, but there should always be some creditable reference to a qualified or experienced higher-level teacher.

- Ask! Go to look at a class. A creditable teacher will not mind you watching or taking part. They should also be glad of any potential new student who asks questions, giving good answers or even demonstrating certain points.
- Talk to friends, or friends of friends. There may be some who are still participating in classes, or have done but have stopped going for some reason, such as work or family pressures (the wrong thing to do!) and can recommend a good instructor.
- This book. Look carefully. This book has a lot of information pertaining to both Taijiquan and the history or foundations of it. This information can be used to find a reputable school.
- Tai Chi for Health. This is a phrase I coined around 2001, but is now being used widely by others. It usually refers to a "Simplified Form" or otherwise modified style, like "Tai Chi for Diabetes" as taught by Dr. Paul Lam. These classes can be a great way to be introduced to the true Art of Taijiquan and many newcomers go on to learn more traditional styles afterwards. Again, qualifications are important. For over four years I studied the "Tai Chi for Arthritis" system and still have the teacher's certificates to prove it: just like my old Grade Books from Professor C. Chee Soo's teacher training classes; you never discard such things as they are important.
- Finally. Try a local, or not so local, Health Centre. People in health centres may know of a reputable school or group. However, be prepared to travel. You will be quite unlikely to get lucky enough to have the ideal group on your doorstep. Our school has students who travel 20-30 miles to get to the classes. Never rule out the possibility though that there may just be something closer to home, so check out local Community Centres, Sports or Health Clubs too.

Chapter Three

武當山
Wu Tang Shan

Five Peaks Mountains.

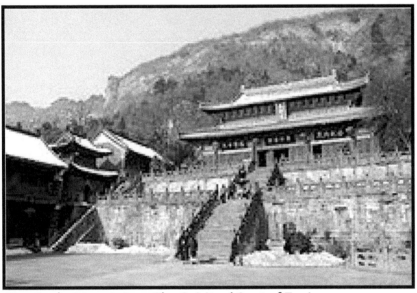

Five Peaks Mountains - The Spiritual Seat of Taoism

My Old Taoist Master, when asked about how we attain the right "shape" in life (Tao) and T'ai Chi Ch'uan replied, "A great sculptor starts with a huge lump of crude hewn rock. The rock is slowly chipped away by the sculptor, removing everything which is unnecessary, finally revealing the true beauty of the Form."

History of Wu Tang.

Wu Tang (Wudang) is located in the Province of Hubei, roughly central in China. The mountain range and Taoist complex are to be found in the North-West corner of the area, situated near to Shi Yan (堰Shiyan) City; geographical map location 320 38 0 N, 1100 48 0 E.

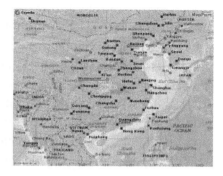

The Taoist Complex began work in the period Tang Dynasty (618-907). During the reign of Emperor Taizong (birth name Zhao Kuangye), the Five Dragon Ancestral Temple was built.

In the Ming Dynasty (1368-1644), about 33 palaces and structures including the Yuxu Palace, the Grand Purple Cloud Palace, the Yuzhen Palace and the Palace of Harmony were all built around this time. The magnificent complex was formed. It covers an area of 400 kilometres around (400 km = 248.548 miles, the equivalent of a journey from Paddington Station in West London to Truro in West Cornwall, if in a straight line!) This idea of scale and size came as surprise to me when I worked it out, no doubt it would cause you some surprise too. The dotted line represents the whole mountain area, *approximately*, it may be much wider!

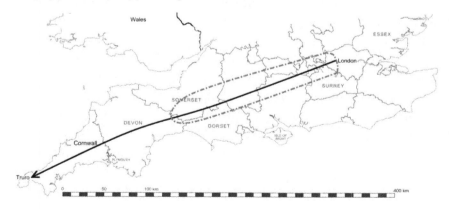

Wu Tang Mountain is also called Taihe Mountain, sometimes Canshang Mountain. It offers a spectacular 800 miles of most beautiful scenery with secluded valleys and picturesque peaks on which are built many "temples" that are designed to complement the landscape and blend in. There are actually around 72 peaks, the tallest being The Sky Pillar at 1612 Metres. The mountains are interlaced by 24 streams, about 11 large caves, many rock-pools and ponds. The forest is home to over 600 known herbs used for health and healing. The main peak is called Tianzhu, which translates as "Heavenly Master", and was the Chinese word used by the Jesuit China missions to designate God. Tianzhu Peak and has an elevation of 1,612 meters. The other peaks surround it and the peaks and streams are very special sights which are enjoyed by many thousands of tourists from China and the rest of the world every year.

The vast complex houses many students of Taoism in every respect. Their main work and studies include Health Longevity methods, natural agriculture, diet, Chinese Martial Arts, medicine and healing (including Ch'i Kung for health and healing), meditation, spiritual development and philosophical study. The Wu Tang complex is truly amazing both as a feat of building engineering and as a dedicated centre for the study of one philosophy, obviously considered to be the most important as no other centre of this size or complexity exists for any other religions or beliefs - at least that I have ever heard of - and far larger even than Vatican City, the centre for the Catholic church. The fact which lodges most in my mind is the 'Golden Top' building as this was obviously included deliberately by the builders and planners as a method of attracting the inevitable lightning strikes to one spot and earthing them out; otherwise they could strike any of the other buildings resulting in major fatalities and damage to structures. This ancient piece of engineering is so simple yet so clever (situated on highest peak, on the left of the image shown below.

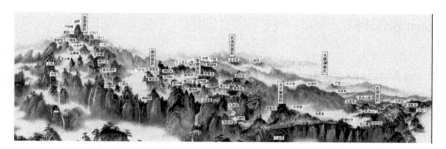

This beautifully painted map (author unknown) viewed from the Western perspective) shows the Wu Tang layout. Far left,: Golden Top. The next upright banner to the right marks the Purple Cloud Temple and on the next high point is Five Dragon Temple. The calligraphy at the very bottom of the picture, one third from the right, is the place of the Eight Immortals Temple and at roughly a two o'clock angle from that Lao Tzu Temple then slightly down and right from there Grind Needle Temple. These are some of the most notable spots but are far from everything there.

Seen from the air the Wu Tang complex is vast, the winding roads like giant snakes curling up the mountain sides. The area is largely covered by thick forest with hewn out terrace farms where the community grow food and study agriculture methods. Where there are waterfalls and lakes there are scenes that are so beautiful and photogenic, where there is unmanaged forest it is teaming with nature, monkeys, birds and snakes, etcetera. Thanks are due to the brilliant artist who painted this picture and gave it to the Internet so that we could all appreciate just how vast this area is.

Modern History.

Wudang Master - Xu Benshan (本善 1860-1932). Born in Ba County, Henan Province. 15th generation of Quanzhen Longmen Pai (真龙门派;. Complete Perfection Dragon Gate Lineage/School) and revered Abbot of the Purple Cloud Temple. Since very young he was educated in the Confucian classics and also studied Chinese medicine and

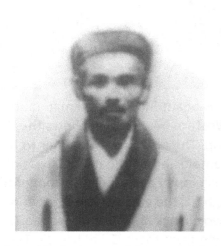

the rudiments of Chinese Martial Arts. His father took him to visit Wudang when he was a boy and many years later, when he was 20 years old, he returned to Wudang and became a disciple under Daoist Masters Wang Fumiao (14th Generation)and Liu Fubao.

For many years he studied the classics of Daoism, medicine and Wudang martial arts. During and after the Communist Cultural Revolution of 1966-1976, the buildings were emptied, damaged and then left in disrepair. According to my source, there were no Wu Tang martial arts being practiced on Wudang Mountain in the early 1980's. This was mostly in part due to the persecution that Wudang suffered during the Cultural Revolution. In the Nationalist Era there was a high-ranking Daoist on Wudang Mountain named Xu Ben Shan. As the Chinese Nationalists (Kuomintang) were fighting the Communists during China's most recent civil war, a Communist regimen leader named He Long suffered a great defeat and the injured who had survived the battle fled to Wudang Mountain. Xu Ben Shan, remaining neutral yet faithful to his beliefs, welcomed the soldiers into the temple and the wounded were cared for. It is also said that Xu Hen Shan and He Long were both accomplished Martial Artists and so the two of them shared their skills with the others. The story of the two of them is recorded in both written Communist history, as well as in Daoist oral history. He Long eventually became known as one of the top ten Communist military leaders, and because of Wudang's connection to this leader, Wudang survived much of the Cultural Revolution with less damage than other sacred sites. Many of the traditional buildings remain to this day. The rest are slowly being rebuilt and reopened.

During the Cultural Revolution (1966-1976) traditional Martial Arts, particularly those related to spiritual traditions, were forbidden. Many Taoists were forced to leave their beloved mountains and hide among the people in the towns and cities. Indeed, many people were killed for having traditional beliefs. A few higher ranked Taoists were allowed to stay at Wu Tang, but were forbidden to accept disciples and share their knowledge. After the end of the Cultural Revolution, the "Cultural Reform" and Opening up of China began. The movement took its time to spread around China, and did not pick up momentum until the early-mid 1980's. In 1980's, the head of the Wudang Daoist Association was Wang Guang De. The Wudang Daoist Association is the organization of all of the Daoist men and women on the mountain, and is not a government organization. The Wu Tang Mountains have since the late 1990's become increasingly popular with tourists from all over China and abroad due to their scenic location and historical interest. The monasteries and buildings were made a UNESCO World Heritage Site in 1994, which has also lead to trails of tourist rubbish there unfortunately as even many modern Chinese seem to have little respect for traditions and places of historic value, just like "modern" people in other countries. Historically it represents the highest standards of Chinese art and architecture over a period of nearly 1,000 years. Noted temples include the Golden Hall, Nanyan (South Cliff) Temple and the famous Purple Cloud Temple.

Taoism, like other beliefs, was banned for several years in the People's Republic of China. Recently, the Central Government of China has supported and encouraged the Association, along with other official religious groups, in promoting the "harmonious society" initiative of President Hu Jintao.

As the Art of T'ai Chi Ch'uan grows in popularity around the world so does the desire for many practitioners to visit its perceived "roots", Wudang area. There is something so special about T'ai Chi Ch'uan that it makes most people feel very humbled by its powers of health giving, levelling or "balancing" and spiritual transformation. The Internet is full of pictures and comments from people who have visited, many who were awe struck by the feelings they got when there. There are now cable cars installed to take visitors to some of the highest spots, but apparently you still have to climb many hundreds of steps to see some of the most worthwhile places; this is reported as being a tearful experience, painful and almost leading to the point of giving up, but compelling and worth it for an experience that is like no other. Of course, feeling that you have made that effort to get to the top must be life changing in itself.

According to my sources, Wu Tang Mountain complex is now quite commercial under the supervision of the new Chinese governing regime, insomuch as taxes and fees have to be paid and that makes everyone responsible to make money. All organisations, temples and the like in China now have to pay their own way, though there may be some slight tax-relief for religious organisations. Apart from the hotels, tea houses and souvenir shops though it is still home to many sincere, genuine Taoists who practice and study with quiet and focused minds amongst the tourist turmoil. As you might expect, if you know the turbulent history of China and the recent destructive past, the mountain and its inhabitants are mainly, but not "entirely", new to both the aspects of Taoism and the practises. By that it is meant that during the 1966 to 1976 period and thereabouts, much heritage and history was wilfully destroyed and lost, deliberately by government directed troops. Only since China opened her proverbial gates to tourism and industry has the opportunity arisen to re-establish Wudang as a seat of important National *and* International heritage.

The aspect of Religious Taoism seems to be prevalent there at the moment, though it is also said that both the religious and practical or "orthodox" aspects seem to merge and blend together, one being barely distinguishable from the other. From my personal studies over the years, it would appear that Wudang was almost tragically and completely lost to the world, then it re-emerged under new rules from the Chinese government in the post-Mao era; If other countries and their governments are anything to go by, only "religious" organisations can receive help to establish centres for practice; and then only under scrutiny and control. Practical Taoism would not qualify, as in practical Taoism or Tao Chia/Daojia there would be no idols, robes or the need for ranking people as priest, abbot, etc. This would not stop the more practical aspects being studied though, so whatever your views, opinions or beliefs, needs, you should still be able to find what you are looking for there. One source tells me that there are still very deep, very traditional practises going on there. Many similar things would be found anywhere else in the world, but perhaps not without a deal of research and effort, but Wu Tang is special.

Note: People often discuss whether Taoism *should* be religious, practical or orthodox. There is no "should" about it as we each see it as what we need. However, it cannot be denied that the original concept of Tao and Taoism was born through observation and philosophy, so therefore it may be stated that the practical aspects came first and were adopted by others later, to create religious or other sects.

In many countries Taoism is still relatively unheard of and even less understood. Many people in the West can be found practising Taoist Arts, to one degree or another, some may be more holistic whilst others may barely know or understand what is behind T'ai Chi Ch'uan, for example.

To me Wu Tang represents not only "the seat of Taoism" but an ideal. It is a symbol of Nature, beauty and dedicated practises and studies that lead to better human life and spiritual enlightenment through becoming more natural, more in harmony with nature, if followed properly. As such I would liken it to a church, where people may go in the hopes that something good will happen to them; or a monastery where those who feel dedicated to spiritual development can live and meditate away from the commercial clap-trap of the so-called modern world; no more modern today as it was 5,000 years ago, apart from technology, that is. Humans have not changed or progressed so well as the gadgets and toys that keep them amused and distracted. Wudang also has not really changed in this respect.

Religion and Tao.

First and foremost a Definition of religion:

Religion: Noun [mass noun] the belief in and worship of a superhuman controlling power, especially a personal God or gods: ideas about the relationship between science and religion [count noun], a particular system of faith and worship: the world's great religions [count noun] a pursuit or interest followed with great devotion: consumerism is the new religion." Oxford Dictionary.

Something often questioned by many lay-people who study Tao is the fact that it is often named as a religion by some but a practical philosophy by others. According to the definition above it seems that it cannot be included under the first category, the "superhuman controlling power" or God version. In recent years the second category has been added to include a faith or system of belief which may be followed in an ordered manner. This could apply, loosely. The third, a "count noun" (A noun that can form a plural and, in the singular, can be used with the indefinite article, e.g., books, a book) is perhaps more fitting; including the witty observation about consumerism.

So it seems that in the modern world, just like the old world, the study of all things to do with Tao is named as a religious practice, something studied with devotion. There are subtle differences though between Taoist beliefs and many others, for example:

• unlike many beliefs Taoism has subjects to practice and study, refine and hone, and all these subjects relate to the same thing or principles.

• Tao studies include diet, herbs and related health matters.

• Tao studies include physical improvement studies, such as yoga, specific "Kung Fu" and other moving exercises designed to improve the body's workings and health.

• Tao studies include mental and spiritual improvement practices, such as meditations, ch'i kung (qigong) and those linked to the physical, like T'ai Chi Ch'uan.

• Tao studies include many practical life skills, like farming, engineering, and relationships, social issues such as morals and manners, etcetera.

• Tao studies include science; many inventions were made by Taoists. One of the most commonly known is Feng Shui ("Fung Shu-ey"), the correct alignments for harmony.

• Tao studies can include medicine, like acupuncture, herbal and dietary corrections, physical corrections and body/mind relationships.

This is what makes Taoism so special and holistic. In our own school we have a holistic syllabus that in itself offers something for many people, whether that is Taoist Yoga, Ch'i Kung, general health, self-defence, philosophical or other study. In Taoism generally we do not hope that the spirit of a kind person will save our soul, or heal us when we fall ill through neglect or disease, Taoists aim for health and longevity by following certain principles with diet, exercise, mental or spiritual guidelines, morals and common sense principles. By studying these things we try to free ourselves from the "clutter" of human errors and or wasted time to become one with Nature and Universal energies. So the Taoist philosophy is more about learning to heal yourself where possible rather than relying on others all the time.

Visiting Wu Tang.

The best way to see Wu Tang (Wudang), for those interested in the Chinese Arts or Chinese people, would be on a training course. These are organised by various groups on Wu Tang and foreigners are welcomed if they have a genuine interest. Wu Tang now has to pay its way, so this exchange of knowledge and tourism is very helpful both ways.

URL Links to Wu Tang Arts Web-sites: http://daoistgate.com/, http://www.wudanggongfu.com/ http://www.daoistkungfu.com, http://www.wudangdao.com/

There are many travel web-sites too; find these just by doing a search for "travel to Wudang", "hotels in Wudang" or similar to find them and then filter out the ones you like. These links are included purely on a random basis and the author has no idea what the places are like or whether what they offer is what you would like. Do your research thoroughly before committing to a thousand mile journey as once there you cannot change your mind. A good tip is to seek out others who have been there; do this from Linked In, Taoism, Tai Chi Network, etcetera, or via Taoist Arts web-sites around the world.

Sincere thanks to Shih-fu Xuan of www.DaoistGate.com for his much appreciated guidance and help.

There are many other tours of China available today, including many that include Peking or "Beijing", as it is pronounced these days. There you will find some amazing blends of old and new, such as there being 18 "Big Mac" places alongside traditional street sold Noodle carts, new cars, old wheelbarrows and a variety of new and old cultural entertainments. Many people there speak English fluently as a second language and are fascinated by western culture; "Culture" isn't that one of things that grows on a Petri Dish? I joke about this as the word culture is a relatively modern term, stemming from the 18th and 19th centuries in Europe and supposedly denoting improvements in society. Nowadays it is taken in a more anthropological sense as being something distinguishing material culture or language, customs, law and everything else which shapes society. Somehow, over the years of studying social changes and people's attitudes, I see this as a meaningless joke at best or a misnomer at worst. It seems that as technology moves forwards at an ever increasing rate of knots that "culture" is diving back into the medieval era where people stoned each other, drowned those who were different, accusing them of being witches, or were encouraged to enjoy public beheadings in the market square (now public humiliations in courts or newspapers), where just like in the stories of Robin Hood, the wicked Sheriff and his henchmen ruled with terror whilst the poor became victims of the Lords; and still happens today in other guises. How can this be described as "progress" or "culture"? This only serves to reinforce my beliefs in Tao studies and confirm the opinion that Taoism is needed even more desperately in today's society to bring back some practical common sense into it.

Tao is Tao.

Great men and women observed life, the world and even the stars. They made deductions based on what they saw and were able to devise simple but very clever symbols to describe how the Universe was conceived and expands. How life amongst animals, humans and all that nature presents around us inter-relates. They even noted the interactions of the elements and how these related to actions or functions within the human body. This was a practical science, a lay science by which the use of representative symbols and simple examples could relate the workings of life to even the poorest of farmers who, in those days, could not read or write. The Great Lord or Yellow Emperor Huang Ti dedicated his life to discovering Tao, translating it into texts and simple teaching methods that would help all his people to gain better lives through "harmony". A great doctor, Hua T'o (华佗), developed acupuncture and all that it entails, helping millions to better health. Many other great men developed systems of health giving or correcting exercises that enjoy more and more popularity today, like T'ai Chi Ch'uan. This is how I like to view Tao and Taoism, or Taoists.

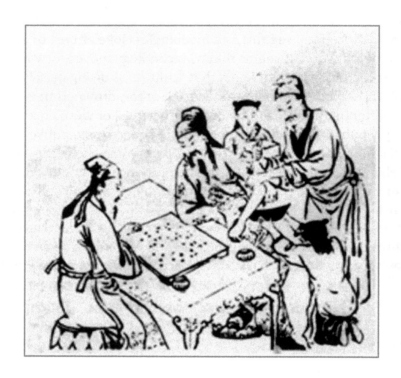

Wu Wei.

Wu Wei is the principle of living,

Live your life like water;

It flows from mountain to the sea,

On its way the water is giving,

And serves all creatures, you and me.

Hills and boulders block not its way,

For water will always flow around

And settle not for it recycles

Even when the sea it has found.

When life you find is dull or dreary

And problems build to make you weary,

Remember Wu Wei, to flow around.

It is not life which blocks your progress,

But the stubborn self-made dam.

Tear down your walls and restrictions,

Lists of what your ideals are,

Rid yourself of preconceptions.

Tao and Wu Wei is the best by far.

©Mike Symonds 23.10.97

Chapter Four

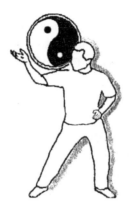

What is T'ai Chi Ch'uan?

What Is T'ai Chi?

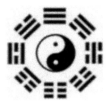

What is T'ai Chi?

This subject will be treated as simply as possible and given a simplified "middle of the road view" so as to adhere to translations and opinions of many T'ai Chi Ch'uan practitioners and experts. Translation from Chinese to English is ambivalent at best; causing the Chinese translations to be just as variable as the Occidental translations are in many cases. One of the basic stumbling blocks in translations from Chinese to English is the fact that Chinese characters are actually pictures, or pictographs depicting a subject. This makes them "variable" according to the context of a sentence; one of the reasons the CCG decided to create "Simplified Chinese" and use one character for the subject and another to categorise it. The second stumbling block is that the subject of T'ai Chi's physical core is philosophic, so again may vary according to subject and translations. If you research enough, you will come across many translations and "supposed" meanings of the same names or phrases; you can decide for yourself which you think is right and this may also take form from your background knowledge.

太 極

The two characters of Chinese, above, are "T'ai Chi" which loosely means "Supreme Power" or "Supreme Ultimate" and refers to The Tao (The Way of Nature/Universe) and its Yin and Yang polarities and elements. It can be translated to mean "Mankind following the path to Oneness with Tao", or similar, implying that this is a method of training and philosophical study. T'ai Chi also means Supreme

Ultimate, Supreme meaning the highest possible form of something and ultimate as it cannot be surpassed by anything else. The Universe is just that, as far as we know, as it cannot be altered, shaped or changed from its course by mankind or any other form that we know of. The Universe is also responsible for the creation of everything within itself. Therefor it must be supreme and ultimate. The Universe is formless – it has no particular shape or form- but it is all things, therefor the old ones decided to call it TAO. T'ai Chi represents the Universe and all it creates in its active form.

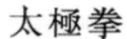

What is T'ai Chi Ch'uan?

Now we add the third character. The third character, "Ch'uan" refers to "boxing exercise" or a physical practice that utilises energy and hands; what we call self-defence or boxing in English translation. In context with T'ai Chi this implies that this is an exercise system that follows philosophical principles of Tao. Because of the nature of the definition from the translation proper of the Chinese name this means that when anyone talks about this particular style of exercise or Chinese Boxing we should say "T'ai Chi Ch'uan" or (modern) "Taijiquan".

Let us look at the traditional translation in detail:

T'ai = Too, very, superlative, exalted. Chi = the extreme limit. Superlative

(i.e.: superior to all others, or eminent, Extreme limit, Outermost limit, most stringent, highest in degree.)

Ch'uan simply means "fist" or "hand" and is a classifier, therefore it is read first to get the context of the other words in the title), also practised Art/Skill, related to hands; another Chinese translation suggests "energy" as the hands are an expression point for energy, so relating again to the exercise factor.

Therefore we can take it that T'ai Chi Ch'uan refers to an exercise, in this case Chinese Boxing by design, which is planned around the concepts of Taoist Philosophy or the Philosophy of Tao. As it is an exercise this implies "physical" to most people but this subject should also include "mental" as the player's Mind plays the lead role in T'ai Chi Ch'uan. As any good psychology student knows, when the mind is used to follow a clear path of development the mind also benefits from using logical or progressive thinking, therefore we may assume that the spirit also develops because of a regime that utilises body, mind and energy. By studying and following the philosophy of Tao many people hope to gain enlightenment, but as Lord Buddha pointed out so clearly, to become enlightened we need to look after both the mind and the body; to this end he rated Martial Arts training and vegetarianism. Legend says that the sagely Ch'eung San-feng was looking for the perfect exercise for Taoists when he developed his routine; which has influenced many other styles since.

In China some people still refer to T'ai Chi Ch'uan as "Cotton Fist Boxing", pertaining to its softness in practice. It is also known as "Shadow Boxing", as it is practiced at first in a solo manner, as though fighting imaginary opponents or "Philosophical Boxing as it follows the Taoist philosophy. Ch'eung San-feng may never have heard of the phrase "T'ai Chi Ch'uan" let alone called the system by that name. In T'ien Ti Tao we just call it Tao Ch'uan - Taoist Boxing - and this covers virtually everything that we do; including what others may call "Kung Fu". Whatever you call it, or anyone you may come across, it is of the same family, shares the same values and more often or not shares some very similar techniques. Commonly in the West people say "Tai Chi" - without apostrophe (') in the first word; which in Chinese is very important as the word would mean something completely different without it! As you can see by the translation on the previous pages, this is totally incorrect as "T'ai Chi" is the active Tao, not the exercise. What you are studying or about to embark on is T'ai Chi *Ch'uan*; pronounced like "Tie Chee

Chew-ann" or "Tai-jee-chew-ahn", or even "Tai- jee-churn", depending on regions and inflections.

As the Universe already has a name, for the convenience sake of mankind who uses words to communicate, Tao. A closer look at the way the original Chinese ideographs are made up suggest that this name "T'ai Chi Ch'uan" might imply that this is a skill that mankind can learn in order to become more in tune with the Universe as the calligraphic character parts seem to suggest a man standing between heaven and earth. Heaven, Earth and Man are originally depicted as a Triangle depicting the relationship between the three. This was the original Triad and was a good triad; much later perverted by a gang leader in much the same way as Hitler perverted the Swastika, a Buddhist symbol for Peace.

So, Taoist Boxing became called T'ai Chi Ch'uan for a reason. It is linked with Tao and the study of practical Taoist philosophy, it is an exercise that revolves around Chinese Boxing (Ch'uan-shu) Skills and it is practised with a mind to becoming more "natural", flowing and spontaneous, like Tao. In using the term "practical" I distinguish between this and the "religious" concepts or perversions in which it is treated like a religion. However, there are also some schools of Taoist study which may appear religious yet are still quite practical! If you see the book 'Practical Philosophy of Tao' (same author) you will see how symbols are used to represent the different aspects or actions of Tao (Universe) so that even those who cannot read could see what was being explained; very clever "translations" indeed. T'ai Chi has a history of well over two-thousand years. The philosophy pre-dates the Art of T'ai chi Ch'uan by at least 600 years.

Chinese classical Taoist philosophy holds that all things are born of Tai Chi. The whole process is stated in detail in the 'Book of Changes' or 'I-Ching' (1100-221 B.C.): "T'ai Chi causes the two opposites (Yin and Yang), the two opposites cause the four seasons, and the four seasons cause the eight natural phenomena (denoting heaven, earth, thunder, wind, water, fire, mountains and lakes)." Logically the eight phenomena then create all things that we know of or can name. Symbols used in training include those illustrated in the text below.

A verse from the Tao Te Ching or "Daodejing" reminds us not to waste time on arguments and falsehoods:

Tao Te Ch'ing: 81.

Real words are not vain, Vain words are not real;

And since those who argue prove nothing

A sensible man does not argue.

A sensible man knows what he knows,

While a fool knows more than is wise.

Therefore a sensible man does not devise resources:

The greater his use to others

The greater their use to him,

The more he yields to others,

The more they yield to him.

The Way of Life cleaves without cutting:

Which without need to say,

Should be man's way.

This verse is so simply expressed by Witter Bynner and Doctor Kiang's translation into poetic verse that it needs no further translation, just study.

And of politics or rulers?

Verse 17.

A leader is best

When people barely know that he exists,

Not so good when people obey and acclaim him,

Worse when they despise him.

'Fail to honour people,

And they fail to honour you;'

But of a good leader, who talks little,

When his work is done, his aim fulfilled,

They will all say, 'We did this ourselves.'

It appears that the majority who aim to get places in governments nowadays are bent on feathering their own nests, making business deals, becoming a Member of the Board or setting up their own International businesses. Politicians study business and politics, the latter being the way to the former. This we all know and see via the news or even more manipulated newspapers. Very little is done for the welfare of the people or the planet. The same things happen on a smaller scale in T'ai Chi Ch'uan, Kung Fu, Karate and other "groups" all over the world; there are those who would manipulate the facts and the public in order to make money; frauds and fakes. This is all done at the expense of the "person in the street" who is treated like cattle; there only to make money pay taxes that are often wasted, keep the businesses running and supply the labour.

This creates negativity, mistrust, anxiety and sickness. There is no need for it. There should be no need for politically active businessmen and women to create such underhanded principles and organisations, like Common Purpose, that destroy people and gives politics a bad name.. Or should I say worse name than it already has.

The very great and truthful comedian, Billy Connolly, loved world-wide by millions, once said "Any ****** who wants to be a politician should never be allowed to be one!" As they say, many a true word spoken in jest. It is the public that makes politicians; the public however keeps making the same mistakes. Being conned by dishonest politicians is akin to being conned by dishonest business man or women who call themselves Martial Artists, members of the public are generally not armed with the same knowledge when it comes to choosing a school of Chinese or other Martial Arts. Unfortunately people who have an ambition or some egotistical desire to be a Martial Arts instructor can just go out and buy a "black belt" from a local sports shop.

The above may seem a bit strong to put in a book but it is done with consideration for the beginner, or would be student, as much as my life-long love for the Arts. It is unusual to include such information in a book, but it is done so with the hopes of helping beginners avoid tragic mistakes in the future, mistakes which could also give an undeserved bad name to the innocent. It also helps with "perspective", the knowledge of what is necessary and what is not, etcetera.

There are hundreds of thousands of good people all around the world. You do not see them on the news, nor do they stand out in the street. There are millions of unpaid T'ai Chi Ch'uan and other Martial Arts instructors around the world who help people become healthier and stronger, some healers too. Realise that within this world culture, sallied by the few, there are the many that offer light and better living. You are in charge of your own destiny and you can vote in a better lifestyle or better still, represent change for better, it is your choice, you can either make excuses or do something positive; we are now even seeing Buddhists in politics. As the well-worn phrase goes, "Time for change!"

Change Begins At Home. This all relates to Taoist Arts and Taoism, as well as Buddhist and other Arts that are taught for the sake of it, because they help individuals to become more fit, healthy and stronger, in body and soul. Martial Arts are not about fighting, winning or self-esteem. They are not about "call me Master" or wearing a belt that happens to be black. Martial Arts are systems of exercise that help body, mind and spirit. The Taoist Arts are more inclined to that direction than most, helping us to take charge of our own lives and come to less harm whilst at the same time helping us to find Tao (that which is, naturally; pure spirit).

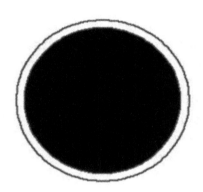

The first symbol used to describe the processes of the creation of the Universe is the Wu Chi. The symbol of Tao, the black and white Yin-Yang sign, has always been associated with the Art and Taoist philosophy from which it stems. Wu Chi came first though; it represents the Universe in a state of "chaos", "randomness", before what we call today "The Big Bang". In our practice of T'ai Chi Ch'uan we begin with this Wu Chi ("Wuji") theory so that we are noncompliant, empty and neutral. Many people find this the hardest part of practice and fail to either achieve or understand the Wu Chi and its importance.

The next symbol is known as T'ai Chi, the Supreme Ultimate. This represents the creation of the Universe, matter and anti-matter, the beginning of "Form" and creation is apparent and emanating from the centre, outwards. The "centre" is important in T'ai Chi Ch'uan. The T'ai Chi is our point of creation, being and organisation. In

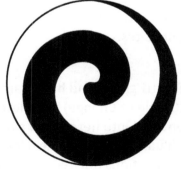

the physical and mental practice of T'ai Chi Ch'uan we move from the perceived "centre"; which is also the centre of our Universe and the point of equilibrium in the human body. To beginners this may seem strange, confusing or even impossible to understand, but in essence it is very simple; and yet another example of just how wonderful this graphic philosophical representation truly is.

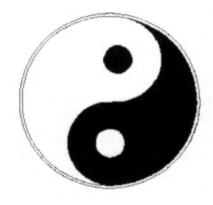

Following on from T'ai Chi symbol we have Yin and Yang. This is the visible expression of Wu Chi and is properly known as "Tao". Do you see the flow? From Wu Chi came T'ai Chi and that in turn creates Tao. Tao is the simple graphical illustration of how the Universe creates the constant change of all things we know. It contains the two basic Forces, Yin and Yang, each of these being influenced by the other. The symbol also shows flow, constant change, balance and harmony, expansion and contraction and many other more subtle perceptions that are both pertinent to the Art of T'ai chi Ch'uan and the study of the Universe or Universal Way.

Yin and Yang can be used to represent opposites that work together, like empty and full, solid and hollow, male and female, still and moving, winter and summer, cols and heat, light and dark, push and pull, static and flowing, quick and slow. There are millions of opposites.

The tri-grams and hexagrams that we know through the 'I Ching' (Oracle of Change) are a later addition and one that shall not all be entered into here. So to summarise the translation of "T'ai Chi Ch'uan" we may make a logical assumption that there are strong connections between the physical practice of T'ai Chi Ch'uan and the mental study of Taoism, combined being a way of tapping into The (Nature's) Way by exercise of Mind and body.

So, what is T'ai Chi Ch'uan in summary?

Simply put it is a form of exercise for health and fitness, but not just fitness training for the body (Wei Kung). T'ai Chi Ch'uan includes mental work (I Kung) and bio-energy work too (Ch'i Kung), this leads to spiritual work (Shen Kung). These are achieved by concentrations of mind, energy and awareness of the same, including full body awareness. If it is called Taijiquan or T'ai Chi Ch'uan then it must contain many deeper elements to qualify.

The legend of "Old Zhang" tells us that he left his well-paid job with the government of the time to do something that he felt was far more useful and rewarding: to study Tao. Having learned Snake and Crane plus other forms of Ch'uan-shu and Ch'i Kung he is said to have dreamed of creating the perfect system of healthy exercise for those who studied Tao.

Ch'uan-shu translates as "Fist Skills", but does not necessarily mean fighting. Fist, in Chinese also means "hand" and it is recognised that the hand can emit energy, so hand and energy can be taken as references to a Boxing Form that gives you energy. If we add T'ai Chi to this then we get a rather long translation that far exceeds the original Chinese three characters for T'ai Chi Ch'uan, being "Health and Energy Boxing Form based on the philosophical principles of the Supreme Ultimate"; translations often seeming "back-to-front in English as the classifiers like "Ch'uan" would be put in front of the subject, which here is "T'ai Chi"; e.g. "The Fist of Supreme Ultimate/Tao" or T'ien Ti Tao translating as "Way of Heaven and Earth".

Is T'ai Chi Ch'uan a dance?

There are many aspects to T'ai Chi Ch'uan that have all been added as afterthoughts. They are adjuncts to training; all to achieve various goals; like T'ai Chi Bang is used to strengthen the wrists for T'ai Chi Jian or Dao, but the 'Bang' is not T'ai Chi Ch'uan itself. The weapons used in T'ai chi Ch'uan practice are merely echoing the Chinese culture for Martial Arts practice as both a way to better health and self-defence, however, be it noted that by practising weapons routines you are using an extension to your body and therefore, extending the mind and the Ch'i*. Therefore the old theory that weapons training in T'ai chi Ch'uan can enhance both the power of the mind's extensions and healing Ch'i projection may be very sound indeed.

* How different this is from the ignorant western perception by many that weapons are just tools of destruction or violence!

T'ai Chi Dance is actually an advanced stage of training. My Old Master would not teach this to just anyone, more often he only taught the more advanced students in his schools. He showed me once and I was immediately awestruck at the grace, beauty and inspiration this caused. Since then, and quite recently on a Forum, it struck me just how many instructors have never reached this level or been shown this aspect by their teachers. The dance is truly a dance, but it is a T'ai Chi dance; you are playing with the Universe and harmonizing with its forces. It is the spontaneous aspect of T'ai Chi Ch'uan training.

In one writing by Chuangliang Al Huang, founder of 'Living Tao Federation', the author suggests the following:

"Once upon a time, anywhere in the world, there was a man (or a woman) sitting on a mountain top, quietly observing nature. He became so inspired by the

54

movements of the world around him that he began to dance, imitating all the natural elements he could easily identify. He opened himself completely to the forces of nature. He became the forces: sky, earth, fire, water, trees, flowers, wind, clouds, birds, fishes and butterflies. Hi dance became ecstatic, completely transforming and transcendent. So happy with himself, he then poetically named each movement [conceptually?]: Bubble of the Cosmos, Yin/Yang Harmonic Loop, White Cranes Flashing Wings, Cloud-waving Hands, Golden Birds Balancing on One Leg, Embrace Tiger and Return to Mountain.

He or she was the originator of the Tai Ji dance. His moment of creation could have happened thousands of years ago or could have happened right now, this moment, somewhere, anywhere in the world. This person could be you."

There have been suggestions in history that the very first form or method of what is now generically known as "Tai Chi Ch'uan" exercise could have been an imitation of the animals and nature in general; which also agrees in theory to the Chinese assertion that all methods of Kung Fu originally came from mankind imitating the animals for fitness and for self-defence. It seems that what Chuangliang Al Huang is doing is to attempt a de-intellectualisation of T'ai Chi Ch'uan and make it something that we can all enjoy, like we may enjoy dancing as a way to express joy and feel better in health and energy. By linking it, and our Mind, with Nature (Tao), we can become more One with the Universe and lose our man-made problems.

As an extra point of interest here I shall mention David Carradine, the actor. As well as an actor he was a lover of dance. It was his ability to dance and do high kicks that landed him the fortuitous role in the TV series 'Kung Fu' (c.1970) During the latter series his guide for the fight scenes became a little known teacher of traditional Chinese Martial Arts. Shih-fu Kam Yuen, who is Student of Seven Star Mantis - Qi Xing Tang Lang under Master Chen Zhen Yi in Hong Kong plus Tai Ji Tang Lang (T'ai Chi Mantis) under Master Chi Chuk Kai, also in Hong Kong. The youngest of eight brothers and sisters, Shih-fu Liang Kam Yuen was born in Hong Kong, where he spent his formative years. Shih-fu Yuen later moved to the USA. There he studied under Master Mon Wong in New York. Over the years he returned to refine his style with help from his teacher in Hong Kong. Shih- fu Yuen studied the traditional Northern Shaolin as well as Hsing-I Ch'uan and Pa Kua Ch'uan styles from Master Wong Jack Man in San Francisco from Master Wong Jack Man. In 1972 he was approached by warner Bro's to become the fight scene coordinator in the Kung Fu series.

David Carradine became a sincere student and was taught many aspects of T'ai Chi Ch'uan and traditional Kung Fu. Not many years before his death, David Carradine starred in a film called 'White Crane Chronicles'; this being one of the finest "Kung Fu films" ever made. In Part Two of the story, he and his two cohorts travel through the countryside where, at one point, they meet three exotic women who offer them refreshment by a lake. The women, thinking that the men might be enemies, attack them. In his own fight scene Carradine uses his own T'ai Chi Ch'uan and also turns his fight with the woman into a dance! This was a magical moment for me and brought not only a smile to my face but all the above thoughts to the fore.

Is It T'ai Chi Snobbery?

Some people around the world can be seen or heard to acclaim that what they do is the best style or method, that is right whilst others may be wrong, or that another person may not be teaching correctly. Is this snobbery, bragging and bad manners? While it may not be best form, especially in public view, it may not always be what it seems. T'ai chi Ch'uan is one of those subjects, one of the few in the world, which is really hard to "put your finger on". How do you identify something which is such a wide variable that it can rarely even be agreed upon by "Masters" of two different family styles? Some teachers may say to their students "That's not right, it should be done like this" or "Our style has proper lineage through Master X... so that's not *real* T'ai Chi!" This can be taken in so easily by the student who then in later years sees something with which he is not familiar and almost instantly casts it aside with a sweeping denial. Life is like that and people allow themselves to act without thinking, or knowing. Just because something looks different it does not mean that it is wrong, or not "real". Keep an open mind and you will find that there is always something new to learn; especially in a vast Art like T'ai Chi Ch'uan; even bigger if you study T'ai Chi itself; Life, the Universe and everything!

The Intellectual Properties.

Part of the problem is human intellect. Carl Jung said that the mind is very complex and that intellect has many levels. If we say that one person has great intellect and another also has great intellect, then we will surely be talking about two different people with two distinctively different intellects. Intellect is a term (a label) which is used to describe the powers of the human mind to reason and come to an intelligent conclusion about whether something is real or unreal, true or false, valid or invalid, etcetera. It is no wonder that agreements on T'ai chi Ch'uan are hard to reach. When the Art is so potentially vast and so complex, often broken up and scattered to the proverbial four corners of the Earth, then there will be confusion.

To illustrate the point made above I shall attempt to list all common aspects of T'ai chi Ch'uan practice; that is, all the subjects that I can think of *easily* that are taught as T'ai chi Ch'uan or one of its supporting role exercises (see three pages below) - please note that these lists may be added to if one digs deeply enough or happens to know more than me, and so this may be considered to be a "rough guide" only!

Some people, especially in the West, may be teaching a supporting exercise, such as Taiji 18 Postures, and call it T'ai Chi Ch'uan. This is obviously misleading and is just a case of ignorance of the facts or even possibly egotism; wanting to appear as though teaching the Art or be acclaimed as such. These people really should not claim to be teachers of anything as they do not know what they are talking about. Misleading yourself is one thing but misleading the public is foolishness and also detrimental to those who wish to be genuine students of the Martial Arts. Readers are encouraged to be wary as there are many fraudulent teachers around, even in China as well as many here in UK or USA, and unless you learn correctly your health can be damaged, even severely. By looking at the lists below you will at least get an idea of what T'ai Chi Ch'uan is and what is merely an exercise that may enhance practice of T'ai Chi Ch'uan Forms.

The main aspect of T'ai Chi Ch'uan is for health, this is achieved through "boxing" because it has been observed that this type of exercise is more comprehensive than any other, generally; The movements cover twists, turns, balance, stretching, aerobic (external) and anaerobic (internal), circulation boosting, use of smaller muscle groups and ligaments, posture, breathing (deeper oxygenation) and breath control, stimulation of the skin and nervous system, massage of the internal organs and more. This is quite comprehensive in exercise terms or comparisons.

Because one has to think about T'ai Chi Ch'uan, or any other Chinese Ch'uan Fa, it also works the mind and the intellect, stimulating logical thought process and spiritual growth; linked with the bio-energies, of course. As in life's many moods, you can sing, dance, be serious, frivolous and express an entire range of emotions through the long term practice of T'ai chi Ch'uan.

The Natural State.

Returning to the natural state is something which is necessary for the survival of humanity. Mankind (which includes women) often think that they can change, manipulate and rearrange the world to suit their plans, this may include many of the despotic rulers, politicians, heads of police and armies. It is not possible to change the world to suit one man's or one group's plans. Hitler failed. Gaddafi failed. Many others have failed or will fail. You cannot change the will of all people and you cannot rule by force or bad example; e.g. acts that go against human nature on the wider scale. In his wisdom, Lao Tzu wrote this observation in the Tao Te Ching.

When we look at the despots, the corrupt and others who seek power over the populace we see people who are disconnected from nature. How did that happen? Was it intense political studies at a college or university, development of greed or lack of respect for fellow humans in a "competitive" atmosphere? Was it that they were raised by parents who were power crazy? Is it a spin-off from what they perceive as a society who only cares about money or positions of so-called power; "lust"? Perhaps it is a combination of all these things. In the world that they live in, in their heads, they see only the greedy, the power-mongers, the corrupt, so it is easy to believe that this is the way of the world. People at street level know different worlds, from those struggling for survival in the slums and ghettos to those who "get by" quietly in the more rural areas on a frugal but peaceful lifestyle. Different again is the rich or political in-crowd who dines richly whilst waiting to be stabbed in the back by their colleagues or other usurpers. This is not true power or purpose, it is allusion, delusion.

Tao is the only power, the only law and the only ruler. Tao is The Universe and no man, woman or heavily armed ruler with bullying police or armies can deny it, change it or stop it. It can stop them though. People, whether they are called white, black, yellow or red are all part of Tao. We are all made of the same particles, the same energies and usually, if we dig deep enough, have the same desires for a better life. This life is short enough, after all, so why live in fear, stress and discomfort?

Tao provides us with the raw materials and examples. T'ai chi Ch'uan is woven by Tao and can save humanity by bringing us closer together; "Harmony Exercise".

T'ai Chi Ch'uan & Common Internal Styles:

- San Shi Fa - Thirty Seven Methods
- San Shi Chi/Sanshiqi - Thirteen Methods
- Mian Ch'uan/Quan, "Continuous Fist", also "Cotton Fist"
- Yang Family Styles - *more than one variation.
- Chen Family Styles *more than one variation.
- Wu Family Styles *more than one variation.
- Wu/Hao Family Styles.
- Li or Lee Family Styles.
- Sun Family Style *recently split into variations.
- Zhaobao T'ai chi Ch'uan - variation of Chen Style.
- Ching-chuan Shi T'ai chi Ch'uan (Wellspring).
- Cheng Man-ch'ing Style - variation of Yang Style.
- Liu He Pa Fa (Six Harmonies & Eight Methods).
- Wu Tang/Wudang Styles - many variant Forms.
- Modern 'Competition' Styles (doubtful inclusion}.
- Various other styles not listed here.

T'ai Chi Ch'uan Extension Training:
- T'ai Chi Kun
- T'ai Chi Dao

- T'ai Chi Chiang/Qiang
- T'ai Chi Chang/Zhang (Cane)
- T'ai Chi Jian
- T'ai Chi Shan (Fan)
- T'ai Chi Chin-na & Chiu Chi Tsu.

T'ai Chi Supplementary Exercise Regimes
- T'ai Chi Bang
- T'ai Chi Chih (Ruler)
- T'ai Chi Ball
- T'ai Chi Shi Ba Shi (Yang Style Extracted Forms to develop Ch'i)
- T'ai Chi Chan Chuang/Zhanzhuang (for developing "rooting")
- Long (Dragon) Ch'i Kung (used for developing Ch'i and Shen; spirit)
- Pa T'uan Chin/Baduanjin (Eight Strands) – Prep' and Warm-ups.
- Silk Reeling Exercises - a few variations exist.
- T'ai Chi Walking - again priming exercise.
- Wild Goose Ch'i Kung / Five Animals / Five Elements & others.
- Wu Chi Ch'i Kung & Standing Posture Meditations.
- T'ai chi for Health - many variants, often based on Sun Style.
- Many variant methods of Ch'i Kung unlisted here.

As stated earlier, this list is far from comprehensive. What this list is included for, lest you have forgotten the thread of the subject after getting lost in a mist of details, is "What is T'ai Chi Ch'uan?" From the above lists even a fresh novice will be able to tell now what is T'ai Chi Ch'uan and what is merely an exercise used to supplement practice of a Form or Style of T'ai Chi Ch'uan. Furthermore, the item before this distinguishes "T'ai Chi" as the philosophy which is 600 years older than the "Ch'uan" or physical Forms but also the philosophy which acts a guide to practice.

Brief Explanation.

The Thirteen Methods are explained herein and should be a part of any teaching professing to be T'ai Chi Ch'uan, alongside other basic principles and specifics. These have a particular way of being taught and at differing levels. The other "styles" mainly vary in appearance only and this can be seen in other books or in videos, as well as going along to see for yourself if local classes are held. Most of these differences are subtle to the casual beholder and are often introduced as a matter of preference; the main reason why there are so many different styles of Martial Arts in the world, the other being "technical" alterations.

The Extension Exercises are all part and parcel of the broader Art. These can help one to learn a specific principle, skill or enhance another. The Staff is an extension of the hands and arms whilst the spear is yet another extension. The Dao or "big knife" is a practical Chinese weapon that has been "adopted" into the T'ai Chi Ch'uan family for extensional training purposes and teaches different coordination skills that the staff or "empty hand" Forms. The Dao also helps develop the body and mind-set differently too. The Dao was an effective weapon on the battlefield and was even successful against the Japanese Katana. There are many other weapons employed by all the major and minor styles of T'ai Chi Ch'uan, including Twin swords, twin sticks and even Chop Sticks! The Jian, or straight double-edged sword, is a very great skill in T'ai chi Ch'uan. It is often called the "Lady's/Gentleman's weapon" as this distinguishes it from the common weapons that might be swung with basic military skills* traditionally. The Taiji Jian requires great subtleness and agility, so it is at a high level of training that this will normally be found.

*Whereas it may take a year to three years training in military circumstances it can take many years longer in T'ai chi Ch'uan.

When it comes to the Supplementary Exercises of T'ai chi Ch'uan most are used to achieve certain goals or enhance development in a way that perhaps the Form cannot do, or cannot lead to quickly enough. Most of these also develop Ch'i; the odd one out is the T'ai Chi Bang; a short stick which some say is like a Rolling Pin for pastry making; the Bang is thicker and smooth. The Bang is "the odd one out" because it does not involve Nei Kung (Neigong) practices like the others. The main purpose for this simple implement is to develop the strength of the sinews, fascia tissue and ligaments of the arms, shoulders and back, so for this reason it can be classified as Wei Kung (Weigong) or "external" in practice. T'ai Chi Chih or "Rule" is a shaped rod that fits between the palms and is used to develop better ch'i flow. Surprisingly this exercise is still little known in the western hemisphere. Other supplements, like Chang Chuan/Zhang Zhuan (standing as though holding a post) are often used in warm-ups and this one is very good at developing "rooting" or "sinking"; there can be contentious

ideas about rooting, sinking, weighting, relaxation and other named elements but my Old Master used to refer to this process in simple terms that required no jargon, technical terms or useless confusions, he used to say "When you are relaxed, 'fang song', you will feel like a Daruma Doll with all the weight sinking to the bottom of your feet".

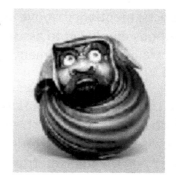

T'ai Chi Ch'uan Walking is a useful supplement as it gives us quality time to think about our placement of feet, knees, hips and head, as well as the interchange of Yin/Yang and other elements of movement. It is like a compact game of Chess - another Chinese invention. T'ai Chi Ch'uan itself is "living chess"! When you employ Taiji walking you must control your breathing and special breathing techniques that can be added into the exercise should only be taught by a competent master-teacher. Adaptations can be made when out and about, taking care of shopping and other menial tasks that require walking. A simple method of this is employed by Monks as they walk from one place to another, so as not to be distracted by daily life.

> Method: Think about each step as you place the heel down first and "roll" the foot. Your eyes should gaze ahead, not focused, or you can gaze "down your nose" at the floor some eight or so yards in front of you. Yet another variant of this is to count your steps whilst walking; a simple meditation. There are many, many variations of "Walking".

Whatever else it is, T'ai Chi Ch'uan is simply a healthy Taoist exercise form which doubles as a method of self-defence and educational philosophical study program; which can also lead to higher spiritual levels; which were seen in the development of this unique style. None of these elements can really be separated from its practice; otherwise it ceases to be T'ai Chi Ch'uan. The other peripheral aspects, mentioned above and those not mentioned, are simply methods employed to assist along the Way; the "path of training". This training can take many, many years, or even lifetimes.

The core principles of the system are achieved by gentle exercises which combine muscle strengthening, stretching and toning (likewise the sinews, arteries, nervous systems and ligaments), improving the bone marrow which in turn improves red corpuscle quality, bettering concentration, balance and self-control, improving circulation of blood (carrying oxygen and other nutrients), developing circulation of Intrinsic Energy (Ch'i/Qi) through the meridians and enhancing the strength of the spirit. Many of the supplementary exercises are used and we also have the common extensions as well. For all those who thought there was just a simple exercise that looks so graceful, of course, there is much more to it than just standing on one spot and "waving hands like clouds"!

The Five Stages.

These Five Stages of training can be broken down into other component parts, so to speak. The basic stage, for example, can be the development of Qi flow to the Dantian, the second to the feet, the third to the crown. This would span sections one and two below. Again it is fair to say that Masters and Methods vary from school to school and the way that one person works may not be comfortable with another. However, the basics are all there and should, in one way or another, be adhered to otherwise progress will never be made. Do not be deluded by frauds or clever advertising, catch-words (" words to catch") or big advertising.

There are five stages to the accomplishment of T'ai Chi Ch'uan;

1. Transforming the physical body so as to generate life energy.

2. Transforming energy to Ch'i which circulates rhythmically.

3. Transforming the Ch'i into Spirit.

4. Transforming the Spirit into Void.

5. Transforming the Void into the 'Great Meaning'.

If numbers four and five seem a little vague to you don't worry. It just means that you learn to calm your spirit (soul, inner-self) and become 'One' with all things, neither clashing or arguing, agreeing nor disagreeing. After reaching this philosophically mature stage of Oneness with Nature (human and otherwise) one then, perhaps, aims for loftier goals and spiritual enlightenment.

Posture.

Postures are very important in T'ai Chi Ch'uan, as are the "weighting" factors. Head your teacher's advice and study the correct postures with the right attitude. Each posture is significant both in its own right and to the next posture in the Form.

Intent.

No matter which Form or style of T'ai Chi Ch'uan you are practicing or teaching the "Yee" is a crucial factor. This method of practice is not only traditional but just happens to be the best way to help you keep mistakes out of the Form and correct applications and postures in. Pay attention to the relationship of the "whip" or "chain" theory in action: Eyes & Mind, Waist & Spine, Hips/Knees/Feet.

Breathing.

There are different ways of breathing for different levels. The minimum method of breathing techniques is two, the maximum four; usually. Beginners will start training with the natural method (Shun Hu Xi - 顺呼吸) and when ready to progress may be shown other methods that compliment practice and raise ch'i levels, etcetera. The length of time it takes a student to be "ready" for advanced breathing and training methods depends on two things; firstly the detail that the instructor goes into, what he or she knows and in what order of importance he/she considers it necessary to introduce it; secondly, the total amount of time the student spends on practice, which determines progress made.

Readers should take note here that if being taught Reverse Breathing (Ni Hu Xi - 逆呼吸) that according to medical reports, it can have dangerous or unhealthy results if done incorrectly! Always seek advice to help counter such problems from an experienced instructor who, amongst other things, should also warn you and tell you how to adjust certain physical aspects to help avoid strain or problems.

Readers who have obtained the book 'Qigong and Baduanjin' will see that I have listed the most important and reliable breathing methods in it. These are applicable in T'ai Chi Ch'uan, at different levels (again, you need to have a competent instructor). Abdominal Breathing is sometimes called "Dantian Breathing" and it seems that "Full Breathing" can be called that too; one expands the abdomen and lower back while the other expands the chest down to the

66

abdomen and lower back, but both have the same aim or point, to develop ch'i. We call full breathing Taoist Breath.

In higher levels and the act of meditation one may come across "the art of breathing without breathing", or "Embryonic Breathing". This again requires careful instruction by a qualified instructor. There are many, many facets to T'ai Chi Ch'uan that cannot be taught by unqualified instructors, so be warned. There are many people out there who claim to teach T'ai Chi Ch'uan but are blissfully ignorant of the Art and the true facts behind it! You cannot learn it if they cannot teach it.

Advanced Level.

Training at an advanced level again depends upon how many hours the student has put in to their training and how much they have got out of it; progress. Only genuine instructors of Traditional T'ai Chi Ch'uan can guide the students through or into these higher levels; generally speaking level 2 to 5 on the Five Stages.

Beginners Level.

Although T'ai Chi Ch'uan may be called 'The thinking person's Kung Fu', it is often grabbed at "willy-nilly" fashion by unthinking people who do not take the time to examine their own words or what they practice. Often this leads to gross misinterpretation and disastrous arguments about who did what to whom and where. No debate which brings T'ai Chi Ch'uan or any past, present or future Master into ill- repute is worth the paper that it is written upon or the breath with which it is spoken. Let it be sufficient to say that real T'ai Chi Ch'uan can only be felt; it cannot be sold in a package or argued.

T'ai Chi Ch'uan is an esoteric and personal system within the midst of many exoteric or external ones. This is just another echo of Nature, the one seed in a few thousand that grows to full maturity whilst others act as a germination compost bed. Does not worry if you are not bothered about philosophical attainments, education or enlightenment; just enjoy the pure and simple exercises that T'ai Chi Ch'uan has to offer. Practice for one full year and see what differences it makes to your health and peace of mind.

For those who do not want T'ai Chi Ch'uan, or perhaps are younger and a little more energetically inclined there are always our T'ien Ti Tao Kuoshu, or "Taoist Style Kung Fu" classes within the Heaven & Earth School. These combine many internal (neijia) principles but with a more obvious external (weijia) approach and livelier exercises; offering both balance and a better understanding of Yin & Yang in Kung Fu. These classes are ideal for those wishing to study the fullness of the Taoist Arts and are in keeping with the principles of Daoquan. TTT's syllabus and structure was tested and accepted by the World's leading Chinese Arts organisation (c.1987) as being "genuine traditional Chinese Arts", it was said by one Old Master of the I.C.K.F. at the time that TTT's practice was (quote:) "... probably more traditional than most traditional systems"; this was not by accident but by design and, of course, years of study and hard work with much spiritual guidance on the way. This situation of development continues and is enhanced with time. The syllabus has been expanded, examined and slowly filled out over forty years, to date (2014) and my studies span another two decades on top of that; my, my, how time flies!

About T'ien Ti Tao System.

The full T'ien Ti Tao, a "system" of three parts, has been built on a foundational studies of, amongst other things, traditional Forms and *methods* of Shorinji Kempo (derived from ancient Shaolin which varied very little from Wu Tang methods in those days, before it converted to Buddhist) and principles of "Traditional Ju Jitsu" (derived from Chiu Chi Tsu, originally Chinese grappling and throwing skills), the "essence" or essential principles of Hsing-I Ch'uan, T'ai Chi Ch'uan and some Chang Ch'uan (Long Fist Form) and some core techniques and methods of traditional styles with traditional values plus the all-important, if to a lesser degree, animal

68

styles. This makes TTT even more unique and desirable to those who wish to gain a more in-depth and profound experience of traditional Chinese Martial Arts (the foundation and inspiration for many other country's Martial Arts) within a traditional Practical Taoist philosophical structure. The objective of T'ien Ti Tao was to develop and old style traditional school rather than "another" modern offshoot. Go back to go forwards!

The student is taught exercises and techniques from ground level up, gradually reaching more complex methods or techniques. This is where a well-structured syllabus is needed. A syllabus is a "ladder" of training. Towards the upper end of the syllabus lay the more difficult and involved Forms or Ch'uan (Quan), these can take several years to master and even then the student can learn more from it later. After a student reaches the prestigious Instructor level, he or she will then go on to learn more "internal" Forms, then weapons, Forms; these are seen as an extension to the body and require new skills and thinking as well as extending the effects of ch'i. Each Instructor then has the options to choose a specialised section to teach, this could be Taoist Yoga (K'ai Men), T'ai chi Ch'uan, Taoist Ch'ang Ming Diet, Ch'i Kung or T'ien Ti Tao's general health and healing skills. This is a yang to Yin process.

So the student begins training with the more Yang techniques and ends up with the more Yin techniques. This method develops the body (Li) then the mind (I), the energies (Qi) and the Spirit (Jin). In theory the individual comes out the other end, so to speak, as a well-balanced person and their personal skills serve as a useful tool to the community by being able to offer self-defence, exercise and fitness, health and healing as well as a clear and uncluttered mind which can resolve issues that may have others confused or fighting unnecessarily.

Putting a system like this together is not just a matter of "cutting and pasting" a few fighting moves together from this and that style, T'ai Chi Ch'uan is a real science and takes many, many years of study, development and testing: I can honestly say that I have grown with the system and that every time I discovered one thing it made everything else more expansive (the 'Big Bang' effect), truly a system of Tao - the Universe - and I still have much to learn!

What Is Traditional Style?

This explanation I have taken from a thread on Linked-In about the same subject. This is included here because this is a subject question often raised by those who claim to be traditionalists, usually in defence of a style and criticising another they may call "modern" or "made up".

The "Style" is the name of a school. In our case, T'ien Ti Tao (The Way of Heaven & Earth) forms "the style". The syllabus, written or unwritten, is the true essence of the school and in this case it is a holistic syllabus (including basic groundwork, grappling and floor defence/counters and basic weapon defence in foundations, etc.). Our school is not a modern off-shoot but has been "taken back", by careful and long-term development and study, to the "traditional" and holistic days of the 15th/16th centuries in China when Shao-lin and Wu Tang were almost inseparable by nature, apart from certain approaches to Ch'uan; until later when Shaolin became predominantly Buddhist and eventually changed to what it is known as now; traditional Shaolin Chan can still be found in the world today, as can traditional Shaolin Ch'uan. Some people are too lazy to train or study, so they break away and form their own clubs after a short period of time or just one or two basic Grades; often proclaiming a "new school" or "style" of their own and promoting Black Belts, at a financial cost rather than at the cost of many years hard work and study; making their so-called Black Belt both worthless and meaningless!

My theory is that:
(a) It is impossible to develop a system if you have not studied a system or two, in full! You need to know what basics are, what

foundation is and what it leads to, more importantly, how to get there.

(b) A system has Parts and Methods; the parts are like bricks, the methods are the skills to build with. If parts and methods don't "marry up" then progress will be lost. If there is no firm foundation then all crumbles.

(c) Traditional or not, a good system should have many hidden techniques that will not be discovered until after many years training. Even then, more will be discovered later; even by the experienced teacher!

(d) Traditional is a concept. It is not ruled by age or lineage (line-age). In Ch'uan-shu there are "traditional" elements which may not be found in Wu Shu, for example. This can be philosophy or the reasons why we train or what we train for.

(e) It is not necessary to slap a good student's face for asking questions. Personally, the more questions my students ask the more I respect them. However, if they need to do some hard work I will say "Enough explanations. Let's do it!" Some of my students have "grown" with me for over twenty and thirty or more years and I still can't get them to leave me and start their own clubs. They are happy to learn; and ask questions, which I am happy to think about and answer; it reminds me of training aspects or other things which I may otherwise overlook or push to the back of my mind with lack of use. This approach also makes me think and progress. You can never have a deep enough understanding of what you practice.

(f) 'F' is for "Finally!" Tradition is a concept; as said. It is in this case, not lineage but method (Fa) and Essence. To use the old analogy again, it is like building a house. First a strong foundation is required, the bigger the house the deeper the foundations must go. Then you start to build, brick by brick. Like a house, and the "empty cup", substance is only useful for its absence, so "tradition" is a proverbial window here or there to let light in. Doors are needed so that you may enter different rooms. In each room, on each level, you will discover the traditions that previous people have left for you; these are treasures in a living museum!

In a world where many people strive to create a new system in their own image, it has been said by some to be "refreshing" that Tiandidao is a system which has "gone back to revive" in the era when Chinese Arts development was at a peak of development and many, many Masters cooperated and developed systems which were based on sound universal principles and suitable therefore for all. This period was around the fifteenth to sixteenth centuries AD and before human error lead to splits between Wudang and Shaolin. These "wounds" should now be healed, so let us go back and enjoy the Traditional Chinese Arts for what they truly are, "living treasures in a living museum" which we all look after and admire.

T'ai Chi Ch'uan/Taijiquan is one of those traditional Arts. Despite efforts by the few morally corrupt politicians and business people who have tried and failed to de-cultivate it, deface or degrade it, "Traditional Taijiquan" has grown stronger and stronger. Like Tao, and because it is Tao, it is an unstoppable force, the force of true nature. Whereas some unscrupulous and manipulative international politicians would have people behave like trained monkeys to fulfil their own political desires for them, the practice of Tao liberates the Mind and betters the health. Taijiquan is Tao and Tao is a path of impenetrable and un-destroyable perfection. Enjoy.

A Note on Politics and Practice.

Taoist philosophy is open to all styles, all people and all opinions. Those who are negative or abusive will no doubt reap what they sow. Those people who try to cooperate and promote the positive usually succeed. Tao provides and Tao takes away. Whilst I am not a politically motivated person, or what the government sarcastically nickname these days an activist, I am like many millions of other good intentioned people around the world who are sick of underhandedness, greed and destruction. Governments may be controlled by greedy and destructive people. This is not Tao. The vain words of politicos or self-boosted players are of no consequence to anyone but themselves and the same applies in Martial Arts; nobody who is a genuine instructor of Martial Arts ever addresses themselves as "Master". There are verses within the Tao Te Ching (Daodejing) that explain all of this and should be studied alongside all else.

Quote: (When asked about Taijiquan, the author said) "It's not the Form that's important, it is the understanding. To understand the Form is to absorb the essence. To do this we need to be taught and shown how, practice with our heart full of Taijiquan and our mind's empty so that it can be filled. Then we need to practice more, until it becomes embedded in our bones. In class my old Daoist Arts Master, Grand Master C. Chee Soo, used to have saying about practice too, 'Practice makes *almost* perfect.' That's it. Simple."

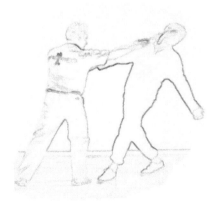

Chapter Five

T'ai Chi Ch'uan: the true History?

T'ai Chi Ch'uan was recorded as far back as the Liang period (502-557 A.D.) of China's Northern and southern Dynasty. We have no record of the person's name that developed this Form, or what he actually called it. For these reasons it does not appear on the Family Tree, below. This, if factual, probably makes it the oldest recorded Martial Art in the world, if not one of the oldest or at least the oldest of the "complete" systems; if it was a complete system.

The oldest we have recorded on the Family Tree below is 'Sanshiqi' (The Thirty Seven Forms, sometimes referred to as '37 Ch'uan' or Sanshiquan). This dates back to the Tang Dynasty and therefore connects with the term "Tang Te" (Tang Dynasty Hand) which was at one point exported via Fukien Crane Style Boxing to Okinawa and eventually the basics of this were copied and then altered in japan, making Japans first formal Martial Art style, which was renamed from Tang Te (Tang Hand) to Kara Te (Empty Hand). This example also shows us how flexible just one character can be in Chinese writing, with "hand" serving to describe a whole multi-faceted and broad-based system of Chinese Boxing and general exercises.

After this, unless there are any gaps that I/we are not aware of, came the Forms of Lidaozi. These became known as 'Long Fist', for their long and flowing movements (joined up without breaks). This implies that the principle of having flowing, joined up movements in one's Boxing at the time was possibly quite unique and remarkable; there are still traditional styles around that use separated Forms and in fact Lee Family Style of Grandmaster C. Chee Soo's 'Hand of the Wind' Style was one of these.

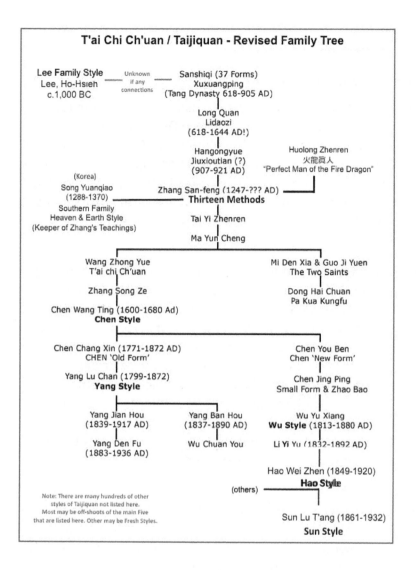

T'ai Chi Ch'uan / Taijiquan - Revised Family Tree

Lee Family Style
Lee, Ho-Hsieh
c.1,000 BC

Unknown if any connections

Sanshiqi (37 Forms)
Xuxuangping
(Tang Dynasty 618-905 AD)

Long Quan
Lidaozi
(618-1644 AD!)

Hangongyue
Jiuxioutian (?)
(907-921 AD)

Huolong Zhenren
火龍眞人
"Perfect Man of the Fire Dragon"

(Korea)
Song Yuanqiao
(1288-1370)
Southern Family
Heaven & Earth Style
(Keeper of Zhang's Teachings)

Zhang San-feng (1247-??? AD)
Thirteen Methods

Tai Yi Zhenren

Ma Yun Cheng

Wang Zhong Yue
T'ai chi Ch'uan

Zhang Song Ze

Chen Wang Ting (1600-1680 Ad)
Chen Style

Mi Den Xia & Guo Ji Yuen
The Two Saints

Dong Hai Chuan
Pa Kua Kungfu

Chen Chang Xin (1771-1872 AD)
CHEN 'Old Form'

Yang Lu Chan (1799-1872)
Yang Style

Chen You Ben
Chen 'New Form'

Chen Jing Ping
Small Form & Zhao Bao

Yang Jian Hou
(1839-1917 AD)

Yang Ban Hou
(1837-1890 AD)

Wu Yu Xiang
Wu Style (1813-1880 AD)

Yang Den Fu
(1883-1936 AD)

Wu Chuan You

Li Yi Yu (1832-1892 AD)

Hao Wei Zhen (1849-1920)
Hao Style

(others)

Sun Lu T'ang (1861-1932)
Sun Style

Note: There are many hundreds of other styles of Taijiquan not listed here. Most may be off-shoots of the main Five that are listed here. Other may be Fresh Styles.

This represents the mainstream lineage of development and not "all styles" or "all variants".

Xu Xuanping (Hsu Hsuan-p'ing. 許宣平)

Hsu, Hsuan-p'ing, is recorded by Chinese historians as a notable Taoist poet and practitioner of Taoist Tao Yin: a precursor to what is now called Qigong. He lived in China during the Tang Dynasty. Legend says that he left the city of Yangshan to become a recluse and build a home in Nan Mountain.

According to the open-source public dictionary on Wikipedia, "His legendary description is that he was very tall, perhaps more than six feet tall with a beard that reached to his navel and hair down to his feet. He walked with a gait like a running horse and that each time he carried firewood down from the hills to the town to sell he would recite this poem:

> 'At dawn I carry the firewood to sell
>
> To buy wine today, at dusk I will return
>
> Please tell me the way to get home?
>
> Just follow the mountain track up into the clouds!"

This seems to paint a picture of a rather enthusiastic old man living a hermitic life on the mountain slopes, amidst the animals, trees and mists.

Another version reads:

> "'I bring firewood to the market in the morning
>
> Bringing wine back at sunset
>
> Where is my home?
>
> It is in the green woods, through the clouds."

Whilst both versions tell us virtually the same thing this also serves to illustrate the difficulty of accurate translation from Chinese to English, something which affects all fields of knowledge coming from China to the west.

Xu is thought by some historians to have taught Tao Yin to Zhang San-feng. This possibly had some influence on Zhang's thinking when he created his Wudang Taoist Boxing Form later. Other schools hold that Xu himself was a Tai Chi Chuan practitioner, and that the style Xu Xuanping passed down was simply called "37", because it consisted of 37 named styles or techniques. During this time it was also known as Chang Ch'uan (長拳) or Long Boxing as a reference to the flowing power of the Yangtze River(揚子江}, (which is also known as the Chang Jiang (長江) or Long River). He also is quoted as having a disciple called Song Yuanqiao (遠橋), who lived in Beijing during the early part of the 20th Century. He practiced an ancient Daoist Martial Art said to have been passed down through the generations to Song Shuming (書銘).

Li Dao Zi

Li Dao Zi (Lidaozi) lived before Zhang San-feng. An early "Taoist style" was created by him and was called Xian Tian Quan (Xiantianquan). The words "Xian-tian" translates to "the stage before the universe is created" or "Before Heaven" style. This is the Daoist concept of Wuji, which reflects the Taoist philosophical principles of returning to the pure state of Wuji, the "original state" prior to Taiji. Wuji is the state prior to Taiji. Lidaozi is one of the first people to use the term "Taiji" in relationship with a Martial Art. He taught his student Yulianzhou a poem about Xiantianquan:

"Taiji is so subtle

To embody it you must be empty as air

Its movements are innate

As the chime is to the bell

Hanging from the ridgepole of an old temple:

Natural as a tiger's growl,

Or a monkey's cry.

Sometimes like the current whirling deep within a still pool,

Sometimes rising like waves at sea!

It makes the body sound,

And also it makes resonant the Mind."

This is just one of many poems which are aimed at teaching students to find less physical ways of practising health and to look for the subtlety of the unique principles of Taoist Boxing, especially those which take us back to an infant-like state; no expectations, no hard muscle, no plans, just experience life as you wander the paths! This carefree sentiment was later echoed by Hujingzi with his poems.

Han Gong Yue.

Han Gongyue lived during the Liang Dynasty (907-921CE) and was accredited as the founder of the style named "Nine Little Heavens" (Hsiao Chiu Tian): The Little Nine Heaven system consists of three skills: Ju Kung (Nine Chamber Fist), Chian-kuan jen (swordsmanship); and Shih Shui (Bone marrow washing). Its theory is based on yin/yang, five elements and the constellations and positions of heavenly divinatory symbols. Its aim is entering Tao by way of physical and mental skills.

The 'Nine chamber fist style', according to Shih-fu James McNeil, "has both the characteristics of strengthening the body actively and in a pessimistic manner for self-defence". It is mainly based on the Confucian thoughts of the merging of Heaven and Man to transform one's disposition. In skill, it is based on the Tao's practice of the balancing between Yin and Yang to relax the tendons and bones, and to perform marrow washing. Even though its name translates to fist, it is actually an exclusive literature and a rich inheritance passed down through the centuries by word of mouth. This style has fourteen postures including lift hands, single whip, big and small punch and grasping the sparrow's tail. Each of these postures are found in present day Tai Chi. In addition, fist under elbow and

80

repulse the monkey are included in Nine Little Heavens but referred to as flower among the leaves and cloud on monkey's head.

The basis of Little Nine Heaven has been recorded in Chinese historical books as originating from the Nine Chamber Scriptures written by the Yellow Emperor, Huang- Ti (2698 B.C.-2598 B.C.). Huang-Ti is credited with improving upon the art of wrestling to defeat the rebellious tribal chieftains, thus bringing all corners of the land under control. This victory laid down a solid foundation of unity for the Chinese nation. Huang-Ti's military feats and tactics were the beginning of China's Martial Arts. He was accredited with the invention and developments of many things, from agriculture to healthier lifestyles and even more practical clothing. He was the "Great Leader" of China.

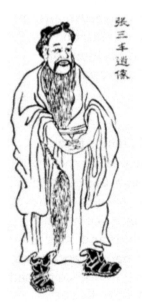

Zhang San-feng (Ch'eung San-feng) developed what is these days generally called 'Wudang Gongfu' (Wu Tang Kung Fu or Chinese Boxing Training of the Wu Tang Mountains). It may have been known simply as 'Thirteen Methods, Tao Ch'uan, T'ai Chi Kung (Supreme Ultimate [TAO] Training) or Taijigong, according to one researcher, not T'ai Chi Ch'uan (Supreme Ultimate Boxing) which was a name used much later in history; after the Chen Style was developed. The new name has since been applied to almost any style of this art. Anyone liking the health and fitness context may have called it T'ai Chi Kung, or even Tao Kung. Who knows the original name? We can only guess.

(Above Left: Ch'eung San-feng from an old wood-block image)

On a previous page you will see the T'ai Chi Ch'uan family Tree. I have tried to make this as accurate as possible with as much up to date information as I could get: with huge thanks to all the dedicated Chinese Arts Masters and researchers around the world who make this possible.

How lucky we are nowadays to have the use of word processor programmes, storage media, Digital Versatile Discs (DVD), the World Wide Web and the likes. Because of this media even more information is coming out of China and to the West. We are possibly much more fortunate than the Chinese themselves, for many in China cannot get access to such traditional knowledge so easily; although changes are happening and public pressure is building up (World news March 2012).

The history of Taoist Boxing is often debated, sometimes written differently and sometimes changed, altered in translation or rewritten. Not even the majority of Chinese historians or practitioners can agree. Nor do they all understand it in the same way. There is no hard and fast way. It is open, it seems, to interpretation. There are, dare I say it, some prejudices and personal ideas* about the history as well as the Art itself but one thing remains that is undisputable, that is the Taoist philosophical core principles that are the guidelines for this most popular life skill. (* This is "Human nature".)

In 1727, Emperor Yongzheng circulated an "official" edict which directed local officials to strictly prohibit individual teaching of "boxing and staff", as the Martial Arts were called then. Emperor Qianlong later directed a severe literary inquisition which destroyed many scrolls and writings from the period 1550-1750. An anthology of Huang Zongxi's writings containing the Epitaph to Zhang San-feng was earmarked and designated for destruction, but fortunately it survived to become a major source of controversy in the history of Chinese Martial Arts. Since then Chinese Boxing styles have been illogically labelled as being either of the Shaolin or "external" school, or the Wudang or "internal" school and, ultimately, Tai Chi Ch'uan was labelled as an "internal" style and identified with the Zhang San-feng legend. This has led to many misconceptions about Taijiquan and its practice. It has also led to misconceptions and jumped upon pre-conclusions about Tiandidao, as many people wrongly assume that an "internal school" should not exhibit "external methods" in training. True Taijiquan practitioners will know that Tao is both Yin *and* Yang, so therefor is T'ai Chi Ch'uan, and so it can neither be internal or external in substance but its effects are truly internal.

The reader must make up his or her own mind about the truth and what is right. I can only say at this point in my studies that it appears to me that the biggest changes in latter day T'ai Chi Ch'uan came along with Yang Lu-chan, family servant and later official student of the Chen Family but later developing Yang Style after moving to Beijing (Peking). It appears that Yang developed his style to reflect the Yin (softer) aspects of training and thus concentrate on the development of spiritual ch'i (transforming Ch'i to Shen); Yang Lu-chan used the Chen Style set known as "Old Frame" - featuring higher stances and wide sweeping movements. His original style today is said to be only known by a few. It is also clear that many original Form or Forms have been lost to time. It has been a common trait in China's feudal past not to trust your "family treasures" (your secret boxing set) to strangers. Like many villages of the UK and other so-called "developed" countries, you can remain a stranger for at least fifty years! Many styles died with their keepers, so much history has been lost and many good skills left to be rediscovered.

Author and scholar Jou, Tsung Hwa in his worthy book 'The Dao of Taijiquan - Way to Rejuvenation', said that in order to understand T'ai Chi Ch'uan (in the modern world) one should study Chen, Yang and Wu (presumably in that order; their order of creation). In his educated view these three styles hold the key factors which relate to the classics and would therefore give the student the best overall view of the original principles if all three styles were studied and "essential principles" extracted. Of course most people neither have the time or the resources, let alone access to three reputable masters of three traditional styles. Therefore I whole-heartedly recommend that you, the reader buys Shih-fu Jou's book and study that also.

Most of the historic styles recorded below have movements (Forms) in them which resemble those found in the three "classical" styles listed in the Family Tree (below) today. There were movements named, Single Whip, Grasp Sparrow's Tail, Looking at Fist under Elbow and Step Back to Drive Away Monkey (Repulse Monkey). Although the author is not aware of any source material which can confirm exactly what the original Forms of the ancient Masters were like, it is said that they varied in length from eight to seventeen or more.

From what documents can be found, from various quarters, we can trace the history of T'ai chi Ch'uan to around the T'ang Dynasty (618-907 A.D). My Old Master said in his book that the Li Family's Arts can be traced back to an Eight Forms practice of Li Ho- Hsieh. Although this has not been verified by any written history which I have personally viewed, I have no reason to doubt this; there are many books around today in which the author omits, deliberately or not, the facts which are recorded by another and historically recorded in China; we may not see it but it can be out there. There are many grey areas in between and you will have to fill in those for yourself as much recorded history in China as well as elsewhere has been lost or destroyed.

The original style's name, as created by Zhang San-feng, has been lost, as stated earlier. I shall personally concede to Shih-fu Wong Kiew Kit's theory and call it "Wudang Kung Fu", after the legendary events in the foothills of the Wudang Mountains. Later it got the name T'ai Chi Ch'uan by a developer called Wang Zhong Yue. Other styles of T'ai Chi were later developed or created, many of which incorporated Snake and Crane plus other animal stylised moves, like

Golden Cockerel, Dragon, etcetera; the reader is asked to note here that the reference to Snake and Crane in Wellspring is deemed as an important reference to Zhang San-feng and his creation after the said witnessing of the fight between these two creatures; animals have always been imitated in Chinese Kung Fu and I have no reason to believe that Zhang San-feng would omit the importance of these creatures' actions in his fighting system if that is indeed what he saw. In all areas of Taijiquan development within Tiandidao I remain unconsciously guided by the spirit of Wudang whilst in the general Taoist Kung Fu syllabus of T'ien Ti Tao both Forms and technique were developed by long term study of traditional principles dating back as far as the 15th century - China's "golden period" of Kung Fu; hence T'ien Ti Tao was said by one old I.C.K.F. Master in R. o. China to be "Probably more traditional than most traditional systems!"

It is recorded that Wang Zhong Yue (author: Wang is reputed to have authored The T'ai Chi Treatise, alleged by the Wu brothers to have been found in Beijing as part of the Salt Shop Manuals in the mid-19th century. This treatise records many T'ai chi Ch'uan proverbs) said words to the effect that one should study the I-Ching in order to understand T'ai Chi Ch'uan. Perhaps it was this which has led to many people intellectualising about T'ai Chi Ch'uan. The study of the I-Ching ("Yijing" - Book of Changes) is important as we should understand its relations. In the T'ai Chi Ch'uan Forms we go from "Wu Chi" to "T'ai Chi" and back again, crossing the various "Pa Kua" as we do so. T'ai Chi Ch'uan is all about understanding the philosophy and applying it to body, mind and spirit, yet its goal is to be set free from the man-made intellectual whilst being true to Tao.

T'ai Chi Ch'uan or Taijiquan is an "energy art". What that means is that any system pertaining to be T'ai Chi Ch'uan, Taijiquan or even named by the abbreviated "Tai Chi" should adhere to certain principles that govern the body and the Ch'i/Qi. We must not forget here also that it is an exercise for health, relaxation, self-defence and all the other benefits that accompany it, not just an intellectual challenge.

Emperor Fu Hsi.

Taoism is thought to have been widely established by Fu His ("Fuxi" with the "xi" sounding more like a "zee"). Fu Xi taught his loyal subjects to cook, to fish with nets, and to hunt with weapons made of iron: which could well have led to the origin of one verse or part of the Tao Te Ching/Daodejing, with a phrase "A wise ruler sets his subjects free, therefore they follow him." Thinking out loud on paper, how true that is. Nobody appreciates anything more than being shown how to be independent. Although this was a rare situation for olden day leaders, emperors or kings, it was not entirely uncommon. These days it seems that the world is full of little dictators, in one way or the other, milking it

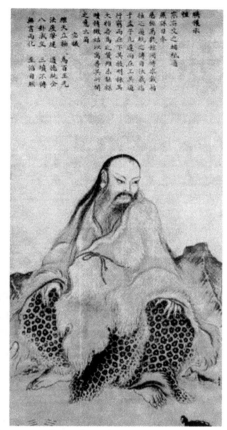

for all they can get and enslaving the populace for their own gains; con men and con women using politics for business and financial gains.

Traditionally, Fu Xi is considered the originator of the I Ching (also known as the Yi Jing or Zhou Yi), which work is attributed to his reading of Yellow River Map. According to this tradition, Fu Xi (pictured right) had the arrangement of the trigrams (卦 Bāgua) of the I Ching revealed to him supernaturally. This arrangement precedes the compilation of the I Ching during the Zhou dynasty. He is said to have discovered the arrangement in markings on the back of a mythical dragon-horse (sometimes said to be a turtle) that emerged from the river Luo. This discovery is also thought to have been the origin of Chinese calligraphy.

King Wen (1152-1056BC and his son, Duke Zhao also figure in this preamble leading up to the "invention" of T'ai Chi Ch'uan Taijiquan as accredited to Zhang San-feng. Each of these figures had contributed to the thoughts and processes of the Taoist Philosophy which gave the philosophical foundations for what Old Zhang created by means of development of the '64 hexagrams' and the 'I Ching' (Book of Changes).

This leads me to further discussion of important aspects relating to the "T'ai Chi Ch'uan Family Tree". The Family Tree, as we know it today, may be accurate or may be educated guesswork and some key figures left out through being unknown. It is an attempted modern day record created by many historians to replace "hearsay, rumours and educated guesses" or destroyed or lost historical records. To have such a record is truly remarkable though and we can, or must, assume that it has reasonably accurate lineage. However, we may never know the lost or left out information on people who were in-between one tree's marker and the other. For example, what or who influenced or lead Wang Zhong Yue to call the skills "T'ai Chi Ch'uan"?

A few of these questions appear to be answered within these pages, if we can trust the often revived and re-recorded historical records. There is no reason to disbelieve them but at the same time there is little proof except for the alleged appearance of an old book in someone's family here and there.

Generally we can accept the Family Tree and the fact that all these people were involved in the lineage development of Taijiquan somewhere. Whether or not other people were and were not recorded we shall never know. Below you will see my researched and revised version of the T'ai Chi Ch'uan Family Tree and below that a brief description of who did what to contribute to this line of developments. This, I have found personally, benefits a better understanding of Taijiquan and its full history of development and emphasises just how worthy a system of health giving exercise it is; for body, mind and soul.

"The only thing which is both predictable and constant is change."

Old Taoist Proverb.

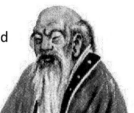

Chuang-Tze / Zhuangzi.

Zhuangzi/Chuang-Tze or Zhuang Zhou (369 BC - 286 BC) is also referred to as "Master Zhang". Accurate detail is lost, but as far back as the 4th Century BC, a Taoist wrote passages in the 'Zhuangzi' (a book in his own name), pertaining to the psychology and practice of martial arts. Zhuangzi claimed that knowledge was limited by life, but knowledge itself is unlimited. Chuang-Tze was renowned for his observations and was, according to one ancient text, unable to be bought by bribe or positions in any social structure. The Record of the Grand Historian says "Chuang was an admirable writer and composer [of argument], and by his instances and truthful descriptions hit and exposed the Mohists and Literati. The ablest scholars of his day could not escape his satire nor reply to it, while he allowed and enjoyed himself with his sparkling, dashing style; and thus it was that the greatest men, even kings and princes, could not use him for their purposes. [Example of this is that] King Wei of Chu, having heard of the ability of Chuang Chau, sent messengers with large gifts to bring him to his court, and promising also that he would make him his chief minister. Chuang-Tze, however, only laughed and said to them, "A thousand ounces of silver are a great gain to me; and to be a high noble and minister is a most honourable position. But have you not seen the victim-ox for the border sacrifice? It is carefully fed for several years, and robed with rich embroidery that it may be fit to enter the Grand Temple. When the time comes for it to do so, it would prefer to be a little pig, but it cannot get to be so." He then said "Go away quickly, and do not soil me with your presence. I would rather amuse and enjoy myself in the midst of a filthy ditch than be subject to the rules and restrictions in the court of a sovereign. I have determined never to take office, but prefer the enjoyment of my own free will."

Zhuangzi's proposition that life is quite short and therefore does not hold enough time to learn everything, is of course quite practical. He said "to pursue the unlimited is foolish", which logically can only be correct. His way of thinking was refreshing in a time when many followed blindly and read constantly the works of others, trying to fathom it all.

This further example of Zhuang-zi's logic and wit is to me one of the funniest because of its simplicity and reminds me of the many critics and time-wasters that one might encounter these days, whether that be in the street or on Facebook, Linked-In, or whatever:

"The Happiness of Fish".

Zhuangzi and Huizi were strolling along the banks of the dam at Hao Waterfall when Zhuangzi said, "See how the minnows come out and dart around where they please! That's what fish really enjoy!"

Huizi said, "You're not a fish, how do you know what fish enjoy?"

Zhuangzi said, "You're not me, so how do you know I don't know what fish enjoy?"

Huizi said, "I'm not you, so I certainly don't know what you know. On the other hand, you're certainly not a fish, so that still proves you don't know what fish enjoy!"

Zhuangzi said, "Let's go back to your original question, please. You asked me how I know what fish enjoy — so you already knew I knew it when you asked the question. I know it by standing here beside the Hao (observation)."

"The traditional interpretation of this 'Daoist staple', writes Chad Hansen (2003:145), is a humorous miscommunication between a mystic and a logician. The encounter also outlines part of the Daoist practice of observing and learning from the natural world."

Zhuangzi's "Dream" where he asked, "Was I a man dreaming that I was a butterfly, or am I a butterfly now dreaming that I am a man?"

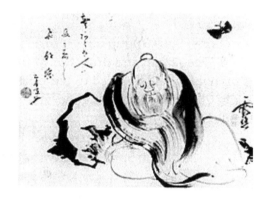

The Song Family.

During the Song Dynasty the Song family of ancient China was well known and highly respected in regards to their moral integrity and values. These reputations lead to the influence of Chinese Martial Arts into the Song family traditions. Hsu Hsuan-p'ing/Xu Xuanping was a very well- known practitioner of Chang Quan or "Long Fist". Hsu Hsuan-p'ing passed his knowledge on to the Song family because they had such a worthy reputation. They were the only known keepers of his Arts. These teachings have been preserved and still pass from generation to generation this day. Song Yuanqiao (1288 - 1370) inherited these Song family traditions and became a disciple of another master. That master was Ch'eung San-feng who then developed an Art based of his previous knowledge and skill; referred today as T'ai Chi Ch'uan.

Song, Yuanqiao was selected by Ch'eung San-feng to preserve the "Tai Chi Chuan" traditions. Song Yuanqiao wrote a famous T'ai Chi Ch'uan manual called "The Origin and Branches of the Song Style T'ai Chi Practice". This manual would be used to pass this particular family style of T'ai Chi Ch'uan down from generation to generation within the Song family. This Southern Group style was called

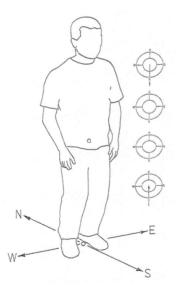

'Heaven & Earth Style'. It is in the history of the Song Dynasty that the Song family of modern day Korea is rooted. In ancient times, there were no hard boundaries between present day China and present day North Korea or South Korea. During these times, the Song family would freely travel between China and Korea.

(Ref: http://chunseungwon.com/about.htm)

Hujingzi.

Apparently "a lost page in history" style is Houtian Fa - "The stage after the universe (Heaven) is created, method", created by Hujingzi. This is said to have had 17 postures and emphasized elbow strikes; which appears to the author to be a matter of personal preference rather than philosophical importance to the Form or Method. The major postures of this style were of course ward off, roll back, press, push, pull, split, elbow strike and shoulder strike. These postures are the eight methods (Ba Fa) which also became the foundation stones of Chen and Yang style Taijiquan.

If you "dissolve" these predecessor styles into to Zhang San-feng's Wudang "T'ai Chi" Boxing proverbial mixing bowl, then add the acclaimed history of his training *Zhang is thought to have met and trained under 'Jinoyuanshangren', a Shaolin warrior monk for ten years. He became expert in Shaolin Martial Arts systems: "The Change of Tendons", "The Marrow Washing" and "18 Buddha's Hands". As well as these classical styles Old Zhang also mastered the six postures of the original Five Fist- forms (Quans - five fist): Dragon, Tiger, Snake, Leopard and Crane Forms of Shao-lin Ch'uan, so had excellent training and knowledge of many varied boxing styles and methods of health) then we can actually get some idea of what Zhang's style may have looked like.

(*Zhang is thought to have met and trained under 'Jinoyuanshangren', a Shaolin warrior monk for ten years. He became expert in Shaolin Martial Arts systems: "The Change of Tendons", "The Marrow Washing" and "18 Buddha's Hands". As well as these classical styles Old Zhang also mastered the six postures of the original Five Fist- forms (Quans - five fist): Dragon, Tiger, Snake, Leopard and Crane Forms of Shao-lin Ch'uan, so had excellent training and knowledge of many varied boxing styles and methods of health) This story is not at all improbable and the history of the Chinese culture denotes early similarities or shared interests of the (earlier) Taoist cultures and (later) Buddhist culture and the Shao-lin Monastery.

In an article by Salvatore Canzonieri, in an old edition of Inside Kung Fu magazine, he states "Oddly enough, the Shaolin fighting arts came from a pacifist beginning: the merger of the spiritual philosophies of Buddhism and Taoism". The first, most famous and main Shaolin temple was located in Henan (Honan) province, along the north side of Shao Shih mountain, and built by the royal decree of Emperor Hsiao Wien [Xiao Wen] during the early Northern Wei dynasty (386 - 534 AD) for an Indian Buddhist monk named Batuo (or Fo Tuo in Chinese). (He is most remembered today by his statue, which depicts a fat and jolly seated monk, a.k.a. the "Laughing Buddha.") It was only then that Shaolin became a Buddhist centre. In one legend they say that Zhang returned to Shaolin briefly, but was not interested in what they were doing there, he wanted to pursue the Tao and Taoist Arts. It seems very likely though that Old Zhang was still impressed by the Shaolin Five Animal Forms and when he saw the snake and crane fighting and that influenced his "new" Form of Taoist Boxing.

Zhang was thought to be about 67 years of age when he met the Daoist hermit called Huolong ('Fire Dragon') in 1314. Huolong taught Zhang one of the pre-T'ai Chi Ch'uan styles as a means of reaching enlightenment and immortality. After four years of training without reaching his goal, Zhang moved to the Wudang Mountains. There, living in an abandoned hermit's hut, he practiced and meditated for the next nine years until he became enlightened. After the snake and crane incident and created his own "complete" Form based upon the movements of the Snake and Crane, but utilising the snake's ability to avoid and use "soft" methods to overcome "hard" attacks. This is the origination of the "soft" element of T'ai Chi Ch'uan, not using "hard" or bone type strength.

Wang Zongyue (宗岳) .

Wang Zongyue (1733-1795) is historically accredited as being taught by Ch'eung San- feng, before himself going on to teach Zheng Song Ze (sadly there is no history or record found for this man who then taught Chen Wang-ting at the original Chen Village; now moved to make way for a Dam).

Chen Wang-ting.

The Chen Family Style (家 氏 or 式太極) is the oldest recorded style and is considered by some to be the "parent" form of the "Five traditional family styles" that are generally recognised today as the "traditional; remember from earlier that much history has been lost or destroyed. Chen style is characterized by Silk reeling (Chan si jin; 纏絲勁), alternating fast/slow motion and bursts of power (fa jin; 發勁).

Chen appears to be the most identifiable point where the term "T'ai Chi Ch'uan" started being used in reference to Boxing Forms that contained Yin/Yang and other Taoist principles. Therefore we can safely say that Chen Wanting's own interpretation of the Wudang Gongfu Forms or Methods he learned, make the first truly identifiable point recorded in the modern history of Taijiquan.

According to information placed in the public domain: "The origin and nature of what is now known as and incorrectly written as "Tai Chi" is not historically verifiable until around the 17th century. Documents of this period indicate the Chen clan settled in Chenjiagou (Chen Village, 家溝), Henan Province, in the 13th century and reveal the defining contribution of Chen Wangting (1580-1660). The informer then goes on to say "It is therefore not clear how the Chen family actually came to practice their unique boxing style and contradictory histories abound." The Chen family style is said to have most of its roots in Chang Ch'uan or "Long Fist", a style of Kung Fu which was generally characterised by its very low stances, jumping kicks, spinning crescent Kicks and joined-up Forms (hence "long"). In terms of the principles that are generally accepted as essential in Taijiquan, Chen style is different to the majority. However, it has produced some good fighters as being able to hold composure and remain centred whilst in such low stances is beneficial to the abilities of a combatant.

Wikipedia information states: "Whether or not Chen invented the earliest form of T'ai Chi Ch'uan is in dispute. Traditional folklore and many lineages name the semi-mythical figure of Zhang San-feng, a Taoist monk, as the progenitor of the art."

Two widely-documented theories of Chen's martial arts work exist: the first is that he learnt his arts from Wang Zongyue and the Wudang tradition developed by Zhang San- feng. The second theory (seemingly accepted by the Chen family, and supported by historical evidence) is that he combined his previous military experience and the theories of Jingluo and Daoyin with the popular teachings of Qi Jiguang.

His complete work contained five smaller sets of forms, a 108-move Long Fist routine, and a Cannon Fist routine. Chen is also credited with the invention of the first push hands exercises. Chen also practiced a few Shaolin forms, and some historians postulate that Shaolin arts also had a significant influence on Chen Wang-ting's T'ai Chi, though none of the Taoist influences on Chen family T'ai Chi Ch'uan exist in the Shaolin tradition; only in recent years has Shaolin been taking on some Taoist Styles, like T'ai Chi Ch'uan, although some people say this is just for commercial reasons.

Chen Wangting's next well-known successor was the 14th generation Chen Changxing (1771-1853), who was the direct teacher (see Yang Lu-chan's story below) of the founder of Yang-style T'ai Chi Ch'uan: Yang Lu-chan." (Pic. Right)

Yang Lu-ch'an

The Yang family first became involved in the study of T'ai Chi Ch'uan in the early 19th century. The founder of the Yang-style was Yang Lu-ch'an (露禪), a.k.a. Yang Fu-k'ui (福魁, 1799-1872), who studied in the Chen Village, whilst working as a servant in the Chen's family home, and tutelage of under Ch'en Chang-hsing (Chen Changxing) starting in 1820. Legend has it that one day a challenger came to Chen's home whilst he was away. In his absence Yang accepted his invitation so as not to embarrass the Chen family by the visitor saying that they were unable to meet him in a challenge.

Yang beat the challenger, to the amazement of the family, using the "secret" Chen Style that Yang had learned by mainly spying through a hole in a fence late at night! For this he could have been killed; stealing a family Martial Art Style was like taking the family treasure! Chen spared his life and was impressed with his skills and abilities. He taught him the full Chen Arts and later allowed him to leave.

It is thought that when Yang got to Peking/Beijing, he found that many older people wanted to learn Taijiquan but could not manage the low stances and high kicks. Yang worked on developing a higher "framed" style by removing all difficult low stances or high kicks. It is thought that when he asked permission from Chen Chang-hsing, Chen was upset that he wanted to alter his system and refused; also disowning Yang. Yang later became a teacher in his own right, and his subsequent expression of Taijiquan became known as the "Yang Style". This directly led to the development of other three major styles of T'ai Chi Ch'uan (see below). Yang Lu-ch'an (and some would say the art of T'ai Chi Ch'uan, in general) came to prominence as a result of his being hired by the Chinese Imperial family to teach T'ai Chi Ch'uan to the Elite Palace Battalion of the Imperial Guards in 1850, a position he held until his death.

Li Ruidong and Li Style

Li-style Taijiquan was created by Li Rui-dong (1851-1917) from Tianjin and Wang Lanting (Wang was a students of Dong Haichuan, the founder of Ba Gua Quan – Eight Diagrams Boxing) from the basis of Yang-style T'ai Chi Ch'uan. Many people have since contributed to its development. Li style has multiple Forms, instead of the usual one or two. The usual idea behind multiple Forms is that each will teach a different aspect of the training and or principles.

The Li-style combines T'ai Chi Ch'uan concepts with the Jinchan style that Li Ruidong had learned from his master, the Buddhist monk Longchan, as well as containing elements of Hsing- I Ch'uan (Xingyiquan) and Pa Kua Ch'uan (Bagua Quan), like the later Sun Style does. The primary techniques of this style are the five fist

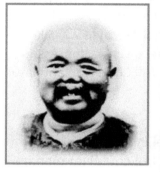

strikes of Taijiquan, and it is also known as "Wuxing Chui" or "Five-Star Fist". The style includes both empty-hand forms and a variety of weapons forms. Most of the movements of this style require a very low stance, like Chen Style, so strong legs are necessary. The low stances of Li Ruidong's style that are used similarly by Chen Family Style, are the only two systems to use this low stance method. There is a deep-rooted (no pun intended) tradition in some areas of Chinese Boxing which prefers low stances to develop better leg strength as well as keep the centre of gravity lower than the opponents.

Wu Chan-yu or Wu Style

The Wù (pronounced with a staccato style "Wu") family style (simplified Chinese: 氏) T'ai chi Ch'uan (Taijiquan) of Wu Ch'uan-yu (Wu Quanyou) and Wu Chien-Ch'uan (Wu Jian Quan) is the second most popular form of T'ai Chi Ch'uan in the world today, after the Yang style, so they say, and fourth in terms of family seniority. This style is different from the Wu style of T'ai Chi Ch'uan (氏) founded by Wu Yu-hsiang. While the names are distinct in pronunciation and the Chinese characters used to write them are different, they are often Romanised the same way.

Wu Ch'uan-yu or Wu Quanyu (佑, 1834-1902) was a military officer cadet of Manchu ancestry in the 'Yellow Banner Camp' (see Qing Dynasty Military) in the Forbidden City, Beijing and also a hereditary officer of the Imperial Guards Brigade. At that time, Yang Lu-ch'an (露禪, 1799-1872) was the Martial Arts instructor in the Imperial

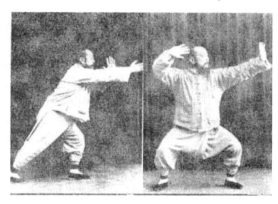

Guards, teaching T'ai Chi Ch'uan, and in 1850 Wu Ch'uan-yu became one of his students. This style is said to be developed from the original Yang Form but placing less importance on the development of ch'i and more on technical ability. The low stances may have been inherited from Chen's "Second Form" which of course Yang knew. Movements are mainly small and done in a slow and even manner with some variations in speed or size. With an emphasis on correct posture, application and technical use, it is hardly surprising that many Wu style practitioners have done well in contest. Wu Family Style is therefore thought to be more "Kung Fu" by some and less "T'ai Chi Ch'uan". Movements are smaller than Yang Style but not quite as small as "Woo" Style; when we say "small" we mean that steps are shorter and arms do not reach so far out, this is "frame", the distance in which we work.

Wu Yu-hsianq – Wu/Hao Style.

The Wu (pronounced like "Woo") or Wu /Hao style of T'ai chi Ch'uan of Wu Yu-hsiang (禹襄, 1813-1880), is a separate family style from the more popular Wu style (氏) of Wu Chien-ch'uan. Wu Yu-hsiang's style was third among the five T'ai Chi Ch'uan families in seniority and is fifth in terms of popularity.

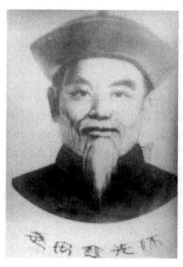

武禹襄　祖师

Wu Yu-hsiang was a scholar from a wealthy and influential family who became a senior student (along with his two older brothers Wu Ch'eng-ch'ing and Wu Ju-ch'ing) of Yang Lu-ch'an. There is a body of writing attributed to Wu Yu-hsiang on the subject of T'ai Chi theory, writings that are considered influential by many other schools not directly associated with his style. Wu Yu-hsiang also studied for a brief time with a teacher from the Chen Family, Chen Ch'ing-p'ing, to whom he was introduced by Yang; Chen Ch'ing- p'ing changed the Chen family system to create a smaller framed version called Shao Gar, Wu Yu-Hsiang studied this along with Yang Lo-sim's style and later created his fusion ("Woo Style").

His most famous student was his nephew, **Li I-yü** (李亦畲, 1832-1892), who also authored several important works on T'ai Chi Ch'uan. Li I-yü had a younger brother who was also credited as an author of at least one work on the subject of T'ai Chi Ch'uan, whose name was Li Ch'i-hsüan. Li I-yü taught Hao Wei-chen (郝為真, 1842-1920), who taught Li Xiang-yuan, Li Shengduan, Sun Lu-tang, Hao Wei-chen's own son Hao Yüeh-ru (郝月如) and a few others that are not named.

Hao Wei-chen and Wu/Hao Style.

Hao Wei-chen (為真, also spelled Hao Weizhen, 1842-1920) was a Chinese T'ai Chi Ch'uan teacher. Hao became a well-known and influential teacher of Wu Yu-hsiang style T'ai Chi Ch'uan, his teacher Li I-yu was Wu Yu-hsiang's nephew. Hao passed the art to his son and grandson, who all became respected teachers in their turn, so that the style is sometimes now known as Wu/Hao style; to avoid confusion with the other Wu Style. One of Hao's most famous students was Sun Lu-t'ang.

The "Woo" (Wu/Hao) style differs from Wu in that it has very small circular movements of the arms and feet with very few fast or "fa jing" movements. The old Wu/Hao style seems to have been lost and the closest teachings found today are those of the newer or more current Wu/Hao family style which has been created to assimilate the old principles as much as is possible.

Sun Lu-tanq (Right) / Sun Style.

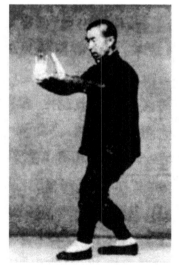

The Sun style (氏) T'ai Chi Ch'uan was developed by Sun Lu-tang (祿堂, 1861-1932), who was considered expert in two other internal martial arts styles: Hsing-I (Xingyi Quan) Ch'uan and Pa Gua (Bagua Quan) Ch'uan and some Qigong before he came to study T'ai Chi Ch'uan. Today, Sun Style ranks fourth in popularity and fifth in terms of seniority among the five main family styles of T'ai Chi Ch'uan; accepted list of styles by mainland China's educational and Martial arts facilities. It is the oldest of the modern styles yet is not "new" entirely. Sun learned Wu/Hao style T'ai Chi Ch'uan from Hao

Weizhen (為真), who was Li Yiyu's (亦畬) chief disciple. Sun Lu-tang mixed elements of Xingyiquan, Bagua Quan and Wu/Hao style Taijiquan and then added elements of Qigong to make "health" a priority.

It is also said that Sun Lu-tang was also the first "traditional male Chinese Instructor" to teach women's self-defence; an odd coincidence as the author of this book was the first Instructor to teach women's self-defence in his home region, c.1976. Today popular variations of the Sun Style Forms are being taught under the various "T'ai Chi for Health" banners around the world; a trend started by Dr. Paul Lam, a Chinese GP in Sydney, Australia with "Tai Chi for Arthritis". Dr. Lam's use of the Sun Style movements has been responsible for a surge of interest from people who would otherwise perhaps never have considered taking up Taijiquan. He achieved this by taking out any movements that may be difficult or risky for older people with balance or muscular/skeletal health problems. This in itself has done no harm to the more traditional styles as quite a decent percentage of people who regain health and balance may go on to learn the more traditional and "full" styles of T'ai Chi Ch'uan.

Note: Whilst Dr. Lam's T'ai Chi for Arthritis Form is based upon the modern Competition Styles of Beijing; these being made suitable for judging and devoid of most original principles. T'ien Ti Tao's "T'ai Chi for Health" Form and Sun's Dragon schools in South Wales, for example, are based on the traditional principles and movements of the "Sun *family* style" and these differ slightly from the Competition Forms, mainly in that they are much more relaxed and natural in movement.

Soo, Clifford Chee and Lee (Li) Family Style.

Soo Shih-fu (right) learned the Li Style from Li, Chan Kam (English: Chan Kam Lee). He in turn had learned from his ancestors in China and they could be traced back (through the above Taijiquan Lineage) to Li Ho-Hsieh who lived around 1000 B.C. (see above). Soo Shih-fu claims that these Arts have been in the Li (Lee) Family for over 3,000 years and that the "original" Li Form was of just eight movements. He wrote, "Originally Ho-Hsieh Lee (Li) and his family lived just outside Beijing (Peking), and it was here that he first started his practice devised the first eight movements. It was in his middle fifties that he took his family and settled down in Wei Hei Wei (see map below), a fishing

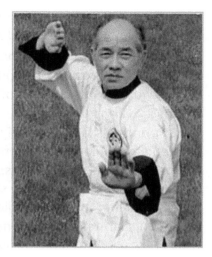

village about 200 miles east of Beijing on the coast, and there they remained in that district up to 1934" (extract from Lao Bah's book, "The Chinese Art of T'ai Chi Ch'uan" - Seahorse Books). From what little research is possible, the place is in a very busy shipping area of China.

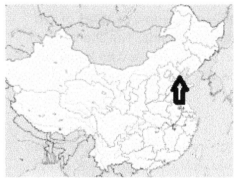

(Map: Wei Hei Wei is situated SW of Beijing, in the top of the Bay to the right side of the map)

It seems that Lee Family Style may possibly derive from Wu/Hao Style with its Northern roots and higher postures with small frame movements. Not only are there similarities in postures but, given the history of Grand-master Li, Chan Kam who also hailed from Wei Hei Wei, there would be even more likelihood of connections. Try as they may, family and senior students have attempted to find history there but so much has been lost or destroyed that this has proved impossible.

As we can see from the above synopsis of the most popular, well documented "family systems" of Taijiquan, there are many changes that have taken place since the days of Zhang San-feng and his disciples. In this respect we could say that T'ai Chi Ch'uan has become just another branch of Chinese Kung Fu but with an emphasis, variable in the differing styles, that revolves around the Taoist principles laid down originally (we can only surmise) by Zhang San-feng; or someone else before him but which he again changed and passed on in his teachings. The truth about all these changes is a bitter pill to swallow by some stylists who like to claim that their style is "original" or "pure Taijiquan" and others who try to claim that Zhang San-feng possibly never existed. The latter is something which is easily disputable through the great work of modern historians, who have gone to great lengths to trace the "real" Zhang San-feng (born 9th of April, 1247); the world now celebrates this with "World T'ai Chi in The Park" day close to his birthday but on the last Saturday of April every year and in almost every country.

One World Wide Web page owner used to show pictures of Wu Style postures and Lee Family Style side by side. The similarity of postures was remarkable and, of course to those who know, an indication of the links between the Wu Style of old and the Li Family Style of old could be likely.

According to Shih-fu Soo's daughter, Lavinia Soo-Warr, the family tree of Lee Family Style is structured as the lineage "tree" below. Rightfully added here, on the "tree", is the resulting branch that is T'ien Ti Tao and in its historical place on the "tree", plus the main Master Grades of Li/Lee Family Style that Prof. Chee Soo taught and who still carry on the lineage to this day.

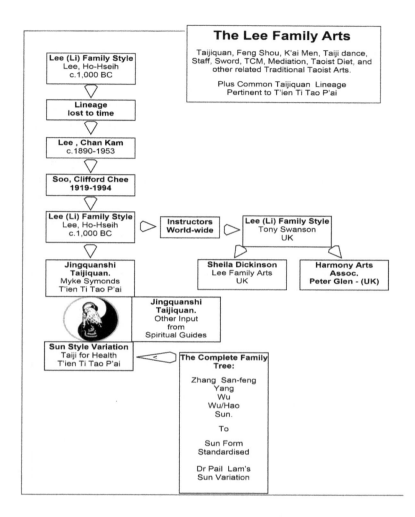

The Lee Family Arts

Taijiquan, Feng Shou, K'ai Men, Taiji dance, Staff, Sword, TCM, Mediation, Taoist Diet, and other related Traditional Taoist Arts.

Plus Common Taijiquan Lineage Pertinent to T'ien Ti Tao P'ai

Lee (Li) Family Style
Lee, Ho-Hseih
c.1,000 BC

Lineage lost to time

Lee , Chan Kam
c.1890-1953

Soo, Clifford Chee
1919-1994

Lee (Li) Family Style
Lee, Ho-Hseih
c.1,000 BC

Instructors World-wide

Lee (Li) Family Style
Tony Swanson
UK

Sheila Dickinson
Lee Family Arts
UK

Harmony Arts Assoc.
Peter Glen - (UK)

Jingquanshi Taijiquan.
Myke Symonds
T'ien Ti Tao P'ai

Jingquanshi Taijiquan.
Other Input from Spiritual Guides

Sun Style Variation
Taiji for Health
T'ien Ti Tao P'ai

The Complete Family Tree:

Zhang San-feng
Yang
Wu
Wu/Hao
Sun.

To

Sun Form Standardised

Dr Pail Lam's Sun Variation

An article on the development of Taijiquan in the UK suggests that "His daughter, Lavinia Soo-Warr, gained recognition from the Tai Chi Union for Great Britain (TCUGB) for his 'Li style', but the practice of other former students of Chee Soo has not been accepted as Taijiquan." (This is odd as I seem to recall that in the 19070's it was rejected, unrecognised by them.) This article is probably well-meaning but ill-informing and ill-informed article just goes to show the personal prejudices that are rampant when it comes to "style and lineage". Not that long ago the TCUGB refused to recognise Lee Style, alongside many others. Being personally aware from training contact of the fact that Shih-fu Soo taught his daughter, then she moved away to do modern Peking/ Beijing "people's style" with Peter Warr, and then began to recognising her father's great achievements after his death – which naturally made her the hereditary family style head by default but not necessarily the most knowledgeable about the system; Pete Warr, by the way, was involved in earlier days with another self-styled Chinese organisation in the UK so it was felt by many people involved in the Chinese Arts that the "recognition" was more political than practical. There are other practitioners of the Li family Style that should probably have far more recognition than they get as they were Shih-fu Soo's top Master Grades at the time of his death and who studied with him continuously for many years; so they actually know the style inside-out. At least one of these men, based in the Midlands of UK, still forges links with China and the Li Family Style and veraciously promotes the system "intact", as far as I can tell, as Shih-fu Soo, taught it to him and many others over many years. They are included on the "tree".

I can only say that the reader needs to know more, far more, about the true history of T'ai Chi Ch'uan, the petty politics and egotistic jostling for pole positions that have and do go on; all against the teachings of Tao, by the way! (Let go!) This seems to be the way of humans in all walks of life and in all countries. There were family rifts and my Old Master was visibly upset and unhappy - something that most of us go through at some time - which eventually caused him to move to another area for some peace and quiet, enabling him to get on with his life without the strife. Shih-fu Soo taught many people to a "Master Grade" level and these should all be recognised for their own contribution in preserving the Lee Family Arts as well as the smaller satellite groups that still exist.

Having been a student of his, witnessed (and felt!) his skills personally, having studied Tao for many years (with many more to go) and knowing many people involved in Martial Arts from many styles and walks of life, I can honestly say that articles like the one mentioned above do nothing to clarify the true aspects, history and acceptance of Taijiquan. It was a difficult decision to write about such things as this but the so-called facts are scattered, often random and biased. Readers should not take anything that denounces a life-time practitioner and dedicated teacher so flippantly. Please bear in mind the human frailties that make some people and some organisations "lick boots" and strive for higher positions and some individuals to make false statements to raise their own imagined status or even bite the proverbial hand that feeds them.

As a student of Shih-fu Soo, I have also fallen foul of comments made by others, *who do not know* me or anything about my training, on a web-site forum that was claiming to carry on his traditions. They even made childish and churlish comments about other teachers of Li Family Style. Hopefully, after being made aware that they were not only undermining themselves but the style they were saying *they* practised; these unthinking comments have been deleted. Sad. This is common not only in Taijiquan but all other Martial Arts. Heed this information but do not be put off. Human frailty includes "leaking ignorance". There are many good schools and good practitioners of Taijiquan and other Martial Arts around and the student has to attend regularly, practice fervently and digest thoroughly and then the truth will be known. In what I say I have to be honest. There is no other way.

Out of interest I shall mention here something which struck me profoundly one day. The day in question was at one of Shih-fu Soo's teacher training classes in Dunstable. As always happens with notable instructors, someone had cast aspersions about him. One of his senior students, perhaps un-tactfully, brought up the subject of lineage and teachers. Shih-fu Soo, I could tell, was not at all happy about discussing this subject, but went on to explain some basics about family and lineage. He concluded with a figure on the chalk-board and said "My first name was given as Clifford", and drew a large 'C' on the board. He continued, "My second name is Chinese and is Chee (he drew another large C, this time back-to-front against the first, making a large circle), my mother's name, which I have kept, is Soo (and then drew the 'S' in the middle of the two C's and two small 'o's shapes either side of the S, which of course makes a Tao symbol! He continued). Quite apart from anything else, T'ai Chi is my birth right" he concluded.

T'ai Chi Ch'uan, I could tell, was something he held in far higher importance than petty human arguments. He was great man and I have never met any other with as great an understanding and ability of Tao Chia and I would be honoured if I was considered to have as much skill in my whole body as he had in his little finger. This is just one reason why I am saddened when sick and mercenary people make false claims of lineage to him and his style, such as one man in Norwich who has never learned any of the Lee Family skills. Personally I think that Clifford Chee Soo was one of the greatest Taoist Arts Masters this world will ever see.

Today, amongst all the many other beautiful styles of Taijiquan we also have Tiandidao 'Jingquanshi' or 'Well-spring Style' which is based on studies and lineage of T'ai Chi's basic principles and has gratefully received much spiritual guidance. It also includes some elements of the Li and Wu Family (Rolling the Boulder, Turn the Great Wheel, Ward off - Roll Back - Press & Push, and others), as well as elements of Sun (the "follow step") and Yang ("Yah-ng"), as well as completely original movements; e.g. not influenced by any other style, but only the Taiji philosophy and spiritual connections or guidance. The odd or strange effect of this is something which although lived with for many years is still something that surprises and is hard to get used to. Why? Because when you study and meditate these "ideas" seem to spring out of nowhere and a new Form (as in Technique) "appears". It is not until some years later, when teaching and studying, that some of the true "meanings" come out of these Forms and genuine surprise is still registered. T'ai Chi Ch'uan has always had a special place in my heart (soul) but as I grow older so it grows too.

To simplify matters the many students of Master Soo and T'ien Ti Tao's Wellspring Style, or Jingquanshitaijiquan, has been added at the bottom of this tree noting the development and continuation of Wellspring Style (Jingquanshitaijiquan): Readers please note that we do not claim to teach the Lee Family syllabus, although several aspects remain, but that distinctly Taoist System has had great influence on our own and is a great part of the foundation of Tiandidao.

The Li or Lee Family T'ai Chi Ch'uan has a very close resemblance to Wu/Hao style, as mentioned previously. As all of the great masters are now dead and left no accurate history we can only hazard wild guesses as to the real history and development of T'ai Chi Ch'uan. I can only add to this that as I see more and more of the traditional or classical T'ai chi Ch'uan "secrets" coming out of China I realise that my Old Master's teachings were indeed very special, spectacular and way ahead of any other in the UK or elsewhere, visibly. Although up to 2004 I had not stated any "lineage" behind T'ien Ti Tao, it is with pride and deep respect that I mention it now in this humble book. The breaks in the lineage of development labelled as "unknown" are

108

Moving Onwards, or Backwards.

Jingquanshitaijiquan was not developed from an amalgamation of Yang style, Chen Style or any other, even though in honour of my Old Master, it does include a handful of moves from Lee/Li Style in respect; they are also very practical. Instead of creating another off-shoot style the Wellspring Style has been meticulously created from the ground up using the basic stances of traditional Taoist Boxing, snake and crane movements and other essential principles; the same way that T'ien Ti Tao Kung Fu was developed. The secret "added ingredient" was spiritual connection, which thankfully provided much guidance at the right times and without which the author would have possibly been "lost" and unable to complete such a complex Form (and Sub-Forms) without the help of the Old Masters; whomsoever they were! This is not uncommon in Taoism or Taoist Arts and many Old Masters had help from their spirit guides when the energy channels are opened. It is only in certain parts of the West where spiritual events have been replaced by commercial events that spiritual side of human nature has been lost to a great degree; so much so that some people get scared at the idea and call it "freaky" or some such reaction to the notion that something exists outside of the tangible, physical or mechanical. It is not mystical either but a natural part of human life. If some people have not experienced this then they are losing out on the wider scene and a quite beautiful view.

There have been many spiritual encounters on the path to learning the history, philosophy and true essences of the Chinese Internal Arts. On many occasions the author was drawn off-course on travels by some unseen force, like being pulled by the spiritual ear-lobe in a direction that one had no intention of going in. In this manner many books, magazines, impromptu training and meetings took place that formed important parts of the development and learning. Such spiritual encounters are not uncommon in the Internal Arts and even in Japanese Ai Ki Do; the founder, Morihei Ueshiba, had a special spiritual moment where he became enlightened as to what his system should be. Perhaps ranking as some of the strangest have been when encountering practitioners of Chinese traditional styles, on these occasions, if techniques or Forms were shown (which often is the case as we like to talk about our favourite things!) The term "spiritual encounter" covers a very wide variety of happenings that were just too unlikely to be coincidence as in many cases they represented the next "door" opening in the journey. One such spiritual encounter was where the author was inexplicably persuaded to switch on the PC and write, although having no ideas what to write. Faced with a blank page and wondering "What the heck am I doing here?" The mind was relaxed and allowing the "spirit" to guide the process fingers started typing. A verse appeared, as though written in the style of Lao Tzu. It was not until the verse was written that it was read and met with incredulity. It also answered an old conundrum, "If Tao is unspoken" why does anyone say or write anything about it, let alone so many people?

The TAO has no name, no form.

No words can describe it, so vast is The Way,

So immense The Universe.

From inaction comes action.

The Tao is action.

Action has no fixed form.

Form has creation. Creation has meaning.

The Way is my tool.

I am a tool of The Way.

Where Tao cannot be heard,

Then I am its voice.

Where Tao cannot be seen, I can paint an image.

Where Tao cannot be touched, I can touch and be touched.

Where words fall upon the ears,

And then fade away,

Ink flows to paper,

And words stay.

Tao is there for everyone.

Tao has much to say!

Another experience, around 1974, took place when the author was walking to the usual Bus Stop in Great Yarmouth by the Market Place. As I walked along King Street, by M&S, I was suddenly drawn off-course again by my Spirit Guide, as though being pulled by the ear, this time to walk along Regent Street to Howard Street. Wondering why this was happening, I was drawn to a small antiquarian book shop and entered. Feeling bemused, I hesitantly asked the bookshop keeper, who was sat in front of a lectern reading and then enquired if could help, "Er... Tao Te Ching?" The shop keeper raised his glasses to his forehead, said, "Mmm, Lao Tzu or Lao Tse?", much to my surprise. The shopkeeper alighted from his wooden stool and led off to the back of a rack of dusty old books hidden in a recess. There he rooted around two or three dusty old books that looked as if they had been there for years. He plucked a small brown book from the shelf that had the title "The Way of Life, according to Laotzu - An American Version by Witter Bynner." This was the book that had been sought for several years! A big thank you was said to my spirit guide on that day! Obviously it was the right day to get that little book. Verses from that little treasure of a book are used in here to elaborate points or ideas. The Tao Te Ching ("Dao-deh-jing") is a key part of Taoist studies and practises, as is the I-Ching ("Yee jing").

Such occurrences have been common, as most long-term practitioners of Taijiquan will no doubt concur. What most people would call "incidental" or "random" appearances of information or guidance are very common, like being mysteriously guided to a bookstore where a previously unknown or unseen book will be opened at a random page, this page displaying text that is pertinent to the reader's current studies or quest for answers. Some people will try to dispel ideas of spiritual guidance and say that there are no "scientific facts" to prove such claims; though they are not "claims" just "happenings" factually reported. Choose as you wish for it makes no difference to what has happened or the path trodden.

Another incidence of the wonderful world of connecting spiritually with books is when the author wanted to know his purpose in life and chose to meditate upon this whilst holding a copy of the Tao Te Ching (The WAY of Nature) by Lao Tzu, the following verse was the one it opened at, reflecting many things that have affected the author's life and development of the Chinese Arts without ever having travelled to China in this life:

Verse 47.

Without leaving the house,

One can know the world.

Without looking out of the window,

See Tao in Nature.

One may travel very far

And still know very little.

Therefore evolved individuals May know without going far,

Recognise without seeing

And achieve without acting.

Lao Tzu suggests in his life study verses that not all is obvious and that there are subtle forces at play which the average person may not have experienced, "touched" or "contacted" yet themselves. One suggestion on Zhang San-feng's Form of Taoist Boxing is that he experienced a spiritually guided vision or dream which gave him directions in his Art's development. Such things are common in history. This is not what we are here to discuss though it is relevant to the development of Taijiquan overall.

With the above chapter in mind let us look at the basics of T'ai Chi Ch'uan/Taijiquan. These principles are generally accepted nowadays as being proper and having rightful place in any style claiming to be Taijiquan.

Note: Basics are more than ink on paper or an image, in any form, of a stance or posture, more than a basic punch, for example, as there are many ways of punching. Knowing this forces study and also bars any imposters from claiming they teach a certain style as that style may be authenticated by anyone in the know; an experienced, long-term practitioner of traditional Chinese Martial Arts and, in this case, Taoist Arts.

Al of the above discussions and reports should be giving you, the reader, a hopefully wider viewpoint about the wonderful Arts of T'ai Chi Ch'uan and Taoism in general. Many westerners seem to think that for anyone to achieve high levels of spirituality they must end up levitating on a purple carpet or something! This is nonsense, of course and is probably derived from all the "holy" images that we see from youth in the churches, on television and, of course, in schools in these parts. Taoism is about Nature and being natural, or achieving oneness with nature. Through the many forms and methods of T'ai Chi Ch'uan we can be helped to achieve this. If a degree of spirituality is developed along the path then this is good, good for the practitioner and good for humanity. Ignorance is darkness and knowledge is illumination. Be light.

The Rough History of T'ai Chi Ch'uan in UK

There have been many differing styles of T'ai Chi Ch'uan in the UK and the USA. At the moment the USA is very lucky as many Chinese ex-pats and traditionalists have uprooted, if you will pardon the pun, and moved to the "land of the free", where they can not only live more comfortably but also make a tidy living. Nothing wrong with that, we all have to live and if we can find something which we enjoy doing and which also imparts health and development skills to others then so much the better. In the UK we have not been quite so lucky, although we do now have a handful of traditional masters over here. Since the 1970's we have had an assortment of T'ai Chi Ch'uan styles and what was nick-named "The Chinese Waiter Syndrome"; various men or women from Hong Kong who had maybe done some T'ai Chi Ch'uan or Kung Fu but set themselves up as teachers which later were discovered to be not so knowledgeable; "Wei Con Yu", as it was nicknamed by one magazine.. Of course, this was long ago before the floodgates of trade opened between China and Europe and we were literally flooded with fake produce! Chinese who want to buy western products now fly to London, Paris or Rome to make sure they buy the real thing!

This is of course not representative of the majority of good and honest Chinese people I might add. This small but unregulated invasion of fraudulent teachers not only caused bad feelings but damaged the "face" of genuine Chinese Arts and genuine Chinese people; all those who were good teachers had to tread carefully and make sure that they were both recognised and registered. This was when a provable lineage became more important amongst Westerners. We had one Chinese man who around 1984 visited many cities in the UK offering a course on genuine Chinese kung Fu. He then took £120 deposit off many, many unwary people after showing them some ineffective techniques and he disappeared.

We also had the British frauds too. These were almost invariably men who had done little or no training in Martial arts and decided they wanted to jump onto the "new" Kung Fu Bandwagon. One such man was in Norwich, Norfolk just before our first club started there at what was the 'Crome Centre', then Duke Street Centre and another actually named his club after the street where he practiced in an old people's home hall, something *like* Red Lion Street. Many people told me horror stories about this man, some of whom had met him at parties, saying that he seemed to derive pleasure from dragging innocent and quiet looking younger people (male or female) off settees at parties and applying punches or locks that hurt the unwary "victim". His bad reputation must have led to his downfall as when proper clubs started to appear he seemed to disappear into the woodwork as quickly as he had appeared. We still have frauds around to this day and some actually have more members than the genuine clubs; their members obviously do not seem to check their credentials or know the facts.

In the late 1960's to early 1970's Master Chee Soo was discovered by many, including myself. He had actually been teaching around London way, albeit on a small scale, since before 1950 and had practiced many Martial Arts since his youth and especially after WWII. It was not until much later that his Chinese Cultural Arts Association and International Taoist Arts Association became very popular. In 1975 he became my Master after I wrote to him politely asking some questions about practice and experiences. He then invited me to his teacher's training seminars in Dunstable. The "Choi Kung" was held in the huge canteen of the Dunstable Bedford Commercial works. There often between thirty and seventy students of his used to gather for further education under his guidance.

One of the most commonly found styles in the UK is a variant of Yang Family Style. This is probably because one of the first popular books available in the UK and written in English was the book by Robert W. Smith and Cheng Man-Ch'ing, T'ai Chi - the "Supreme Ultimate" exercise for Health, Sport and Self-defence. Many people tried to learn from this book and failed dismally. Learning from a book is not possible of course. As my old Master used to say, "The picture shows this position here, this one here and this one here. What you can't see is all the twiddly bits in between". Many people tried to learn all sorts of Kung Fu from books in the UK and USA but their movements, hardly surprisingly, looked jerky and very unlike real Kung Fu or T'ai Chi Ch'uan.

It was not long before some who were lucky enough found the opportunity to travel to China, Hong Kong or Taiwan, some to Malaysia where many traditional Chinese had fled to get away from the "cultural revolution" and threats of death to them and their families.

Dan Docherty was one of those who were lucky enough to have the opportunity. He purportedly travelled to Hong Kong where served in the police for a while and then says he learned a style of Taijiquan from a man called Chu King-Hung. During the 1970's Dan Docherty set up his own 'International Tai Chi Ch'uan Association' in London. He taught Yang style Taijiquan, Xingyiquan and Baguazhang and, unusually for this period, weapons training in sword and sabre.

As already mentioned, there were those in the UK who were already teaching the Chinese Internal Arts, like Shih-fu Chee Soo.

A third notable presence in the foundation of the Arts in the UK was Rose Shao-Chiang Li (1914-2001), an "upper middle class Anglican from Beijing with a background in missionary and educational work". From around 1975 onwards, she taught Taijiquan, Xingyiquan and Baguazhang in Durham and in Manchester (at the invitation of Danny Connor) and later in London. She was also said to have "de-emphasised Martial aspects as well as focus on the artistic and philosophical dimensions, urging her students to understand Taijiquan as a way to access Chinese Culture". During these early days in the UK T'ai Chi Ch'uan was only available in small enclaves, and the general orientation appears to have been more towards self-cultivation and discovering

Chinese Culture more than Martial Arts practise or pursuit of wisdom, personal development or spirituality.

When very limited videos became available (c.1985) many more people tried to learn from videos. This was still ineffective as when learning from a video one cannot see all details correctly and, more importantly, does not have a competent observer (teacher) to tell them where they are going wrong; and there are many, many places where it is more than easy to go wrong!

The late 1980's to 1990's saw few others started up T'ai Chi Ch'uan schools or clubs, including the now fairly abundant UK Wudang T'ai Chi School which seemed to expand quite rapidly from 1998 to the current time. Only two or three individuals sought publicity in the magazines of the time and stood out from the crowd. A quest began to discover and teach T'ai Chi Ch'uan in the UK and some apparently managed it on weekend courses whilst others took two to five years; an old Chinese saying is that "it takes at least ten years to make a T'ai Chi Ch'uan instructor, twenty to make a good one!"

The laws of probability dictate that somewhere in the veritable crowd of ill-informed instructors that there would be at least few whose movements looked acceptable to a novice. A few people with little knowledge made their own videos; some of these were still in circulation in 2005 and claiming to offer insight into the state of Chinese Taoist Arts in the UK. When compared with Chinese Video CD's or DVD's available today; bearing in mind that most of the latter are also quite limited in their content, but usually more accurate technically at least.

The early to late 1990's saw some of the first influx of visiting or newly residential Chinese practitioners. Some of these men or women still come to visit from China for weekend seminars organised by students they have established here. There is now a Chinese Taiji centre in Manchester and individual Chinese instructors holding regular seminars; some traditional, some not.

Various organisations began in the UK. Most of these did not last. There are some of notoriety who were accused of being "cowboys", like the farcical 'MAC' (Martial Arts Commission) and others who it was said became a closed door club, others still who overstepped the mark and tried to assert their self-assumed authority forcibly on all others, like the "....British ******** ****** mob", as more than one associate has described them to me; apparently trying to rule by force or coercion is never a good principle, as stated in the Tao Te Ching: e.g. it was said that letters were sent out around the UK that told hall hirers "if they are not members of B**** then these people are not genuine and should not be hired a hall", etcetera, as well as upsetting quite a few people who had been trained by very respectable Chinese "Masters" in the East and were told apparently that the organisation "did not recognise them" so they could not join. This is the kind of petty and egotistical behaviour which gives Martial Arts a bad name and whilst it is not confined to the West, it is something that we can do without and replace with a spirit of cooperation and education for the betterment of these wonderful Arts. However, this is life and human nature, so unfortunately, in Chinese Boxing as with all things in life, the reader or seeker has to learn how to distinguish between the fakes and the real so as to make an informed decision for him or herself. Of course the Chinese have long had a saying that covers this, "If it works then use it. If doesn't work, forget it!"

In China, because the Boxing Arts are part of the culture, they have only a handful of organisations, some family style orientated whilst others may be linked to national Associations and Sports Universities, et cetera. It seems that because the UK had never had a set organisation for Martial Arts that many people have seen it as safe to start their own. This has caused much confusion and damage. Even the government linked Sports Council organisations have come under great ridicule and disapproval from the overall Martial Arts community. The majority of Martial Arts schools or clubs are very withdrawn and parochial. Many of the organisations which currently exist take carefully chosen members, not always accepting those with legitimate lineage or unknown Masters, or otherwise some others appear to take just about anybody who makes up their own style and grade. Neither of these factors has been conducive to strengthening the structure and public faith in Martial Arts, T'ai Chi Ch'uan nor other style; let alone generating any faith or support from within the traditional Chinese community. Personally I have experienced break-ups even within a traditional Chinese organisation because of petty personal politics and the desire for kudos.

There are now (from 2010) a few centres in the UK which offer instruction from genuine Chinese Masters who have both family lineage or style lineage and in-depth knowledge of particular family systems. So few though that you could probably count them on one hand. There may be a few instructors out there who take a reclusive type approach and never make public (advertise) their whereabouts, taking on just one or two keen students. Generally though the state of T'ai Chi Ch'uan has taken a turn for the better since 1990, having more well informed instructors either coming over here from China or UK resident instructors/students going to China; some may learn parts of the more traditional styles whilst others may learn the new Beijing Competition Forms: discussed earlier in this book. This introduces a split in the proverbial UK T'ai Chi Ch'uan market place where there are those on the one hand performing competition routines, like 'Yang Styled 24 Routine' or '42 Compulsory Set' and those on the other hand performing more traditional sets.

The old original Maoist Chinese Communist Government attempted to kill off all the traditional Arts in P.R.o. China and replaced them with "squared off" or stiff looking "competitions style" Forms that have no traditional connections and are judged on postures alone. Those who conformed were given titles of Professor and Director, etcetera, and handed the task of bastardising every mainstream style of Taijiquan or Kung Fu that could be found, especially if popular. Many who did not agree were allegedly whisked away to prisons, or killed, amongst those who died either of starvation or other means, a total nearing 36 million in all (Recommended read:

"Tombstone: The Untold Story of Mao's Great Famine" by Yang Jisheng).

Conform and Reform.

Madam Sun (Sun Lu-tang's daughter) was approached and told that she must create a Competition Form from Sun Family Style 97 Steps, she was disgusted and refused and was told that she could not refuse. She then taught one of these new leaders the original Form and said, "There, now you have it. You can do with it what you must!" Peking (Beijing) is the epicentre for these so-called "modernisation" activities and some are an off-shoot of government run university schemes apparently aimed at "de- culturing" the Chinese people and instead developing the love of competition 'gold medals' and the spirit to win or be rich; this obviously works, but is stripping the Chinese of their heritage, true identity, spirit and soul. In short the government are treating people like cattle, a work force they can drive in any direction;, we have a similar thing happening here in UK, also in other Western and Eastern countries, with family values being destroyed and culture lost whilst young people idolise passing fads, games and "fifteen seconds of fame" TV "celebrities", mindless drug culture and worthless fashions, all driven by a few ruthless businessmen or businesswomen and their political puppets. You can chase this one up yourself on Google by searching for "common purpose exposed" and then work out for yourself what is happening in the world.

You may be well and truly flabbergasted at how such a small minority of corrupt and mentally unbalanced people can cause so much harm to others. The way that nations are run has a direct effect on the lifestyle and health of the populace, as well as the economy. It is this effect that causes so much stress, ill health and unhappiness. It is the government ministers and their various business advisors who cause the problems, probably because they are focused on money and power, not happiness and natural stability.

It is for these reasons that ill health ruins so many people's lives. It for the same reasons why practising Ch'i Kung and/or T'ai chi Ch'uan on a daily basis is so important for it will help restore "balance" within the individual, health and happiness (from within, as opposed to from outside/environment). Now you can see why politics has a place in this little book. What a shame that politicians do not practice the Taoist Arts each day, maybe they would become better balanced, more in tune with the environs instead of "out of touch" and maybe, just maybe the world would slowly become a better place to live in.

Dr Hua, T'o.
The creator of Acupuncture and Five Animals
Frolics qigong.

Dr Hua was perhaps one of the greatest and most significant doctors that ever lived. His legacy lives on today in Acupuncture, but he also contributed many other aspect to the Internal Arts through is studied and notation of Ch'i/Qi. He developed the Wuqinxi (Wade–Giles: *Wu-chin-hsi*; 五禽戲; lit. "Exercise of the Five Animals"), derived from his studying the movements of the tiger, deer, bear, ape, and crane.

One historic account says that it was he who performed a dual-heart transplant using acupuncture and herbs. Another says that it was Doctor Bian Qui (circa 401 BC). Dr Hua was executed by an ego maniac "Lord", Cao Cao, who would not excuse the great doctor from his presence as he wanted him for his own selfish needs. Most of his great works were lost due to this shameful act.

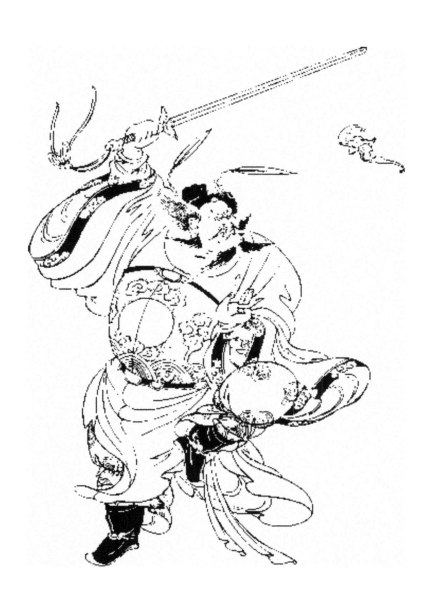

Chapter Six

HISTORY OF TAOIST BOXING

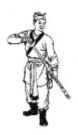

Chinese Boxing Exercise in Harmony with the Way of Nature

The History of Taoist Boxing

Chinese Boxing (Quanshu or Ch'uan Shu) can be traced back to around the Ch'in Dynasty period of 221-226 B.C. as a precious comb was found in a tomb dating from around this time. It had engraved upon it two bare-chested wrestlers depicted competing with each other with a Referee present. There could have been earlier fighting skills but historic records do not appear to exist beyond that time. In the following Han Dynasty the popular wrestling skill was given the name of Xiangpu, which means "to rush against each other". The Japanese pronounce Xiangpu as "Sumo" and the wrestlers of the Han dynasty wore the same type of loincloth. By the Tang Dynasty wrestlers had taken to wearing a strongly made vest so that grappling moves could be used in throwing and controlling. Modern Chinese Grappling has developed into the very refined Art of Chin Na, some of which can be found in Taijiquan. In this book I am concentrating on the Art of "Chinese Boxing (Quanshu), the Way of The Supreme Ultimate (Taiji)."

Xu Xuanping (Hsu Hsuan-p'ing. 許宣平)

As well as wrestling in the T'ang Dynasty (618-907) this was the period when a man called Hsu Suan P'ing (Xu Xuan-ping - 618-905 AD) invented the Thirty-seven Tun Chuen or Sanshiqi - 37 Forms, a Taoist Boxing Exercise Set. It is highly unlikely that this was the very first Taoist Boxing Set as Taoism has been around since probably before Christ was born, though we do not know for certain and modern historians give a time span of around 1,700 years. The Yellow Emperor reigned from 246 B.C. to 210 B.C.; his given name was Huang Ti (or Hung Di). During this time he was said to have created many changes in "Unified China" and is remembered very fondly in folklore for his work in collating and disseminating information about Tao and Taoism. His most famous work was a canon on Traditional Chinese Medicine. This dates Taoism as being at least 1,803 years old but logically a lot older; the reasoning I apply being that Huang Di collated information from across China, which must have taken some years and whilst he was in his peak years.

Therefore I feel that it reasonably safe to say that Taoist theory and practice has been around for over 2050 years.

There appears to be a six-hundred year gap until Ch'eung Sam-feng came along and developed the famous Taoist Boxing Set which was said to have been the inspiration to develop Taoist Boxing further along the lines of the Taoist philosophy and eventually became known globally as "T'ai Chi Ch'uan".

History of the factual kind leaves us uncertain about T'ai Chi Ch'uan's ultimate roots, as we have already discussed earlier, and we are not even sure that Ch'eung Sam Feng's style or Form would have been called "Wu Tang Boxing"; this is again a modern naming. What is known is that the man claimed to be at the head of modern T'ai Chi Ch'uan is Chen Wangtin (Ninth generation of Chen family in Chenjiagou Village), 1771-1853. However, our legend at the beginning is said to pre-date Grandmaster Chen. Grandmaster Chen is named by convention as the accurate history that predates his family system has been lost. It is still claimed today that Chen Family Style is "the original T'ai Chi Ch'uan" and this may infer to the naming (e.g. "T'ai Chi Ch'uan"), not the invention of the techniques or principles. The historically recorded hard facts remain to be found, if they still survive, for they alone hold the keys to our quest:

Who first associated boxing sets with the Tao? What was the name and nature of that boxing set? Has "it" been lost, fragmented and/or converted?

Was it a Form invented by Taoist Ch'eung Sam Feng? Did it hinge around the principles of the snake vs. crane and the Thirteen Methods?

Perhaps some of these questions will never be answered factually, as much literature and documentation was wilfully destroyed by some of past China's rulers and invaders, including in the more recent Cultural Revolution.

As much as "assumptions" can be vague or misleading, the "educated" assumption here has to be made due to the lack of historical facts. Scholars have reasonable faith that the Arts and Styles which have influenced or led to the development of what we call T'ai Chi Ch'uan nowadays would be those listed on the Family Tree (fond later in this book). Taoist Ch'eung Sam Feng did exist, according to the latest studies, and has been accredited with the development of Taoist Boxing with his "Thirteen Forms", or "Shisan shi" (十三式) "thirteen techniques"; as there were and still are thirteen foundation techniques that are essential to practice.

We must also assume that historically the term "T'ai Chi Ch'uan" is irrelevant, to a larger degree and that the name for this style of Chinese Boxing known commonly as Taoist Ch'uan-shu (Daoquanshu/Taoist Boxing Skills) applies more accurately. Whether, or not, this is agreed with, whether or not it suits personal preferences it remains better than arguing over petty naming differences. Taoist Ch'uan Fa include many forms of health, fitness and self-defence, including those that use the philosophy of Tao as a guideline; which also means that T'ai Chi Ch'uan perhaps is not that unique and that [mainly] Western hype over the past few years has raised this Style (or these styles) head and shoulder above all others that share common philosophical principles. Perhaps Tao Ch'uan is a better name?

Having said all that it occurs to me that through the practice of this Art, long term, we gain a better insight into ourselves and an increasingly better insight into humans, nature and the Universe as well as having spiritual development "thrown in" as a free added extra. In this light it would seem more appropriate to me to name it in two sections, the first being Tao Ch'uan (Daoquan) where we learn the basic Forms, principles and procedures and at a later stage, when the effects start to take shape and we choose to learn advanced methods, T'ai Chi Ch'uan (Taijiquan); as an indication that we are now heading towards harmonisation with the Universal Principles (T'ai Chi).

Immortal Legend of Ch'eung Sam Feng

The earliest written reference to Ch'eung San Feng ("Zhang San-feng", in simplified Chinese: 三丰; traditional Chinese: 三丰; pinyin: Zhāng Sānfēng; Wade-Giles: Chang San-feng and sometimes written as "Sam-feng") as a boxing master is found in the Epitaph for Wang Zhengnan (1669), composed by Huang Zongxi (1610-1695 A.D.) His real name was thought to be Zhang Junbao (君宝 - Guardian of the

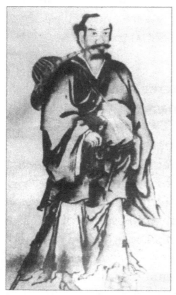

Mountain Ch'eung), born at midnight on April 9, 1247 AD, in the area of what is known today as Liaoning, near Dragon Tiger Mountain in Kiang-Hsi Province in the southeast of China and just bordering North Korea today. Later he became better known as a Taoist and became known as Ch'eung San-feng ("Three Peaks" Ch'eung).

In an article posted as 'Everymartial', an on-line source, the writer says, "The real significance of this piece at the time laid not so much in its reference to boxing but in its anti-Manchu symbolism. The Epitaph is the first reference in the history of Chinese martial arts to describe boxing in terms of a Shaolin or 'external' school versus an 'internal' school of boxing, originated by the Taoist immortal from Mount Wudang, Zhang San-feng." He goes on to define, "While the Epitaph accomplishes its intended purpose of eulogizing Wang Zhengnan, it conveys two additional messages as well, one reflecting trends in thought on boxing and the other political defiance".

According to the history written by Shih-fu Jou, Tsung Hwa (which we have no reason to doubt due to his many years of in-depth scholarly endeavours), Ch'eung Sam Feng (Pronounced like "Zhang San-feng") was born on April the 9th 1247. He was also apparently known as Chang Tong ("Zhangtong"). Shih-fu Jou relates to "Ch'eung Sam Fung's ancestors who were from the Dragon-Tiger Mountain region and his grandfather who moved Yizhou in Liaoning, a province in the north-east of China. His father was an intelligent man by the name of "Zhangjuren".

Ch'eung San-Feng passed the Emperor Taizong's Government Examination and became a highly revered Official of the Emperor in the Yuan Dynasty. He was not a man of worldly titles or possessions and after the death of his parents he resigned from his government post and decided to return to his birthplace, just for long enough to give away his property to his relatives. He set off to roam the mountains and countryside for thirty years accompanied by two young boys; probably family "donated apprentices" as was the custom to donate sons to Monasteries and such in the hope that they would gain an education and become wise; also making them less of a burden to poorer families too! He visited many Temples in the hope of meeting a very wise man. He finally settled in mid-western China near the "Baozhi" Mountains, also known as "Sang feng" as they have three peeks and from whence his nick-name came. He is supposed to have already mastered the Five Fists ("Wuquan") of Tiger, Crane, Snake, Leopard and Dragon and other Shaolin Kung Fu by that time. This was at Shao-lin (Young Forest) Temple before it became a Buddhist only centre and the seat of Chan.

After the Yuan Dynasty gave way to the Ming Dynasty he was worried that the royal family would need him, as he was by now a famous Taoist and they might wish to capitalise on his fame. To escape this unwanted burden and going back to work he did not want anymore he pretended to be mad. It was with his act that he earned the nickname of the "Sloppy Taoist". In 1385 he was ordered to serve the government but he returned to the Wu Tang Mountains to see his friend ("Wanpuzi"). It is then said that in 1407 the Emperor Cheng Tsu sent men to find Zhang San-feng but they failed to bring him back. It would seem that with what follows there is some indication that his exploits in searching for "Tao" had been noted by the Emperor. The Emperor sent high ranking officials to supervise the construction of a Temple in Zhang San-feng's honour on Wu Tang ("Wudang") Mountain. The Emperor bestowed the title of "Immortal" on Ch'eung and thus it was said in legend that he lived for over two-hundred years through three dynasties!

Exactly how Zhang San-feng created his famous Taoist Boxing Set we do not know for sure but there exist at least three versions of the story in legend:

1. As he slept on night he dreamed about it and when he awoke remembered the formula. Not improbable as famous people have dreamed the answers to questions and the subconscious can work on resolving issues whilst we are asleep; the mind being less cluttered from daily distractions.

2. It was possible that he saw some monks boxing on the Wu Tang Mountains and thought that their movements were too external and lacked balance. Then, working on the principles of Taoist philosophy, he refined Forms to be more balanced and in harmony.

3. Early one morning he was awakened by the most piercing screech. He sprang to his feet and peered outside. Not many yards from his shack, were a Crane and a Snake in close proximity. The Crane's actions were very Yang, whilst the Snake's actions were Yin. He was impressed at how the Snake used coiling and evasive actions to counter the strong and aggressive Crane. Old Zhang observed that this was the perfect reflection of Taoist philosophical principle in Boxing and set about creating a new Form using these basics and other Tao essences.

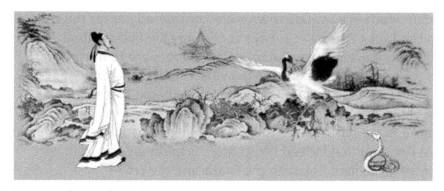

Personally I believe in the last theory. Why I do not know, call it "gut instinct" if you like, I just do. Part of the reason is because that when I was a small child (around four to five years of age) I used to "play fight" around the house. At times I would create ways that I could practice, like using a large pillow, which then was as big as me, as a punch bag or substitute body by throwing it over my shoulder. At other times I would wander around the house thinking of "What happens if....?" situations. Each one would be a response to a specific attack or threat. The movements I used - not that I knew it then - were all "classic T'ai Chi Ch'uan" style, using the attacker's force against themselves, evasion, takedowns and even Chin Na (grappling and joint locking) against attacks, and practiced in slow motions, just like T'ai Chi Ch'uan. Consider also the fact though that at that time there were no books about T'ai Chi Ch'uan, 'Kung-fu' or any other Martial Art available to me, not even any films or television programmes as we had no TV then anyway. The only explanation possible could be, as it has been suggested by others, is that it came from a past life experience or from some other source, like a spiritual guide.

Wherever it came from it was as natural to me as breathing and by the time I started school certainly came in handy to deal with the bullies! Later, in my teens, I felt that most of what people would call "normal life" was in fact not normal at all, if not downright abnormal. My favourite games with my friends all involved fighting, not just "scrapping" but using a more refined technique. This was very handy as it was used on many occasions in later life to ward off attacks; which in a seaside town were considered par for the course! Thus the Taoist Arts have always been in my life and spiritual encounters were as common to me as holidays are to most other folks. Then, when I was around ten years of age came the "snake and crane" incident; mentioned next in this book. This and many other things that are too frequent or numerous to be called "coincidences" has lead me to believe that my destiny is within Taoist Arts and that indeed Old Zhang's inspiration was from witnessing the fight between the snake and the crane.

The Snake & Crane Symbol.

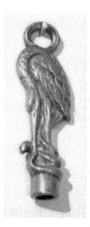

Around ten or so years of age our family used to have coal fires. There was always a brass fireside set on the hearth; brush, dustpan, coal shovel and tongs. Usually these had cast brass sailing ships as decorative handle ends. They never lasted more than a year or so before the handles started falling off, usually due to poor screw threads and the brass wearing. I used to love to come home from school in the winter and sit by the fire whilst I awaited my evening meal. One winter's evening I went into the front room where there was a roaring fire. As I sat by the fire I noticed with amazement that we had a new fireside set and was immediately mesmerised by it. It was brass. It had decorative handles, but not the usual old sailing ships. The new set had handles that depicted a snake and a crane locked in combat (a picture of the original is shown on above). The bird was standing on one leg and had the snake in its beak, but the snake was entwining the carne and its tail was about to strangle the bird whilst its body coiled around the bird's legs; stalemate. Mentally I was both stunned and in awe. Quite clearly I remember sitting there for ages just staring at the snake and crane. It meant something very deep and profound to me, then a young boy, but it was not until much later that it became clearer exactly why. The image shown above is a photograph of the actual piece.

The Symbol – continued in later life.

It was not until long after my father died and I was in my late forties. On one of many occasions I visited my mother's house, during the course of conversation with my mother about my problematic sister 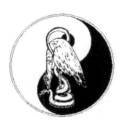 taking my dead father's treasured personal items and selling them, that I requested that I safeguarded some of my father's old belongings to keep as family memorabilia. I was told to look in a kitchen dresser drawer where I would find a small black tin cash box which held his old driving license and a few others of his personal objects. Imagine my sheer surprise and delight to find one of the brass Snake and Crane figures from the top of that old fireside set, after all these years. It was like my fate had been sealed from birth. In fact it seems it was as everything in my life led me to the practice and teaching of the Chinese Internal Arts. No matter how hard I sometimes tried to change the course of my life I was always steered back by some unseen force. Today, through my father's (unbeknownst to me at the time) safe keeping, I still have this brass image and it forms part of our school's logo (see left) within the Yin and Yang sign of Tao. The question always remains with me as to how my father knew to keep it and where it came from in the first place as such a fireside set is so uniquely Chinese! In the 1950's was there any trade with China and such items made for the West?

As a note here: in becoming a Taoist one seeks to find Tao, the Way. This is also translated as finding your true self. As stated before, since childhood my entire life has revolved around Tao and Taoist Arts, so in seeking Tao I have learned to "let go" of false or artificial things or ambitions and become what I am, who I am, doing what I do and going with the flow "Wu Wei". This is what Old Zhang did in the end and many, many thousands of other Taoists like him. In this day and age I consider it all right to use technology, for it is common and can help us to study or communicate. It is no more unnatural than olden day's scrolls or letters.

The Battle!

The legendary story of Zhang San-feng witnessing the Snake and Crane from his window goes something like this:

> After being awoken by the noise of the Crane screeching, the hermit watched transfixed as the battle commenced. The Snake coiled, writhed and twisted around whilst the Crane stamped, pecked and flailed its hard-edged wings. The Crane's wing has enough strength to break a man's leg. After quite some time the two appeared to be equally matched, neither one gaining the advantage. Then the man watched with curiosity as the Crane appeared to drop its guard leaving it wide open to attack. The suddenly weary looking bird hung its wings and raised one leg as if it had been paralysed by the reptile. Snake raised his head and then in subtle motion edged closer, his head slowly pulled back and then in a blur he struck at the bird's chest. Like a graceful dancer the Crane hopped from one foot to the other spinning and extending his wings, one wing caught the reptile across the back of its head and almost at the same instant the beak of the bird made a stab and pecked out the Snake's eye! As the counter-attack came to the Snake's head his tail lashed out to ensnare the Crane's leg. There was an almighty screech from the bird as its leg was broken by the force of the ensnaring snake, and hissing from the Snake. The snake countered the bird's aggressive direct attacks with subtle evasions and softness. This inspired Zhang as he watched. They had both injured each other, the crane was tired, and so they both retreated to a safe distance and ceased the fight.

Old Zhang noticed that the snake had lost one eye while the crane had a broken leg. And although the fight was futile in the end he was in awe at the well matched tactics of the creatures. He was, we believe, impressed with the snake's ability to overcome hard, fast and direct attacks with subtle, evasive and soft counters, often delivering a strike at the same time.

He spent much of his time after that incident in devoting his creative talents to developing a form of Taoist Martial Art (Boxing) exercise based upon the movements of the Snake and the Crane. So, it is said by many scholars that, with this revelation "the true Art of T'ai Chi Ch'uan was born", even though it was not called by that name at the time.

To this day we do not know exactly what his new Boxing Form was called, possibly just "13 Methods", even though a few historians have made guesses, like "Thirteen Methods". It was not "T'ai Chi Ch'uan" though as this came later from the general observation that it followed the principles of Tao: Yin, Yang, Five Elements, Eight (Major) Directions and other aspects of the philosophy.

T'ai-chi (Verse)

Peerless was the Immortal Zhang San-feng,
Travelling all domains,
His Great Dao was unmatched,
Later generations, for fame,
Bungled the boxing art,
Altering my Tai-chi,
Sullying my name.

Accredited to: www.PureInsight.org

(Unknown author. July, 1996.)

There is a Form being taught in Wudang Shan this day that they name after Zhang San-feng, but it is not the original as that has been lost to the annals of time. Like all of us, assumptions and educated guesses have to be made. We do not know how much Zhang San-feng knew about Tao and Taoist Philosophy - Tao Chia (or "Daojia").

Did he understand the Pa Kua (Bagua)? Bagua Quan, the Martial Art, was developed in the 19th Century, so is it possible that anything was developed before this using the Eight Directions and 64 Symbols? It seems doubtful, unless it was never spoken of; unlikely, given the fervour that surrounds all other historic styles. May we assume, or guess, that Zhang San-feng knew well and understood the actions of Yin and Yang and the importance of the Eight Directions of the Compass? This may have been the limit of general knowledge in those days, some 500 years or so before Bagua Quan (Note: Quan is sometimes written as Zhang; to avoid confusion with Zhang San-feng I have used Quan here. All we do seem to know for almost certain is that Ch'eung developed a set of exercises that involved Thirteen Principles and Taoist philosophy, plus very probably, many Snake and Crane techniques.

It was Chinese philosophers who first closely observed and interpreted the patterns and structures of Nature. This they called Tao 道, meaning "path" or "way", as in "the natural way of things". This gradually formulated and became infused into different aspects of everyday life, from geomancy to medicine and education to exercise. In time Taoist philosophers applied the principles of Tao to health giving exercises that are "natural" and therefore will help practitioners to live a longer like than those who follow unnatural ways.

Taijiquan is not just a health exercise though. T'ai Chi or Taiji means "Supreme Ultimate" (Tao) whilst Ch'uan or Quan means "Boxing Exercise" - roughly translated. It is a Martial Art based exercise, Kung Fu (Gongfu, meaning "Trained Skills Person") and is a deep way of making something of your life as it has profound effects upon the thinking processes, internal body development and spiritual development. T'ai Chi Ch'uan is Kung Fu/Gongfu, and Gongfu is Taijiquan, they are just different Forms (Practice Sets) with different "style" influences and varied backgrounds; some militaristic, some influenced by the family practitioners and developers, others influenced by philosophy, like T'ai Chi Ch'uan. The philosophy of Tao has been used in other Ch'uan-shu styles which exhibit the Yin and Yang aspects as well as other elements of the philosophy applied to both the movements and actions. Hsing-I is a linear method in theory, but uses "internal" principles. Pa Kua Chang uses circular methods and close-quarters applications, but hinges around the visualisation of the T'ai Chi and the Eight Diagrams and their meanings. All methods are slightly different; which makes it very hard for most outsiders to fathom.

T'ai Chi Ch'uan uses mainly rounded movements, like the Snake in combat or defence, but some may be direct, linear or even angular. One of my initial surprises on learning my first style of T'ai Chi Ch'uan was how forty-five degree angles and "triangles" there were! The wisdom of the snake's defensive tactics certainly seem be creditable to Zhang San-feng, if the legends are based upon any truth; and why should they not be? The title of "T'ai Chi Ch'uan" is not his doing. The Chen family created their own version of whatever was shown to them by Zhang Song Ze and this has be the pattern since then, but the philosophy remains the same and was then passed down to Yang, Wu and the other "families" who created Forms of T'ai
Chi Ch'uan.

It seems that whilst there are many disagreements about who invented this name, that technique or that principle of training, the main factors are being overlooked in a typically human form of mental blindness real inventor of T'ai Chi Ch'uan was not Chen, Ch'eung or any *one* person or family, it was a whole succession of people who devoted the best part of their lives to the study of it. We can only trace its roots back on paper to Xuxuangping and his Sanshiqi (Thirteen Steps). This, from my own experience and observing similar others, was probably influenced by one of his peers or teachers, but who it was and what he saw we shall possibly never know. My theory does not exclude that the roots of T'ai Chi Ch'uan could go back to The Yellow Emperor, after all, much Chinese folklore, legend and written history points to this man being responsible for collating much information about Tao and Taoist beliefs and so on, as well as instructing the people to whom he was responsible in many life skills and even authoring a book on Martial Arts. It seems logical that such a powerful influence could have helped develop a form of exercise based on Martial arts and using the philosophical principles of Taoism. Just like nowadays, trends and new ideas spread, only faster now. Then perhaps just a handful of people would have taken the idea and nurtured it, perhaps only one or two adding further contributions and helping it grow over the centuries; until it gets to Zhang, Chen, Yang, Wu, Hao and Sun and still now goes on, flowing and changing like a great river, ever supplying the even greater sea.

Our question at the beginning of this chapter was "Who invented T'ai Chi Ch'uan?" It seems the correct answer may be "They all did!"

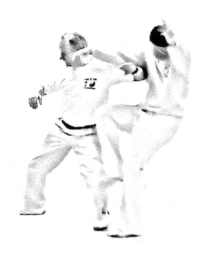

Applying the Yin and Yang in Wellspring T'ai Chi Ch'uan

FINDING TAO

Follow the Way
And you will find home,
The path is wide,
The view complete.

Atop highest mountain
You'll sit alone,
But in the Market Place
Your friends you meet.

_____

Shih-fu Myke Symonds c.1997.

Development of Taoist Arts

It is said that Taoism developed from the 'School of Naturalists' or "Yin Yang School"; this being a school of belief that all things followed the natural patterns of Yin and Yang and Universal principles. The study and development of the Taoist Arts, Traditional Chinese Medicine and other health, healing and exercise methods followed on and were later collated and developed by the Yellow Emperor. The reader should realise that the Chinese mind (collectively) has been responsible for the greatest and most useful inventions in the world, regardless of how they are used later; e.g. gunpowder and armoured ships. Many Taoists gave their entire adult lives to discovering the science of living, like Dr. Hua To (right), the famous physician, and possibly the best the world will ever see, he developed a set of Qigong exercises called Five Animal Play, around the third century B.C. He is also accredited with the systematic development of acupuncture, with which he later performed the first ever successful heart transplant: approximately 750 years before Jesus Christ was born and using bamboo needles on twin brothers who had volunteered.

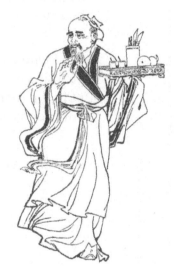

Physical exercise plays an important role in Chinese history because in the past people had to be reasonably fit and able to defend themselves in order to survive. If it was not marauding Mongolians it was bandits they had to worry about, and if was not bandits it might have been the local War Lord's army that was plundering and pillaging or even greedy Europeans trying to take over and control them. After a hard day's manual toil farmers would don their sack cloth belts and practice their Ch'uan-shu (Chinese Boxing) to develop their Kung Fu (Trained Skills). This probably became even more popular after the introduction of Buddhism, as Siddhartha Gautama (the son of a warrior Prince) recommended martial Arts practice as a great way of sharpening the mind as well as making the body stronger; an important concept of Chinese philosophy and echoed by Confucius as well as Taoism and others.

The original Temple at Mount Wu Tang/Wudang ("Woo-dahng") (当拳) or Five Peaks was built during the Tang Dynasty, called 'The Five Dragon Temple. The Emperor had this built in the belief that it would lure a legendary Taoist Priest who meditated there to him in the city. The Emperor thought that the old Taoist's wisdom would help him run the country more successfully. The old priest never showed up but the idea of seeking the peace, spirituality and wisdom of the Wu Tang Mountains certainly took off.

T'ai Chi Ch'uan/Taijiquan Evolves

As Wudang grew more people were attracted to the area to study Taoism, so the skills mixed and bred. Many forms of Chinese Boxing were developed over the long and complex history but one of the richest and everlasting has been T'ai Chi Ch'uan or Taoist Boxing. Many forms of Taoist Boxing existed before any Form was called T'ai Chi Ch'uan. It took more than one style or one man to make the history of China what it

is today, likewise, it took many men and many styles to create T'ai Chi Ch'uan - Self- defence in accordance with the Tao (Universal Principals, or Supreme Ultimate). However, one man was responsible for a turn in developments which led him to create a suitable Boxing Exercise for Taoists which became not only popular but legendary. Ch'eung San-Feng ("Zhang San-feng"). The man they called, "Three Peaks" Ch'eung (San-Feng can also translate as "Heaven and Earth" (三丰) in the 8 trigrams of the Bagua, San (三) represents heaven, or qian (乾) whilst Feng (丰) represents earth, or kun (坤); in traditional Mandarin the Romanization would be T'ien Ti or pronounced "Tian di". Ch'eung had previously studied some

Chinese Boxing already at the famous Songshan Shaolin Temple and in other places. He was intelligent and accomplished at his organisational and administrative skills; from this we can assume that he was also a good communicator, otherwise he would never been offered an important post as a government official.

What led him to believe that what he saw was lacking? What was so different in his Forms? These things we shall never know. It may be as simple as he just wanted to leave his stamp on the Chinese Boxing Arts. This he certainly did, maybe not in the way he expected, if he expected to. May be he wanted to develop something which was less physical and more philosophical? Who knows what he thought. What we do know is that his great study and efforts made Wudang famous and respected. Wudang Kung Fu is now known as one of the two major types of Martial Art form in China and enjoys the parallel position with traditional Shaolin Kung Fu in Chinese Kung Fu listing.

A book now in China State Library called 'Taiji Masters Lineage' has the following entries: "Sir Zhang Sanfeng, surname Zhang, first name Sanfeng... went to Mount Zhongnan when he was 61 years old. There he chanced to meet one immortal called 'Dragon Fire' who late transferred his knowledge regarding inner alchemy to him after knowing Zhang became a competent practitioner."

Later, it is said, Zhang San-Feng travelled a lot to famous resorts in the south, possibly holidaying or sight-seeing, and finally settled down in Mount Wudang. Then, ordering the disciple Qiu Yuanqing to stay in Five Dragon House, Lu Qiuyun in Southern Cave and Liu Guquan in Purple Heaven Palace, Zhang San-Feng is thought to have constructed a house in the place where Immortal Encountering Palace now stays. After many years spent cultivating "true self", for as long as nine years, Zhang San-Feng finally succeeded in achieving Tao (Oneness). People called him an immortal who could exercise unimaginable power to restrain the bad and promote the good, and transform all material things into different forms as he wished.

Later, Zhang San-Feng taught one set of boxing forms to Zhang Songxi and Zhang Cuisan, which was said to be the very original form of "Taiji boxing". Because there are only thirteen forms people call it 'Thirteen-Form Taiji Boxing'. Among these 13 forms were the techniques or methods of stretching out, stamping, squeezing, chopping downward, picking up, changing place, using elbow, leaning against (or "butting") which symbolize separately the eight trigrams, while moving forward, retreating backward, watching to the left, turning to the right and staying in the centre indicate the five elements. Together these are known as the Thirteen Methods. From these specific sayings there came the name of Thirteen-Form Taiji Boxing.

Based upon the Yin-Yang-Qi theory and aimed at regulating operation of the inner organs according to five-element theory, T'ai Chi Boxing styles often incorporate many soft movements imitating cats, birds, snakes and monkeys, thus gaining the effects of soothing the inner mental state, harmonize the operation of inner viscera, strengthening the immune system, etc. T'ai Chi Boxing developed very quickly among general people and later different branches came out to develop into different forms after long-term evolution. Nowadays, Chen style, Yang style, Wu Style, Wu/Hao style, Sun style T'ai Chi Boxing are said to be the mainstream styles to represent themselves amongst the modern day world-wide community. However, a common mistake made by many is to think that the practice only contains soft or slow movements, internal and placid. T'ai Chi is, by name and nature, Yin and Yang.

Why Does T'ai Chi Ch'uan Follow Tao?

Tao is Nature, life, the Universe and everything. Nature is subtle in most respects. We cannot see the changes in Nature but only see or feel the effects. T'ai Chi Boxing originated from the study of Tao, this creates subtle changes within, what people who follow Tao call "inner alchemy". Such key movement points as lowering Qi into

Dantian, hollowing the shoulder, keeping spine erect are just as same as the requirements for inner alchemy. These are in fact quite natural but many of us loose these principles as we grow up. Nowadays, people begin to forget their relationship to Tao and often treat T'ai Chi Boxing as a separate entity. That should not be the case at all. When we were born we had no identity, save that of the genes that built our physical body and the spirit inside it. As children grow older they are often given, or forced to take, an identity that may not be in-line with their natural rhythm. In T'ai Chi Ch'uan – the exercise of Tao – we strive to be in touch with Tao and become "One", not separate, not false, not fake or forgotten but "pure" in the sense of untainted and natural.

What is inner alchemy? Quite simply, or not in practice, Inner Alchemy is the ability to change the "base substance" into something more precious. The example of turning lead-to-gold is commonly used as humans tend to value gold above lead but do not readily it seems, be able to connect this figure of speech with human life and development. Inner Alchemy in the pursuit of Tao by a human is to become realigned, purified and rid of all falsehoods, becoming as natural as the Universe itself; if you contemplate this within the idea that the Universe is self-regulating, non-stagnating and constantly in flux, then you may well answer your own questions about this subject.

Chinese people prefer to use former experience and tend to know the lineage for anything in a long run. Yes, under such circumstances, the consecutiveness and unification gained an important position. Yet, in the same time, qualitative changes often gained not enough attention. Therefore, regardless it is Shaolin School, Wudang School, or if it is Da Mo, Zhang San-feng, people should go to the very root after getting rid of the superficial phenomena. In other words it is not the lineage but the foundation of the style which is truly important; lineage chasing can be just plain snobbery.

Ch'eung San-feng, who we might call the founder of Taoist "formulated" inner Kung Fu, has stayed there in history like a flying flag. Under the direction of this banner, Wudang Kung Fu began to develop and gradually became rich in contents and looked mysterious from outside after many Kung Fu masters' hard working and donation. After hundreds years of development, Wudang Kung Fu incorporates much useful nutrition form ancient Kung Fu defence and offence theory, from the theory of I Ching ("Yee-jing"), from the practice of achieving stillness and emptiness widely adopted in inner alchemy, and thus forming its own special features as summarizing the essentials, detouring to reach the core, nourishing Qi, concentrating attention, getting free of any frivolousness and rigidity. Accordingly, Wudang Kung Fu seems more to aspire for the full inner strength, the tremendous harmonization between hardness and softness, the ever-changing position adapted for different circumstances.

Wudang Taoism Association of China and other organizations have published books on more than 30 schools of Wudang boxing forms, 18 schools of Wudang weapon forms, 9 schools inner Qigong practice forms. Among them the popular are as following below:

'Wudang Taiyi Five Element Boxing', 'Wudang Pure-Yang Boxing', 'Yin Yang Ba Gua Chang', 'Wudang Sword', 'Wudang Original T'ai Chi Boxing', 'Taihe Boxing', 'Zhaobao T'ai Chi Boxing', 'Wudang Heavenly-Gate Qigong', 'Wudang Moon-Watching Qigong', 'Wudang Southern School', etc. These lists may be taken with a proverbial pinch of salt as the criteria under which they were accepted is not generally known. Logically any style or school that teaches a majority of Taoist principles is categorised under "Wudang", by what degree is another matter. The questionable blind acceptance of lineage again raises its head. Wudang is not the heart of Taoism, it is the "seat" of Taoism, the heart is Tao and the main person said to be responsible for correlation and promotion was, according to the information available, The Yellow Emperor and his team.

A Cultural Heritage.

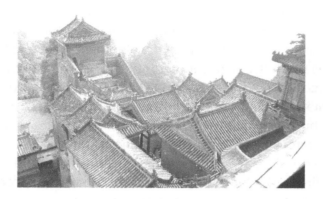

Wudang Kung Fu is excellent cultural heritage for Chinese people and not just because it is Kung Fu (Hard earned trained skills) but because it is Taoist and as such promotes many things from physical health to spiritual health and development. No other form of Kung Fu, Chinese Martial Art or any other National form of Martial Arts offers so many "paths" that the user can choose and so many levels; see the list of T'ai Chi Ch'uan and related Arts and sub-categories. Nowadays, more and more people get involved in the campaign to further treasuring this Art form and making efforts to promote its healthy development. Every year, many famous Taoist Kung Fu masters and Qigong masters go to Shi Yan City to pay respect to Mount Wudang and exchange their experience and skills with each other: not something that occurs so readily in other Martial Arts it seems. Why should the Taoist Arts in particular develop such enthusiasm and respect? Perhaps it is just a reflection of the practitioner's acknowledgements that he or she has gained so much from the Arts.

(Picture above) Golden Palace complex, atop the Tian Zhu (Heaven Pillar) Peak of Wudang Mountain; Wu Tang, Most buildings were constructed during the Period 1403 - 1424 of the Ming Dynasty. Photo by Seth Kramer (public domain).

This spirit of inter-human and even International cooperation is a hallmark of true Taoist Arts and one which help us to create a better world or heal that which is sick. This always reminds me of a great Chinese teaching story:

> In a remote part of China, a man was walking the path home late at night. It was pitch black as the moon was covered by cloud and he could not see where to walk. He slipped and stumbled, tumbling into a deep hole by the side of the path. His leg was hurt and he could not climb out. For over an hour he shouted for help and was getting cold, "Help me. I am injured and in a hole and can't get out!" After a while an old man's voice was heard. He said, just keep talking to me and I'll find you. The old man had a lantern and edged toward the hole and then climbed down to the injured man. He helped him out and then supported him, leading him to his village and the local doctor. "How can I repay you?" asked the injured man. The old man smiled and replied, "Many years ago I too was in a predicament and needed help. My helper told me that he too had been helped by a kind man who then told him that it was his commitment. That man then told me that in return I should help at least ten others. So, I have helped you and I now pass on this commitment to you."

It has taken me forty-one years of teaching (to 2014) and many more of practice and study to bring you this humble book with just the "essential knowledge" in, as a small contribution towards the development and preservation of T'ai Chi Ch'uan and Taoist Arts and traditional knowledge. It is not complete or comprehensive as there are many factors that you need to be taught by a competent teacher on a personal level. Some things cannot be transmitted via a book or video. The basic knowledge herein will help students with a good teacher to track progress and understand relationships between the philosophy and the practice. This work could not have been completed without the help of many other dedicated enthusiasts and scholars around the world and of course the internet.

With this effort dear reader, I pass on a commitment to you, to study well and practice every day, then to help at least ten other people gain from these beautiful Arts. My repayment is that and yours will be seeing the good that comes from it and having the power to change people's lives and health for the better. There is no better reward than that!

Taoism and T'ai Chi Ch'uan.

You do not have to be Taoist to practice, enjoy or benefit from T'ai Chi Ch'uan. In our small school alone we have people of many beliefs, some more dedicated than others. Understanding the practical "lay science" of Taoism is quite necessary to the practice, but not "devotion", per se. As you will see in this book and some others, the philosophical principles are what T'ai Chi Ch'uan derived from. Understanding Wu Chi, T'ai Chi and Tao are fundamental, and then the Pa Kua and Wu Hsing can be studied in even more detail.

There are several "layers" to Taoism and its study. On the surface you have millions and millions of people world-wide deriving benefit from Taoist Arts, be it Taoist Yoga, Ch'i Kung or - the most popular exercise in the world bar none - T'ai Chi Ch'uan or one of its offshoots, like T'ai Chi for Health. Within this layer there are a larger number of good folk who know very little about Tao, Taoism and its foundations or structure. This is fine, there is no reason why they should not enjoy these things as that is exactly what they were invented or developed for, health and enjoyment.

The second layer is a more curious one. These tend to be people who look for a little more knowledge, history and fact behind what they do, but they do not necessarily take it any deeper or further.

148

Many become teachers and help others to better health; another aspect which is fine.

The third layer seems to connect with the first, second and fourth. These are the good folk who also study meditations, healing and the deeper aspects of health and life behind these wonderfully versatile Arts. Diet may well be part of what this group practice and teach; but not by force or in a class, but on a personal level because diet is inextricably linked to personal health. There is an old saying in Chinese Martial Arts circles "Warrior, Doctor, Priest." This indicates that regular practice of a fighting skill can make one more of a warrior, but we are not talking "war like" here, more "justice and humanity". During training one will learn something about anatomy and physical health, posture and strain, and many common ailments. This is when the "Doctor" level may be reached. It used to be very common in China that the village Martial Arts instructor was also the village healer for he or she understood many of the common injuries and ailments and probably a bit about diet and herbs too.

This brings us to the fourth layer. They may communicate more with those on the third and fifth layers; but still have some contact or business with the first and second at times. Matters of a more spiritual nature are more pressing and the higher development of the human soul is equally important to maintaining teachers and providing what you might call a "higher education" for them. Many people in the fourth layer will be far more careful about their diet and lifestyle and will be more outwardly (and inwardly) Taoist than most.

The fifth layer will be hard to find in average society. They may be easy to spot in the street as they may stand out from the crowd as they may appear to have glowing health and an ease of being that makes them look very relaxed and comfortable. These are the "Priest" types who have travelled far and become more devoted to

Taoist Arts and practises for their own enlightenment and the sake of future humanity. They may not see themselves as a "priest" or even religious, yet in some circumstances may be called by such a name. There are many of these in Wu Tang but they also exist in other places too, not just China. These practises are not just for better health, they are a vehicle, or part thereof, which will hopefully carry them far in terms of spiritual enlightenment and universal fulfilment. One may well be your spirit guide and you may not even know it; not all spirit guides are the souls of people who have died on this plane and moved on to some heavenly plane.

This whole sense of "layers" is somewhat like a pyramid, layer one forms the base as it has more people in it. Layer two makes the next level which is slightly lesser, so tapers in a bit. Layer three tapers off even more, and then layer five (or possibly six!) makes the top and, ironically, points to the heavens. The notion of Heaven is not uncommon to any form of mankind; whatever they may call their religions or beliefs. I believe I have written this in another book, but will repeat it here as it is relevant: in a discussion with some students once one asked something like "If my belief is Christian, Muslim, Catholic or whatever, does that mean that we cannot see eye to eye? Is your belief different to mine?" The reply was simple. "No. All beliefs share common thought, common ground and they all seek higher spiritual development, etcetera. Beliefs are like houses alongside a long road, it does not matter which house you live in, it is what is at the end of the road that is important."

At Mount Wu Tang the highest peak is the Heavenly Pillar where old Golden Top resides. This shows us the importance of the connections with that that we cannot see within the Universe and what we do see on Earth. There are many wonderful sights to be had around those seventy-two peaks and all those beautiful valleys and waterfalls, but it is the climb and the view from Golden Top that seems to be the most memorable for most people and the spiritual significance that is most prominent for most "serious" Taoists. People from all over the world make a pilgrimage to Wu Tang Shan and some do it every year. It is said to "top up their batteries" and give them new inspiration. There is no denying Wu Tang's meaning in Taoism.

T'ai Chi Diet.

Diet plays an important role in our everyday life. As stated in 'Tai Chi Diet: food for life' (ISBN-10: 0954293282), a book for the masses. My Old Master said, when asked about what we should eat and why, said, "If you have a car and put poor quality fuel in the tank then poor performance is expected". Levels one and two above may be less concerned about how they fuel their body. Level three and four is more likely to be vegetarian and eat less "junk" food, dairy produce, etcetera. Level five is almost certain to be Vegan. Why? Obviously, to those who know and understand, being Vegan eradicates most of the fats and toxins that come from other foods. There still are Taoists and others in China who eat no meat, no grain and live mainly off natural herbs, spring water and ch'i kung exercises between long meditations. They live to be very old, but wise and spiritual.

T'ai Chi Global Effects.

As well as having a profound effect on the individual who practices sincerely and often, T'ai Chi Ch'uan can also have a positive effect on the rest of the world. There is an old Chinese saying which I used in another book. It states that improvement of one's self will reflect upon those near to you (the home), that will in turn improve those in the "town", by example or influence, and that will help to change the country for the better. This "ripple effect", as it is known, is the unseen, unheard force that emanates from the balance or harmony of T'ai Chi Ch'uan practice. It is like the various forms of ch'i that emanate from space, giving life and nourishment, or support and energy. Have faith in the whole, the balance and the power of harmony; not dwelling on the negative and imbalanced that so often dominate the news.

It is interesting to note that the Chinese system which traditionally governs the training hall hierarchy, names the teacher as Shih-fu; meaning "Teacher-father" and implying head of the family group. His teacher is the "Grandfather", so even wiser. The students are all brothers and sisters, paying respects to older brothers or sisters (those who joined before themselves). This family system of mutual respect seems to be a natural recognition of welfare, not power. The older and wiser members look after the younger and more prone, thus passing responsibility and care down the line and encouraging the act of looking out for each other. Whether or not this was originally thought out or not I do not know, but it is certainly in harmony with the Taoist principles of sharing and helping; akin to the principles of Mahayana Buddhism too, to help yourself become enlightened in order that you may then help others who seek enlightenment. In this day and age of meaningless toys, gimmicks, political greed, butchery and selfishness reigning misery upon the masses, people becoming disgruntled, taking harmful drugs or going "off-course" and committing social outrage, what could be more important than following a path which sets a good example whilst helping yourself to a better life?

The laws of Nature (Tao) are the only laws that a Taoist need follow. There should be no need to follow man made laws, often corrupted, misinterpreted and abused by those who are mentally sick and out of tune; whichever "side" they claim to be on. The laws of nature include human laws; common sense "rules of thumb" which need no books, no explanation to those who are in touch with reality and the path of good natured progress. T'ai Chi Ch'uan is a reflection of Tao, or the principles thereof, so is it any wonder that the effects rub off on millions of practitioners of these Arts world-wide?

How Is T'ai Chi Taught?

In the West T'ai Chi Ch'uan was seen at first as some strange dance-like exercise where the practitioner was in a trance-like state. This awful description was partially due to ignorance and that was partially due to language barriers. There may even have been some doubts at first as to teaching foreigners such a precious skill as no self-respecting Chinese Master would want to see their hard-earned skills being turned into some grotesque form of lifeless exercise.

It was author and ex-soldier Robert W Smith who first published a book on this mysterious Art form. He had witnessed Chinese Arts while on active duty, so the story goes. He later studied, learned and translated as much as possible in his book. This was the first book published in English and distributed world-wide: as far as I am aware. It caused quite a stir and had many a western "Hippy" trying to mimic the postures from the illustrations therein: causing it to look like an early form of robotic dance! It was the actual text that proved more interesting to me though, with many valid points and comments in it.

My Old Master, as mentioned elsewhere, was the first person to teach in UK: again, as far as I am aware. Shihfu Rose Li was not far behind and her school still exists in UK today. In retrospect, having been a teacher for the past forty-two years, I can only say from my personal experience how it was taught in the West.

In the 1970's, after Kung Fu' came onto our television screens and Bruce Lee leapt across our cinema screens, most young men wanted to learn Kung Fu. There were of course many frauds that jumped on the bandwagon and started Kung Fu classes. Some of these were just 1st Degree Black belts in Karate, or even Yellow Belts! What they taught was nothing like Kung Fu, nothing at all. The odd one or two decided that they would teach T'ai Chi Ch'uan and because they did not even know the proper name, it soon became "Tai Chi". In traditional Chinese this has nothing to do with our subject matter here! You can see what the true meanings are in Chapter Four. With little knowledge and a thirst to try to be "the first kid on the block doing…" it was soon bastardised, alongside Kung Fu.

Was it any wonder that many real teachers in China shuddered at what they saw? I think not. In China it has always been accepted as an Art form, a special exercise with very high values and well developed reasons behind the principles. It is not like "exercise" as we think of it in the West.

My first taste of Chinese teaching was c.1967. The instruction was simple, "Stand in Ma Bu for up to two hours." Then there was making a fist, "(detailed explanation then) Stand there and make the fist, then unmake the fist for two hours." Later, after about two or three weeks of this I could extend fingers, clench fist, extend again, all whilst in Ma Bu (Horse-riding Stance). That is how the Chinese train traditionally! In T'ai Chi Ch'uan it should be no different: one week, one posture or one move. If I taught most western students that method they would up and leave, being impatient to learn more of the Form. To compensate for this I teach one move, maybe "leaking" into the next if they are "as one", then correct the steps, the posture, the balance, the way they move until it becomes clear to them that they need to practice more: and get rid of bad habits. It appears that we in the West have more bad habits than most people in the East do, or at least "used to" as many in the East are now falling prey to western lifestyles and learning bad habits at an alarming rate! They are even picking up on obesity, junk food and cancer.

In the western hemisphere there are thousands of self-styled teachers who claim to teach one or another style of "Tai Chi": sorry if you think me pedantic, but I refuse to call my Art "Tai Chi" and shall stick to its proper name T'ai Chi Ch'uan. If you named your child René and everyone in ignorance called it Renal or Ronny, you would be rightfully entitled to correct them. T'ai Chi Ch'uan deserves to be treated with respect.

T'ai Chi Ch'uan should be taught in the following manner, loosely: each Instructor may have differing methods, but the following are important steps.

- Wu Chi and posture: the alignments.
- Song. Correct relaxation and movements.
- Stances and stepping.
- What to do with hands, toes, eyes and shoulders, etcetera. (Or "What *not* to do!")
- Breathing and coordinating.
- Correct application of Spirit, Mind and energies.
- Application of techniques.
- Other aspects of T'ai Chi Ch'uan: later stages.

As stated above, each Teacher has a different way of doing this. In my own classes I have developed a method which may combine two or three elements within one frame. Breathing, or T'ai Chi Ch'uan breathing, can be encouraged in a simply coordinated manner so that the student subconsciously picks it up without too much trouble. Certain methods of movement can be taught by doing T'ai Chi Ch'uan Walking, for example, during the warm-ups.

In china the traditional method of copying the Teacher is perhaps still the most commonly used one today. In the western world we often have to physically move the person's limbs or body into the proper posture: mainly due to tension and bad postural habits formed by a stressful western lifestyle; tense shoulders, arched spine or stiff hips, for example.

These are the basic differences between East and West, old and new methods. Your instructor should fit in their somewhere.

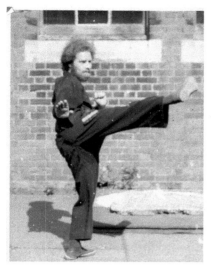

Here is a recently found picture of me from 1974. This shows commonly accepted principles of posture and attitude in Kung Fu and T'ai Chi Ch'uan (same thing!). Look at the feet, the hands and the eyes and see if you can tell what these principles are. I shall be generous and start you off. Look at the supporting foot. It is flat on the floor. Now, work your way up the picture from there.

Bad Western Habits.

There are many bad habits and most are associated with work or lifestyle. Here are few things to watch out for in your life if you are going to (a) learn T'ai Chi Ch'uan properly, and (b) want to improve your health.

1. **Check out your chair**. Does your backside sink into the back of the seat? If it does then this is a common cause of lower back problems. Likewise, many computer chairs can cause back problems. Sit at right-angles, back straight, thighs parallel to the floor and feet below knees.
2. **Walk the Walk.** When walking try to stand upright. Do not slouch or lean. The top of your head should be raised, the spine straight and the hips and shoulders relaxed.
3. **Be relaxed, not lazy!** To be relaxed means to conserve energy. Do not tense muscles unnecessarily or use more energy in a movement unless you have to. This can improve your overall feeling of well-being, but can also prolong your health and life. Stress is a killer. It begins in the mind, then transforms into the physique and appears in movements. Learn to "go with the flow" or "bend like a reed in the wind"

and accept things that make you stressed, but refuse to let them cause stress.

4. **Dress sensibly.** Clothes that are too tight, ill-fitting or even too big can make movements awkward, restrict blood flow or muscle work and breathing.

Men need to wear suits for work quite often, so try to buy natural fabrics, like cotton or wool. Avoid nylon and synthetic fibres. Many men wear tight pants (underwear, not "trousers" in American). Boxer shorts are far better for your health.

Women should buy Bras' that fit, not squeeze into a size smaller. The cup size should be right and the straps not tight. From my years of studying health and lifestyle, I have wondered whether there may be a link between too tight Bras and Breast Cancer, possibly metal wires used in the support structure too. Try to buy those made with plastic supports or better still, pure cotton with well-made cups and straps that fit correctly. Again, avoid nylon and similar fabrics as these can all affect the flow of the body's natural energies.

Shoes are another important health factor. High heels can cause back problems which can get worse or exacerbate other physical health issues. Try to wear flatter shoes, ones which have arch support and perhaps heel cushioning. Why do women wear high heels that make them walk in a funny way and also make their calf muscles go "knotty". It is not attractive, neither is make-up: which clogs the skin, etcetera.

5. **Breathe!** You already think that you breathe, but do you breathe properly? Many people as they get older get shallow breathing. This is caused by shallow or weak movements of the Diaphragm: the muscle that makes you breathe. Get your Instructor to show you Taoist Breathing exercises and then practice them every day, religiously. This alone can improve health by a large percentage.

6. **Empty the trash!** Many people carry problems home from work, or family issues can be prevalent whilst training. When you learn Wu Chi, use it every day, everywhere and in every way. In the Taoist philosophy we call this "Detachment".

However, it is very hard to practice in reality. Do not give up or be disparaged. Practice it and it will become a good habit. Look at problems as what they really are, and obstacle that needs to be overcome. If you carry problems around with you then stress can follow and bad posture, or bad health, so practice Wu Chi in your daily life. Even if your boss gives you a huge problem to resolve, it will do no good to think about it 100% of the time. Look at it. Understand what it is. Then rest it in the back of your mind and *sub-consciously* look for possible solutions that may fit. This works far better than almost any other method. The key to the solution is "understanding".

"I seek not to know all the answers, but to understand the questions." A phrase spoken by David Carradine at the beginning of each 'Kung Fu' TV episode. How true, apt and easily adaptable that is.

Diet is covered in another section. The majority of health problems are caused by either one or a combination of these topics. If you can cure these then you can cure many pathogens. One step at a time though. You can make all changes by recognising one negative factor, then changing it, then moving on to the next one when done.

Lifestyle also includes where we work and where we live. It is a sad fact that many people living in small flats in cities are cut off from Nature. This in itself can lead to depression, low energies and other health problems. Try to get out to the park or countryside as much as possible. You will see a difference in yourself as well as other people when you do. People are much more inclined to speak to each other, even strangers, when out in the countryside. This I have observed by joining a wild-life trust. Watching wildlife can be most rewarding too. There is more on the subject of environment in the accompanying book '"Qigong and Baduanjin'. You cannot always easily change where you live, but you can change your environment or at least improve on it.

Dao Jia - Practical Taoism.
This is the application of Taoist Arts into lifestyle and can be really liberating, refreshing and health changing.

When you begin T'ai Chi Ch'uan you begin along and never ending journey. It is a pleasant journey and gets better with time and age. If you practice diligently and take the simple advice offered you may well say to yourself in the future "How ever did I manage without this?!"

There are many ways that are advertised nowadays which claim to "improve your lifestyle" or "improve your image", the floor in that though is that these things often prove to be cars, furniture, expensive clothes or other inanimate objects that do not really improve your image or lifestyle at all. Many can land you in serious debt. Those debts can cause stress and ill-health. How is that improving your lifestyle? When you take up the practice of T'ai Chi Ch'uan you are, as I am often telling my students, entering "you time". This is for "you" and "your health". It must be highlighted here though that doing one class a week will not give you the results you need or want. Nor will two. You really need to practice it every day, early morning, noon, early evening or night (just before bed). Then attend classes with a view to polishing up. T'ai Chi Ch'uan is not like a pill or magic potion taken once weekly, it is something that you have to port into your life and daily routines in order o get the best from it.

There should be enough simple information in this chapter to work on. In order to make it work though, do not just skip to the "pretty bits", come back to this chapter every so often and read it again. You will then see if you have changed something for the better, then slipped back into something worse.

160

Old Chinese Proverb:
"The teacher can only show you the way. You must walk the path."

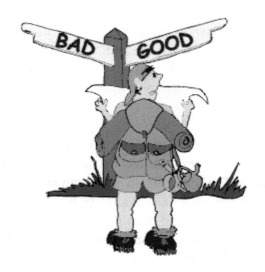

Clothes to Wear for Training.

This subject has been partially covered in topics above about clothing. You need to wear cotton clothing. Avoid all tight clothing, including underwear or belts. Wear flat or low heeled shoes.

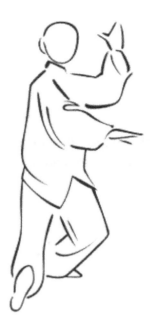

You do not need to wear a Chinese style suit, but if it is both acceptable by your instructor – certain colour or dress codes may prevail with his or her school and you do not want to get off on the wrong foot – then by all means try to find one that is comfortable and made from cotton: they have two types, heavy cotton for winter and thin cotton for summer.

You do not have to wear the black cotton shoes that are made in China either. These are traditionally made for every day wear, not Taijiquan practice. The black plastic soles can mark tiled or wooden floors and are very much an annoyance to hall hirers or those with their own expensively floored training halls. The brown ones are not too bad and do not mark floors so much. The cotton soled or "rope" ones tend to slip too easily but may be alright on certain types of carpet.

Trainers can vary. Many have higher heels built in and this may be detrimental to balance. Try to find some trainers that offer good grip on shiny floors or carpet, but not ones that "stick" on nylon carpet: training on nylon carpet is a big "no, no!" anyway. Flatter sports shoes may be found in squash, tennis or other sporting sections of shoe stores. Bear in mind that if you need to wear supportive insoles then the shoes need to have removable insoles.

What is the best age to start?

There is no prescribed age. It all depends on when you want to start. Most young people do not have the patience to learn T'ai Chi Ch'uan or assume that it is "boring" because it is not fast enough for them to be deemed "exciting". That is often the fact even in China. The irony of that little fact of course that patience is a good thing and can certainly help you out in life. T'ai Chi Ch'uan is learned and practised slowly because there are many things to think about.

Most people in UK who take up T'ai Chi Ch'uan are in their forties to sixties, with another group taking up the less demanding T'ai Chi for Health classes usually after retirement age. It is never too early or too late to take up T'ai Chi Ch'uan. Any time that you do so will be advantageous. However, if you start when younger, say for example in your twenties, then you have a better chance of learning more. If you learn the full Art and intend to keep it for life, then the more time you spend on it the better it will be.

The Relationship of T'ai Chi Ch'uan, Ch'i & Health.
Firstly, note that the word "*Chi*" in T'ai *Chi* Ch'uan is different to the word "Ch'i" used secondly in the title. The first one means "Ultimate" whilst the second one means "Energy".

Whilst almost any movement is good for your health, some types are far better than others. The relaxed and rhythmical movements of T'ai Chi Ch'uan are known throughout history to be beneficial to health. All over the world medical experiments are being conducted, or have been conducted, to establish the "facts" behind these claims. This is ridiculous of course because T'ai Chi Ch'uan would never have gained such a reputation were it not factual and supported by hundreds of thousands of people who have already reaped the benefits!

Stress is a killer. Western type lifestyles cause stress through work and social pressures. Life in "westernised communities" is often far removed from Nature, or to put it another way, natural earthly elements, like trees, shrubs, water flow and wildlife. Anyone who spends time out in the countryside will agree that it can be very therapeutic. So how does T'ai Chi Ch'uan relate to Nature? Firstly it is based on natural principles and movements are "soft", not strained, so also more natural. If you look at how animals move you will see that most look like they are doing it "naturally", without much effort. Secondly its theoretical framework is based on Tao, the creator of all things including what we call Nature. This gives it dynamism almost on par with a scenic highland view or place with cascading waterfalls that energise and support life.

Thirdly T'ai Chi Ch'uan has been very well developed over 1,000 years or so. It has been used and highly recommended by medical practitioners, as well as tested and developed in conjunction with some too. A common phrase echoed across China by Doctors, when confronted by patients with many types of common ailments is "Go do T'ai Chi Ch'uan!"

Ch'i or Qi is a reference to many different types of energy that pervade the Universe and all things. We also create certain types of Ch'i in the body. Certain types of movement help to strengthen the flow of these energies as well as stimulate more, especially rhythmic movements combined with specific breathing patterns. Various medical experiments have already noted that the daily or regular practice of T'ai Chi Ch'uan can improve the strength and flow of these energies, help to control or even eliminate various health problems. In recent times Harvard University has conducted many tests and experiments with T'ai Chi Ch'uan and published the results on its website. In modern times T'ai Chi Ch'uan has been accredited with helping the following:

- General Effects are helping internal strength, toning muscles, boosting the immune system, physical balance and movement control, storing energy and reducing stress.

- Breathing is helped by regulation and diaphragm exercise and the resultant oxygenation of the body cells helping improve overall condition.

- Blood Pressure is reduced by a claimed 10 to 15 mm Hg Systolic whilst at rest.

- Aches and pains reduced, especially headaches and neck or shoulder pains caused by stress and bad posture.

- Mental and Physical Stress levels reduced drastically after practice and with regular practice. Reducing stress can increase life expectancy and reduce likelihood of heart attacks.

- Mental Homeostasis or the emotional effects helped and/or levelled out with practice. Emotions are linked with psychological, physiological and physical effects, all helped by T'ai Chi Ch'uan and acupuncture, etc.

- Rheumatoid Arthritis tests have shown that T'ai Chi Ch'uan practice does not exacerbate joint problems when weight bearing. It was also said that gentle weight bearing exercises can stimulate bone or tissue growth as well as strengthening the connective tissues. The symptoms or pains associated with arthritis can be neutralised, giving pain relief.

- Many more benefits have been claimed including cardiorespiratory health linked with better health through aging, sports performance even in later life, use in support groups for Fibromyalgia, Multiple Sclerosis, Parkinson's Disease, Chronic Pains, Aids and Lupus Migraines.

T'ai Chi Ch'uan movements and methods have been linked with both the Mind and C'hi/Qi for centuries in China. Traditional Chinese Medicine is generally far in advance of anything found in the modern world. In fact, and as you will note from modern research and medical development programmes, many western systems are now seeing the wisdom of incorporating traditional Chinese healthcare methods, including diet, Acupuncture (针灸 – Pinyin: Zhēnjiǔ) and T'ai Chi Ch'uan. The proper practice of T'ai Chi Ch'uan includes special elements that make Taoists refer to it as "Inner Alchemy". This term is also associated with Ch'i Kung/Qigong. It refers to the practice of creating, moving and storing energies in the body and also to transforming them. Your body becomes a laboratory wherein you develop these energies in a specific fashion using time proven methods. These energies are called The Three Treasures: Jing, Ch'i and Shen. Jing energy is reproductive Energy and is associated with the Lower Tan T'ien. Ch'i/Qi is Life Energy and associated with the Middle Tan T'ien. Shen is Spiritual Energy and is associated with the Upper Tan T'ien. Many Taoist practitioners learn how to transmute Jing into Qi and Qi into Shen. This becomes and on-going process and is usually accompanied by meditations and correct diet.

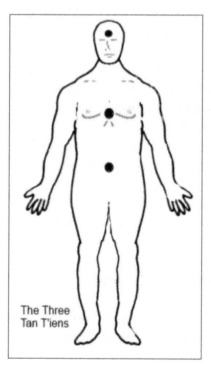

The Three
Tan T'iens

At certain times in T'ai Chi Ch'uan practice, depending on the Style, Form and Methods employed, the students may use either the lower or middle Tan T'ien (Dantian) when moving Ch'i (Ch'i Circulation). The Upper Tan T'ien is used more in Taoist Meditations, along with the others. Depending on what the achievement goal is, various other points or meridians may be used in both practice and meditation. Generally your teacher will guide you on what he or she thinks is necessary at your level.

Addendum: Special Notes for Senior Students.

6.1: Advanced Studies for Senior Students.

One of the best known and perhaps bemusing aspects of advanced practice is "sensing". This is practiced in special exercises, often in Pair Form, that help to increase sensitivity to someone else's ch'i. Given time, this practice coupled with other aspects of T'ai Chi Ch'uan practice can increase a student's awareness of presence from touching lightly to distance awareness. This is a fascinating subject and one that stood out in my mind and studies since many years ago, especially in the early 1970's when I used to train privately with my "Martial Brother", Kevin Addy, at the old church hall near the Hippodrome in Great Yarmouth. Kevin and his two associate Budoka were interested in the Internal Arts, Chinese in particular. In the course of a training session internal elements would be introduced, when the circumstances were right. One such practice was "Blindfold Training". This started of quite tentatively; each person's first attempts were full of fears, doubts and speculation. Once we had done it a couple of times it was not so bad and we were soon sensing, to varying degrees, even te stealthiest of attacker's approaches. One day I recall not hearing, seeing or physically feeling one of the group coming in with a knife, but somehow my hand shot out and grabbed his wrist. He was as surprised as I was!

While out one night a senior student asked how I avoided a man who was, apparently, trying to nudge me as he walked past: a totally futile and childish thing to do, but some men and even some women do it. My reply was "Did I?" as I was not consciously aware of it. A subtle "twitch" of movement had been used to avoid the collision and the man stumbled instead of bumping into me. How does all this work? Is it related to distance healing, or awareness of distant events? This has "bugged me" for years and has be lying in the "Unfinished Work" box on my mental office desk for years. That is until I watched Professor Brian Cox on television one night in a show called 'Life: Expanding Universe'. In it he looked at a small life form that scientists call Paramecium.

According to Free Wikipedia, "Species of Paramecium range in size from 50 to 330 micrometres in length. Cells are typically ovoid, elongate, foot - or cigar-shaped. The body of the cell is enclosed by a stiff but elastic membrane (pellicle), uniformly covered with simple cilia, hair-like organelles which act like tiny oars to move the organism in one direction." In Nei Kung we would call this "using ch'i". All life forms have or use ch'i.

They are found in water, fresh, pond or even brackish or marine environments, so are very adaptable. However, the subject matter of Professor Brain Cox's dialogue about Paramecium was their ability to sense and avoid contact, especially with predators. This is done

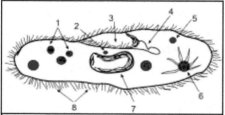

Paramecium diagram. The parts are as follows: 1) food vacuoles 2) micronucleus 3) oral groove 4) gullet 5) anal pore 6) contractile vacuole 7) macronucleus 8) cilia.

using the Cilia – tiny hair-like extensions protruding from the body (see diagram below, left.) According to Professor Cox, the Paramecium manipulates both positive and negative Ions with its membrane by sending out Positive Ions to the tips of its "sensor hairs", the same ones they use for propulsion. Negative Ions are drawn inwards. When the outer surfaces touch any object the Positive Ions surge back across the membrane. This is called "action potential" and causes the cilia to flex the opposite way, somewhat like oars propelling a rowing bot, moving the Paramecium away from the object or threat.

In modern theories regarding Acupuncture and the Energy Channels, it is thought [in some quarters] that the main energy channels are linked, via the brain, to nervous system actions: e.g. by tuning an acupoint, this sends a message to the brain which in turn adjusts the flow or creation of electrical energies within the nervous system.

Traditionally the energy channels have an effect on their related viscera or general health maintenance functions within the body. No relationship to Brain functions was mentioned. Before we get into semantics of this and disagreements between one scientist and another, let us just remember what Ch'i is. Ch'i in the human body is a mixture of energies. The three main energies which we produce, use or store are Electro-magnetic, Low Frequency Modulation Infra-Red Microwaves and Static Electricity. Without going into too much detail and starting a whole new book by itself, I shall say that the Low Frequency Modulation Infra-Red Microwaves may be used for healing. Other energies, or combinations thereof, may be used for other purposes.

My theory on this subject at this point is related to "sensing". We have looked at the tiny Paramecium species and their ability to use energies or Ch'i to sense potential danger and then propel itself away from it. Most people also know that cats are sensitive to energy, more specifically energy resonance or "waves" caused by mood and emotional status. Dogs, "man's best friend", are sensitive to coming events, catastrophes such as earthquakes or even storms. Birds I have noticed usually feed at fairly regular times, as do many other smaller creatures, but when a storm or bad weather is due they tend to feed early and in more of a frenzy. They sense a change in atmosphere, energies. Many humans are unaware of energies, so no time will be wasted arguing pedantic points about diet, health and awareness here. Instead let us concentrate on T'ai Chi Ch'uan and the effects of Nei Kung (Neigong) or Internal Training.

When we strengthen the Ch'i we also circulate it, or to be precise, "boost" the circulation. There is a relationship between ch'i and the central or motor nervous systems insomuch as we can feel ch'i as we circulate it or build it up. When we build up the strength of our energy we build up everything else that it comes into contact with or uses. This is like tuning up a car to race standard; it is no use in putting a powerful engine into a standard chassis with standard equipment; e.g. brakes, suspension, fuel input and extra strong bodywork. The point of this analogy is that anything increased in power needs to be upgraded to suit. In the human body, and in in T'ai Chi Ch'uan, this process happens according to practice, method, inner health, mental condition and physiological condition. The correct practice of T'ai Chi Ch'uan will achieve the higher results multiplied by practice time and other factors. We also learn to harness other energies, like Ions, that pervade the atmosphere as well as create our own energies through correct dietary intake.

A natural emergency state in the human body and probably other animals too, is generally called the "Slow motion state". This is a response experienced by some, but particularly Martial Artists, in a "emergency situation": this could be an accident, a serious fight or even when falling. This is triggered by perception. Perception is a state of sensory protection, usually started by sight, brain response, reaction and action. In the Slow-Mo effect, what actually happens is the eyes (or other sensory organs) perceive a threat, the brain receives this information, sends signals to the body. The Spleen releases the extra pint of blood we carry. The heart rate increases, the Adrenal Gland pumps adrenalin into the blood stream and the nervous system draws blood away from the skin surface and also tightens up the surface of the skin to protect from cuts or blood loss. When this happens we see everything in what *appears* to be slow motion. However, the Slow-Mo effect is a trick of the mind. Because there is more blood, faster heart beat and hence circulation, there is more oxygen going to the brain. The brain, via the eyes and other senses, then responds far more quickly than normal and diverts the energies to where needed accordingly. If ch'i is present, the mind will also divert the ch'i to where it is needed. This effect is often depicted in Chinese movies where two characters fight and you see them leaping high or "flying" in slow motion. As good a representation as one could hope for in a film. When the action is over, the blood returns to the spleen, heart rate drops to normal, the adrenalin soaks away and the system restores its natural state.

Experiences in Internal Training have been interesting, to say the least, but also educational as I could study the effects and do research to find related points. This has led to experiencing such phenomena as the "Blindfold Training" incidents, mentioned above. In the practice of T'ai Chi Ch'uan we use ancillary exercises to promote sensitivity. In the Forms we can develop the power to move the ch'i to different parts of the body or even beyond the body. Self-defence applications are just extensions of these practices but we learn to sense an attacker's energies so that we can react before any blows land. This explains incidents such as the sub-conscious "dodge" in the story above where someone tried to walk into me. It explains these situation and many more that have been experienced, but it does not say *how*. The illustration (right) shows the Three Tan T'ien, Upper, Lower and Middle, all three black circles on the centre-line. The skin has sensory activity through fine hairs (Cilia) on the surface sending messages to the nervous system. We receive signals of "contact" through the hair/skin/nervous system to the brain: just like an animal's whiskers - Neurotransmitters. The grey circles are just to illustrate the presence of secondary energy centres: not all shown. These are mainly related to the Small Orbit and Grand Orbit of Ch'i Kung. Then there are both left and right (L&R), front and back (F&B) Sensory points. These are known in Acupuncture but theories as to the "why and wherefore" are many. Here we are dealing with sensory perception only.

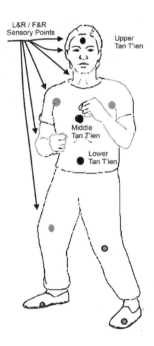

When we practice "proper" T'ai Chi Ch'uan, we stimulate all of the Internal Processes: Mind, ch'i, nervous systems, physical, metal and visceral functions, lungs, blood and even bone. The gains from this are all linked and will increase sensitivity via the skin and small hair follicles to the nerves that connect and send the signals to the brain. We have a slightly different type of hair in the ear which responds to sound waves.

An article on Public Wiki describes this: *"The deflection of the hair-cell stereocilia opens mechanically gated ion channels that allow any small, positively charged ions (primarily potassium and calcium) to enter the cell.[4] Unlike many other electrically active cells, the hair cell itself does not fire an action potential. Instead, the influx of positive ions from the endolymph in the scala media depolarizes the cell, resulting in a receptor potential. This receptor potential opens voltage gated calcium channels; calcium ions then enter the cell and trigger the release of neurotransmitters at the basal end of the cell. The neurotransmitters diffuse across the narrow space between the hair cell and a nerve terminal, where they then bind to receptors and thus trigger action potentials in the nerve. In this way, the mechanical sound signal is converted into an electrical nerve signal."* Those who have read the book 'Tai Chi Diet: food for life' will of course note the connection between Eastern healthy diet and balance of Yin and Yang through intake of Potassium and Sodium. The daily intake of calcium is also important.

Sensing through the hair or skin is base-level. Although close proximity sensing can be achieved this way, the practice of T'ai Chi Ch'uan and affiliated exercises can increase the field of sensing using ch'i – commonly used "Aura" or "Outer Energy Field" which uses the whole body and is controlled by the Mind. The ch'i is moved from one Tan T'ien to another, inwards and outwards, along the main channels and sub-channels until it becomes stronger and automatic. The connections, including "mind power" are also increased, thus being able to achieve higher levels of sensing. In advanced practice the Mind and Body become like a radio transceiver, able to both transmit and receive energy signals from near or far. T'ai Chi Ch'uan stimulates and develops this to unusual levels. Old texts tell us of the power of T'ai Chi Ch'uan to increase the physical, metaphysical, physiological and spiritual. My simple theory strongly connects this to diet, environment and the affiliated exercises of T'ai Chi Ch'uan that boost these effects.

Broaden your study and practice more.

Chapter Seven

Tiandidao Jingquanshitaijiquan -

The Way of Heaven & Earth
Wellspring Style Taoist Boxing

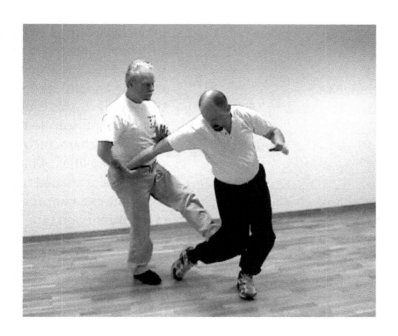

Wuji begat Taiji,

Taiji begat Tao.

From the One came Two,

From Two came Three,

From Three came all things in Heaven.

Tiandidao Jingquanshitaijiquan.

T'ien Ti Tao (Tiandidao) has a lineage of "style and method" which undoubtedly goes back much further than many more modern Martial Arts that seem to capture people's imaginations just because they have a "direct family lineage"; e.g. trained with a previous descendant of a particular style. Frankly though it is not the lineage which is the most important but the knowledge (stored light) held now which is important. Not all Instructors who have lineage are able to transmit full knowledge, or even be good teachers of their subject. This is because of several reasons to do with a person's character and personal abilities; which are more or less shaped before birth and during childhood. Teaching is like landscape or other scene painting, the eye of the beholder is most important and thus followed by the skill to relate and make it transfer to the media; in this case an individual student.

```
Founder (Shih-Jo)
        |
1st Generation Students/Teachers.
        |
2nd Generation Students/Teachers.
        |
3rd generation
        |
4th Generation
        |
     so on
```

T'ien Ti Tao has a simple lineage. The Instructors who learn from the founder, or Grandmaster, are the "1st Generation" of the lineage. Students who learn from them and become Instructors are then known as "2nd Generation" and so on. The term "generation" in this context applies to anyone in a category of learning but in life of humans a generation is just 25 years. Lineage is like a tree, with roots, branches and fruit. The ripest and largest fruit which bears many seeds and falls on fertile ground will continue the strain (family), although this fruit owes its existence to the roots (lineage and foundations) it is the amount of sunlight, nutrients and ch'i which makes it what it is, for those who live in the shade do not grow so well and often perish. It is a fact of teaching, in my forty plus years of experience so far at least, that one can spend a lot of time and effort trying to teach new students and with over 60% of them giving up after a few months. Whatever new skills and confidence they started to gain is lost, dropped or discarded. This shows a massive difference between westerners and easterners, especially Chinese people who may more readily accept the benefits of prolonged practice. After many centuries of Chung Kuo Ch'uan-shu, in all its forms, being a part of the culture, a known health giving and life enhancing formula, a preventative medicine and natural healer, they may take to it like a proverbial duck to water. Here in the west though we, the teachers who know these facts, are struggling to get lazy westerners up off their backsides and into something worthwhile.

As intimated elsewhere in this book and others, the UK National Health Service (NHS) is overwhelmed with patients who need not be there. The doctors, nurses and even the street level General Practitioners (local doctors) are inundated with many cases that are trivial, "minor wobbles" or people who have become dependent on drugs and health care: this is caused by the government who feel a need to control the populace and inform them from birth that they need to see their doctors if the slightest thing seems wrong. This blanket policy encourages misuse, panic, abuse and over use of the system; the system that should be there for more important cases of illness only. This may sound like a harsh judgement, it is just true facts, but allow me get two things straight here:

(1) I do not "judge" or make assumptions. In life I see facts that I have personally experienced and have also been experienced by others and are therefore a more reliable guide.
(2) Practical experience of using Chinese based exercise, health and healing techniques have given me enough sound proof that most illnesses, injuries and health wobbles can be either avoided or cured using TCM; which includes Ch'i Kung and T'ai Chi Ch'uan.

This, however, is easy for me to say because my whole life has been laid out like a sign posted path. Any time I strayed off the path I would be confronted by an "invisible wall" and have to get back on track again in order to progress. My spirit guides have been both kind and cruel in keeping me on this track; I say "cruel" because at times in my life I would have rather done other things, avoided problems caused by other people or become rich and successful to at least the "comfortable" point, but no, this was not to be. Even the gypsy woman who intercepted me that time on Regent Road had my tag marked! The powers of unseen forces are far greater than the whimsical and fragile desires of any mere human.

Many times something would happen that would bring me straight back to *it* would be, what you may deem, a good thing. At other times something happens that is deemed bad, but it makes you think, philosophise and gives you the impetus to drive on in your studies unhindered by any man-made or woman-made folly. At other times the path is bright, warming the soul and pleasingly creative in terms of success, helping others and watching the joy that Taoist Arts can bring. These moments seem to drive humans more than the disasters do; we could call it "getting hooked on good times"!

Jingquanshitaijiquan is one of those things that brings a great deal of satisfaction to many people and being able to show them this humble T'ai Chi Ch'uan Form is a great privilege and a great honour. It also brings people better health, spiritual development, awareness of ch'i, confidence, self-control and much, much more besides.

As previously stated, various persons and spirit guides and such all appeared at the right time, including Taoist Arts Master Soo, who invited me to join his Teacher Training programme. The "unknown shadow boxing" that I used to do when I was very young and all the other things that have happened have all led along a path that is signposted by one simple word "Tao". When I was young and realised which way I was heading, I was quite uncomfortable with any idea of developing a new or unknown system. However, it also struck me that the few mainstream systems that were available were not my proverbial cup of tea either, indeed they were only variations on a theme. This I realised while many others took them as gospel. If I refer to "creating" or "developing" what I should really say, to be honest, is that I was the tool of the Way, the vessel in which the mix was stirred, not the ultimate creator as such. Never did I realise that so much input from spiritual masters would be heading my way. Never in my wildest dreams could I have imagined that I would be sitting there, minding my own business and doing something completely unrelated, would I suddenly be compelled to get up, do a new movement/technique and have the name of it pop into my head at the same time! One just cannot predict Tao and all the unseen forces which operate within it. Some of you may call this God; I just call it Tao, "Way" for want of a better word.

In the history of T'ai Chi Ch'uan there have been many people who have developed their own styles, as you read earlier, that have become well known, Yang, Sun, Chen, Wu, Hao, etcetera. Then the mainstream styles that do not bear a family name but are named after some principle or animal: Hung Gar, Hsing-I, Pa Kua or T'ai Chi Ch'uan, for example. There are of course many more that are not well known but may be equally remarkable. The real point is that all these various styles have helped many people to overcome poor health, caused by bad living habits or an unbalanced diet. There you have the history of T'ai Chi Ch'uan in a proverbial nutshell. Even the styles which were made up by those with a love of a physical challenge and of a competitive nature, those styles still helped many thousands of people to better health; to the degree that in any part of China almost every doctor consulted about common problems would say, "Go do T'ai Chi!"

Did you know: T'ai Chi Ch'uan is *the* most popular form of exercise in the world?

Is Jingquanshitaijiquan a New Style, Made Up?

Neither. All styles are "made up" by someone, Chen, Yang, Wu, Sun and this one too. The word "Choreographed" would be more appropriate, but still not quite accurate, especially in the case of T'ai Chi Ch'uan. The governing factor is whether they are made-up of genuine technique or imitation movements that might "look like" a Martial Art, to the untrained eye. Genuine technique in the case of the subject matter is that which follows the correct principles.

Sorry to digress for a second, but I keep using this term "Martial Art/s". T'ai Chi Ch'uan is not "martial" it is "Taoist" and we really should strive to understand that Ch'eung San-feng wanted to create a balanced exercise system for health, fitness *and* self-defence that was suitable for those studying Tao. It was not for battle or warring, even though it might be superbly effective in self-defence.

Jingquanshitaijiquan or Wellspring Taijiquan Style is based upon years of research into the philosophy and background of Taijiquan and is based on basic principles of Ch'eung San-feng's probable original concept of Yin/Yang, Snake and Crane, plus the 13 Essential Basics. It also contains a few elements or 'Postures' of Lee (Li) Family Style, from respect for my Old Taoist Arts Master and Li/Wu styles out of both respect and practicality, plus traditional techniques like "silk reeling" and Single Whip, with at one point a "follow step" as favoured by Sun Lu-t'ang. Much of the Form came after meditating with a view to contacting Great Masters, either alive or in the so-called "Spirit world" somewhere; I for one would love to know who or where; but at the end of the day this is unimportant. As stated before, the urge to get up and suddenly start moving, the movements followed on from the previous and seemed to flow quite naturally; in some cases the name popped into mind with it, like "Sweeping the leaves off Mt. Hua" which, for some reason that I did not quite comprehend at the time, but *felt*, seemed to be a "Chinese style" joke. In that particular instance I recall I was sitting down and attending to other work. Then I was compelled to get up and do a "strange" new movement; the likes of which I had not done before and seemed quite unfamiliar. Having done the movement, with the name coming through at the same time, it was then stripped (backward engineered) by me, analysed and later seemed quite appropriate as well as practical. Some year or so later I came across an article in which someone said to the effect that "The Taoists on Mt. Hua say that they know nothing of Martial Arts training" and just live a peaceful life farming or studying medicine. The Chinese humour is very subtle at times, philosophical at others.

Jingquanshitaijiquan is a Form which does not repeat moves from left to right; it is a Mono-Form. The "13 Fa" (methods) all present, some are "hidden" and can only be revealed later with practice and diligence; this is one aspect of T'ai Chi Ch'uan that really inspires and encourages me, the fact that practice is like a "time release mechanism". The more you practice, the longer you have trained for, then the more you get from it. Jingquanshi is a practical Form, meaning that there is an obvious self- defence application to every aspect, though some are less obvious than others so again may only be revealed after much practice. It differs greatly to the commonly seen modern "Competition Forms" or "Standardised Health Forms" as it has depth, intention and expression as well as other traditional aspects. Postures are natural and movement complies with the internal principles, not competition rules or exaggerated postures that can be seen by judges from twenty or more yards away.

In terms of performance and character, Jingquanshitaijiquan cannot be allocated a seat in a row precisely, but at an "educated guess" I would say it sits somewhere in-between Chen and Wu, possibly both sides of the middle! However, it does not have to sit alongside the other styles as it has its own character and form (as in "shape") and was never meant to be "like" any other, it is "original" and just happened that way. One of the main things which distinguish traditional styles from modern competition variants is "application", as intimated above; this includes several peripheral exercises, including qigong and special pair exercises, like sensitivity training. Jingquanshi or "Wellspring style" falls into this traditional category.

Without traditional aspects no style calling itself T'ai Chi Ch'uan or Taijiquan is really that but just something that "looks like". You may say that the reflections from water in a shallow puddle look like the reflections on the sea, but there is a huge difference beneath the surface.

There are many styles of Taijiquan, as stated previously, but the oldest traceable Form (via existing paperwork) is said to be "Old style Chen", according to the historians. This is followed by original Yang Style (developed from Chen Style), Wu and then Wu/Hao, all taking something from its predecessor. Each style has their own way of doing things, it cannot be said that one is right and the other is wrong. Chen Second Form is said to be developed using both Tao Boxing and Long Boxing (Chang Ch'uan) principles, hence its low stances. Yang developed his from the Chen First Form, which was more in line with Tao Ch'uan principles. Others followed suit and adapted and adopted.

Tao is Tao and no two trees look exactly the same in nature's rich meadows, though they all have roots, absorb light and bear fruit or "seed". T'ai Chi Ch'uan is not a Form it is a set of principles and those principles conform in one way or the other to the philosophy of Tao.

Is It New?

Not really. It may be new in terms of history, creation or dates of development, but it is old in the sense of both principles and time-span of T'ai Chi Ch'uan. If you think about the lineage of T'ai Chi Ch'uan, right the way back to the Thirteen Methods, then account for all the modifications in between then and now, you will get a sense of change. There are some techniques taken from the newer Forms or Styles, like Sun, Li (Lee) and Wu. However, these are incorporated using the essence of Jingquanshi, not Sun Li or Wu and not just duplications; they all have their own character.

Imagine also the concepts behind the most basic Forms of T'ai Chi Ch'uan; or should we say Taoist Inner Harmony Boxing (TIHB), to save any arguments about history and names! As we apparently have no accurate history *before* Chen Family Style, at the time of writing, we have to look at Taoism and the general history of Chinese Boxing leading up to then. This is what I tried to do here. The most prominent factors of Taoist theory would have included, in simplified terms, Wu Chi, Tao and Yin and Yang and perhaps other deeper translations scattered across China (pieces may "filter through" to be added or retranslated), add to that the Snake and Crane principles of Old Ch'eung's perceived vision and a garnish of smaller developments and classical observations from across the centuries and there we have the basic recipe for not only Ch'eung's creation but also Jingquanshitaijiquan. The "project" was shelved proverbially in the late 1980's due to other more pressing matters and changes in life paths. However, the Form stood at 32 steps then and was more than enough to practice and get feedback from. Later, around the late 1990's the feedback was used and the Form studied in detail again to complete. The records of time were not kept, but as an estimate it could be said that the Form took many years to complete, about ten; not counting the many years study prior to its creation, of course. It is now considered to be "ready" to teach.

There were only a handful of T'ai Chi Ch'uan instructors in the UK during the early 70's, and then with all the arguments about style, lineage, who is right and who is wrong, there seemed only one way to go, study the "roots" and grow a new "stock" from those traditional roots. Does it work? In terms of health, "yes". In terms of self- defence, "yes" again. In terms of "is it really traditional T'ai Chi Ch'uan?" I would say yes and so would my students and other practitioners who may have seen it, including people from China who have a background in Chinese Arts. Some experts seem to think it is traditional, even the Old Masters of the ICKF when we were "tested" by them in the Republic of China, especially the Old Master who said "It's probably more traditional than most traditional Arts!"

In terms of enjoyment, ask the students, but they certainly seem to get a lot from it; and some of those hail from other styles in the past. Just a while ago I asked one of my students "PJ" if he still kept up practice of his Chen Style routines. "Yes," he said "I still like to keep it up but Chen style always makes me feel like I want a fight with all that stamping and Fajing. This one I love because I feel my ch'i flowing and it makes me feel calm." Others who have seen it but do not practice it have commented, in various ways, "That's an interesting Form". One gentleman from mainland China who showed us his Standardised Wu Shu also saw it and was amazed by the fact that he could see Jingquanshitaijiquan had "practical values". In a world where people often make hasty judgements based on the knowledge that they have about their style or their teacher, I am not going to join in; I shall leave my cup empty!

The History of T'ien Ti Tao P'ai.

The School: Officially founded in January 1975.

The founder was not in contact with any Martial Arts but as a small child used to practice holds, locks, throws and "Shadow Boxing" and had Spirit Guides. Later on, c.1951, after starting school, these innate skills became useful when confronted by bullies.

Studies of philosophy, psychology, Eastern religions and beliefs were later accompanied (c.1965) by studies of Eastern Martial Arts: Mainly Korean and Japanese. The "roots" of these to be traced back through their native culture to the Chinese culture, from which most emanated.

Philosophical studies can be linked to principles and methods in Martial Arts, so these were traced back to China and the techniques brought in-line with the cultural principles of the time: as near as possible with information available.

Studies of Indian Yoga, Chakras, Pranayama and cross-cultural meditations and spiritual methods were integrated. Later on, when becoming available, the Chinese methods were also integrated and Compared.

1968 – 1974: Martial Arts Theory was bolstered by (a mix of old school Shaolin and Ju Jitsu) and parts of other Martial Arts.

1975 saw the invite by Grandmaster C. Chee Soo to Lee (Li) Family Style Arts in Dunstable- where the Teacher's Training classes were held. These sessions included Li Style T'ai Chi Ch'uan, Ch'i Kung, I Fou Shou, Whirling Arms, Whirling Legs, Stick (Kun), TCM and Taoist 'Long Life' Diet, to name the basics.

1980 – 1985: Further development and studies including classic Hsing-I Ch'uan under Shih-fu Brad Waldron plus various essence techniques of other styles.

Myke Symonds was at this time East Anglian Representative for Kung Fu with the A.M.A. of Great Britain.

1985 1987: The School was fully tested by the International Chinese Kuoshu Federation (I.C.K.F.) in Taiwan, R.o. China. Committee members at the time included the venerable Master Hung, I-Hsiang and many other respected Old Masters of Traditional Chinese Arts.

At his time Myke Symonds was made East Anglian Ambassador for Kuoshu by Si-fu Raymond Goh of B.K.P.A.

Late 1987 – Accepted as "Genuine traditional Chinese Arts" by the I.C.K.F. One of the Old Masters commented "It's probably more traditional than most 'traditional' systems!"

1988 – Present Day: Further development, testing and promotion of the traditional Chinese Arts, their philosophy and values.

1997 Onwards: Head of British Association for Chinese Arts (B.A.C.A.) And other National Associations.

THE PHILOSOPHY OF THE FORM

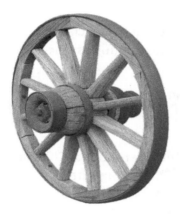

Thirty spokes are made one by holes in a hub,
By vacancies joining them for a wheel's use;
The use of clay in moulding pitchers
Comes from the hollow of its absence;
Doors and windows, in a house,
Are useful for their emptiness:
Thus we are helped by what is not
To use what is.

What Makes T'ai Chi Ch'uan what it is?

In one word, the answer is "Form". In this case Form is of a wider context, like the "Form" in the west that we would call a "mould"; used to make parts. The "parts", in the case of T'ai Chi Ch'uan, are philosophical and physical, physiological, mental and "unknown" or un-nameable. Form does not refer to style or a set of movements that makes the style. The true Form is that of creation in all its glory, all its steps and stages, all its materials and the philosophy that creates the mould. It is the Form of T'ai Chi Ch'uan that makes us One.

There are many views as to what makes a great style, which qualities make a great teacher, which style works best and so on. With regard to style, in my considered opinion, I would think that the style of T'ai Chi Ch'uan (TIHB) ranks high level, as long as it is taught and performed correctly. It is with sadness and dismay that we see many people today practising what they think is T'ai Chi Ch'uan but in fact is only a "watered down exercise" version. Qualifying this remark, made not by me but by many Chinese experts, are these simple Taijiquan facts:

1. T'ai Chi Ch'uan follows the principles of Taoist Philosophy. Seek to understand Tao and you will understand T'ai Chi Ch'uan.

2. T'ai Chi Ch'uan is a system of self-defence, not just exercise and vice-versa. To understand and do it properly one should learn the applications. This also helps develop Ch'i.

3. T'ai Chi Ch'uan follows a pattern of teaching which also teaches Tao through example and has profound effects on the practitioner's mind, body and spirit.

4. T'ai Chi Ch'uan is high-level Art, not base level exercise or just dance; Taiji Dance is an exercise from Taijiquan and uses certain principles from it but is not T'ai Chi Ch'uan by itself.

186

5. In order to understand T'ai Chi Ch'uan one must spend many years learning and studying the complete Art; even then it may not be whole.

6. T'ai Chi Ch'uan is usually taught after other Boxing Arts; because this builds a firm foundation and helps "break in" to a more complex system.

7. T'ai Chi Ch'uan 'empty hand Forms' should be followed by T'ai Chi Ch'uan Sword, Spear, Staff and other weapons, usually in a specific order.

8. T'ai Chi Ch'uan also has complementary or peripheral exercises which help to hone skills and develop specific areas; Dao, I Fou Shou, Jian, Bang and 'Rule', for example (not in specific order).

This brings us to the modern practices emanating from China and the 42 Step Competition Routine; which was replaced in 1999 by another routine. This, in both original and updated versions, is not what experts call proper Taijiquan. According to historians and scholars, this "pseudo" style was "cobbled together from almost random postures... ...taken from the 5 main styles"; two of which are in fact modern and variations of the other mainstream styles, Chen, Yang and Wu. It does not use Taijiquan principles or indeed any of the theory of Taoism in its practice. The movements and postures are regulated by rules dictating trivia for the judges, like having exact finger positions, uniform height of hands or kicks. This is physical or external exercise, not internal Art. There is other, such as a more recent (c.1988) variation upon this theme but claiming to teach basic principles in-line with the old styles; lack of full information prohibits further detailed writing at this time. According to author and scholar Jou, Tsung Hwa, it is a shame that this new Form also lacks the essential principles of T'ai Chi Ch'uan.

With the advent of YouTube™ you will be able to view different Forms just by typing in that style's name and Quan or Ch'uan after it. Many schools that attract tourists to go on courses or "workshop vacations" are actually teaching non-traditional Forms or variations that have names that may sound as if they pertain to ancient influences. There are even schools in UK, Europe or USA that teach modern competition or standardised Forms and try to give the impression that it is "traditional". Some of the people teaching such Forms may be Chinese in origins simply because they grew up in an era where nothing else was known. Others may be just playing on their cultural background to generate consumer faith; this happens in all societies. The reader must study the facts and not be fooled by false claims. T'ai Chi Ch'uan has certain principles, amongst which is the use of the waist, posture and "spiralling", currently made famous by Chen's Silk Reeling methods; although these were taught in Wellspring and Li/Lee Style long before the author had even heard of Chen Family T'ai Chi Ch'uan.

The Yin and Yang

Most versions of Yang Family style in the UK have been taught in a completely "soft" (Yin) manner and completely devoid of any hardness or vigour or even self-defence applications (Yang). The Yang Family system, as originally designed by Yang Lu-chan, is said to have preferred the Yin techniques; done with a slow 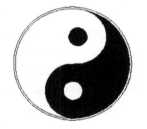 or soft movement; as influenced originally by his training in Chen Village and the Chen family's original First Form or "Yin Form". Although not at first taught outside of close family circles, the Yang Family Style also had some impressive self-defence techniques, or applications. These were obvious in Smith & Cheng's book as some were demonstrated in photographic form at the back of the book. The most impressionable of these was Cheng Man-ching showing an application of Push and Uproot, lifting a man up off his feet. The expression on Cheng's face is placid and his body upright and relaxed. This caused a huge "Wow!" factor amongst many Martial Artists and would be T'ai Chi Ch'uan practitioners who then tried around the 1980's to find teachers who could not only teach them Form but its applications too.

Possibly the greatest influence on Chinese Boxing, due to the spread of Taoist Philosophy, was the counter-balance of Yin & Yang; Chen style uses this in its original Lao Jia "Old Frame" Forms which had five routines known as the "13 move Ch'uan". The Forms, one a Yin (First Form) which was of higher stance and more "internal" was the one that Yang Lu-chan is said to have based his style on; this was, so the story went, because he went to Beijing and wanted to teach there, but most people who wanted to learn were old and could not manage the low stances, foot stamping and explosive movements of the second set. The "Yang" Frame of Chen is said to be shaped more from early Chang Ch'uan and not Wu Tang Ch'uan style. The object of this structure was to teach the student the soft (Yin) Forms first so that they can concentrate on correct posture, relaxation of the muscles, etcetera. After the Yin Form had been mastered they could then learn how to perform the Yang Forms, expressing energy and issuing power, as developed with the Chen variations of the Silk Reeling Exercises. Their body would still be comparatively relaxed and free from tension. In Yang Style, by comparison, the body is kept soft and all Forms are done slowly, except in Push Hands practice where applications may be done later at a more natural pace and speed. As far as I am aware, but cannot name individually at present, there are variations of this where during a relaxed Linked Form certain punches or kicks are done faster, expressing energy, "Fa jing" as the Chinese call it. In T'ien Ti Tao's Jingquanshitaijiquan the same aforesaid principles of softness apply but there are Fajing movements as well as more hard to describe physical aspects; they can be shown but not written; much of the skills are like that and that is one good reason why you need a teacher who knows the Art.

The Wu Style also emphasises the development of ch'i by using "Yee" or Mind's will as a major tool. The Li (Lee) Style is very similar, but with no explosive "Fajing" movements. There are many variations of styles all based on the theory of Tao. Many Chinese Masters are now gathering or collating information from their stylists across China and examining the findings.

(Illustration: Wu Style 'Archer' left, Li Style 'Archer' right.)

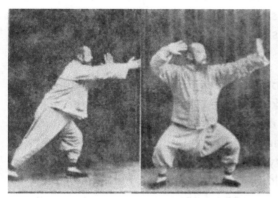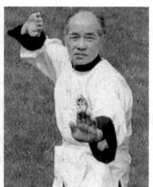

In some cases the full style background and teachings are coming to light for the first time. In many ways the history books are being rewritten and the major styles are being documented properly: but only taught to a select few "inner door disciples" as a complete Art.

Jou Tsung Hwa suggests that if you want to see what T'ai Chi Ch'uan is all about then you should make a long study of the three major styles; Chen, Yang and Wu. He points out that one is more yin than the other, one more yang and one more focused on other elements. This seems to imply that a traditional Form should have all those elements within it to be in harmony with Taoist philosophy and general Taoist boxing practice. Wellspring Style does have the various elements within the one relatively short Form. This varies throughout from Small Gate to Medium Gate, then Big Gate. It has some low stances, some higher and some in between.

Basic Level - Yin & Yang.

Within all styles of Taiji, the principle of Yin and Yang should be dominant. Yin and Yang have many translations and can be translated externally (body-wise) as Yin on the outside and Yang on the inside; meaning whilst the body is still or soft and moving

190

relatively slowly, inside one develops great power and the spirit and mind are actively controlling all performance. Yang Style in the classical sense holds many secrets which modern practitioners do not have access too. Therefore what most people teach may seem incomplete and may not usually contain the fighting aspects, ch'i expression or other factors.

Some traditional stylists hold to the principle of Chang-chuan training for as long as it takes before learning any Form moves. This will develop the body and ch'i for practise. Then the movements may be learned, one at a time and each being held for a certain length of time, this is a very Yin way to begin. Others will teach Forms first, sometimes holding, sometimes not. Perhaps other methods are employed, this is Yang. Either way is correct as long as you achieve the desired results. Either way takes a long time to reach any level of competence and achievement.

One thing that should be noted here is the amount of time spent on practice. Whether your teacher holds sessions once a week or five times, it is you that needs to practice regularly and at home every day. Once a week is not enough, nor will it enable you to learn what is really T'ai Chi Ch'uan.

Harmonising.

There is much confusion being spread about fast and slow T'ai Chi Ch'uan. Some practitioners will always stay with the slow practice. Others will spend years learning the slow method and then graduate to faster practice until it is done at often very fast "fighting speeds" (very rarely seen outside doors). Thus the Yin and Yang become harmonious and flux and flow at a natural pace, directed by the Spirit: during this practice the body remains free of muscular tension, yet the muscles contract and relax; much the same as we would react to a fly bite or reaction to a sudden burn. To graduate to this level can take many, many years and the practitioner must never try to rush the education.

Moving on to Adhering or Push Hands is another stage and without it what you are doing is merely a form of callisthenics with added benefits. It must be remembered at all times that T'ai Chi Ch'uan is an exercise for body, mind and spirit based around the essential system of self-defence. And the core of the system is the philosophy of Tao. Developed to express this philosophy T'ai Chi Ch'uan has had many translations, many of which have expressed the same principles, many others have deviated according to the focus of the Form designer and his focus, background and the depth of his knowledge. The principles of practice and advancement follow the philosophical expressions.

The Philosophy of Practice.

The first actual steps in learning Taijiquan usually start with distinguishing Yin from Yang. This deliberately mindful practice is essential in one's endeavours as without it the "Form" will never feel right. Yin and Yang are the equal but opposite forces created by and found throughout the Universe. Before the Universe was created there was chaos; unstructured elements. Then, following the "big bang" of creation the elements were sent forth, colliding and creating as they went their ways, the basic forces behind all actions being either Yin or Yang.

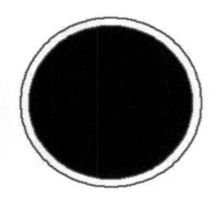

This circle represents the Universe before time. We call it Wuji (Inaction and Chaos).

The black line around the edge is used to denote "within the Universe", whatever that may be, bounded or not. Before we can become "One" with Taiji we must

192

empty our minds and be inactive. Taiji does not plan; Taiji is spontaneous and springs from emptiness.

This image can represent so many things including the "pre-heaven" state, standing posture for preparation and being "empty". This may sound daunting to many beginners, but it is not a prerequisite that you should know all these things before you start. Like all things, time is of the essence and the more you study the more you learn, the more 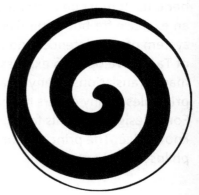 you learn the more is uncovered. This way Tao will be achieved with regular practice and sincerity. This is Tao and Taoism helps develop humanity and better virtues.

This symbol (right) is T'ai Chi, with spirals expanding outwards from the centre. This represents "creation" from the "big bang". It is creation, life and all things ever changing. The forces of Yin (represented by black) and Yang (represented by white) can be seen flowing outwards in a circular way just as it is perceived by scientists that the Universe is constantly expanding, spiraling outwards and changing, and that within it there is death and new life, expansion 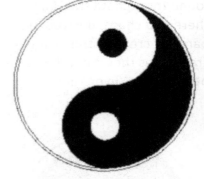 and contraction and all the forces, actions and things we can think of. From the Wu Chi came the T'ai Chi; the One begat Two.

Again the line around the outside is only there to visually suggest that this action takes place within the Universe. Creation can also represent the beginnings of the Form learning, practise and more.

When we take what is natural and create we see beauty and harmony. This is learning to become one with Tao. Creation is not only learning but teaching, an honour and a privilege for those who have already found a true path and wish to help others achieve similar good things. Creation began and has been taking place ever since. We call this Tao.

Tao is represented by the image (right) which shows Yin and Yang in constant harmony throughout the Universe.

Yin and Yang constantly flow, interact and exchange. Imagine that this image is turning clockwise. This symbol is also used to describe the relationships of many other things, like men and women, summer and winter, day and night, heavy and light or full and empty, for examples.

From stillness or chaos came creation; from creation comes harmony, Yin and Yang. It is a blessing to our life if we can achieve harmony and get on with all people; *if* they allow it to happen and do not create problems or "disharmony"; those who are disharmonious or "sick" will often "infect" others for reasons they may not even understand themselves.

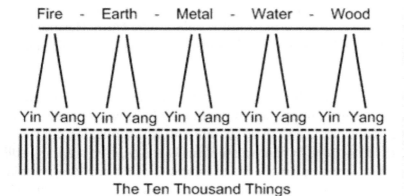

The Ten Thousand Things

From Yin and Yang stem the Five Elements or Wu Hsing, from this flows the 'Ten Thousand Things'.

Harmony is what we see in Nature, all around, like night and day, summer and winter, solid and empty, for examples. The enlightened and educated human should not be wasting time with temporary fashions, trends and trivia, like "fifteen minutes of fame" on some mindless television show. This is not true contentment but mere childish distraction. That feeling that a longer termed practitioner gets at the end of a class, both within themselves and with their classmates, that is contentment, harmony and the pleasure of life. Trying to live by woman-made or man-made rules, regulations and pseudo social laws is a sign of abysmal failure, a breaking from the roots of nature that will only lead to unhappiness, destruction and decay. This effect can be seen across our world where there is bad government or leadership, widespread corruption for money or favours, where technology takes precedent over personal welfare and advertising puerile trivia, make- up, fashion, gadgets, and "wannabe" celebrity fads take over from reason and welfare. This is the result of many people "losing the way" and human relationships breaking down through lack of personal development; personal development is not getting a well-paid job, it is not buying more clothes, handbags or accessories, it is not having a bigger house than the neighbours, a flashy car or exotic holidays, personal development is a course of life-long action whereby one looks after their physical health, mental health and spiritual well-being. Some may find these strong words, but it is only simple truth. Harmony is obtainable, on a "personal level" by the practice of T'ai Chi Ch'uan.

Generally speaking, in terms of physical movements or movements of the body, arms and legs, any movement where we contract - as in draw the hands closer to the body - are Yin, whilst pushing out the hands would be Yang. When we step this is Yang, when standing still it is Yin. There are many more manifestations of Yin and Yang within each Form and peripheral practice. If you cannot find them then ask your teacher for guidance, but once you have a clue you should seek them yourself and not rely on being shown everything. The reason for this is simple, it is like the difference between watching a video of the Form and practicing the Form, only with practice do you benefit by gaining lasting impressions or personally discovered knowledge; knowledge in the video is one-dimensional and shallow, you are unlikely to gain from it but can learn some things about the movements or directions, applications or flow.

We are human; one of the many varied animal forms on this tiny planet in this enormous Universe. We do not know for sure where exactly the centre of the Universe is, so vast is it. Science, like Nature itself, is always in a state of flux. Perhaps we - the human race - shall never know. However, your body is a creation of Tao or Nature. As such it has a centre. This is located approximately two inches below the navel and inside the abdominal cavity. We relate it to the Tan T'ien ("Dantian") or "Heavenly Field" as named in Acupuncture. This point is your centre and is where the centre of your Universe is. Everything outside of you is Universe and you are at centre with your Dantian being your central point. All Yin movements come in to the Dantian and all Yang movements emanate from there.

Although Yang is often associated with "hard" or "strong" it is in this case something else, expansion; like hydraulics or water being driven along a hose pipe, a pressure from within that drives the physical and has great power. For now you can think of Yin as being like when the hydraulics are turned off and the internal fluid settles at base, finding its own level.

Yin and Yang, in Daoist theory, give rise to the Wu Hsing ("Wuxing") or Five Elements. These are, fire, earth, metal, water and wood. Each of these has a Yin side or a Yang side to its nature. Some examples of these can be found in the book called 'Practical Philosophy of Tao, for schools and individuals' (same author); a book which works in partnership with this and any other of Tao subject. Suffice it to say here that, in terms of Taijiquan, if you attack me with a fire technique then I may use a water technique to counter and the same can apply in health related issues. An earth technique may be countered with wood, for example, or wood with metal. In another light, the creation cycle, wood may cause a fire response or water techniques may create wood and so on. The image on the left shows "Duality" and ch'i flow within the Universe.

The Wu Hsing are furthermore linked to directions and basic traits or patterns; templates of life. These are depicted in Daoist philosophy by the simple use of lines, either broken or unbroken, to create what is called a Trigram. On the image here we can see these Trigrams arranged around the symbol of Tao; Tao being the creator and emanating from the centre, all other things move outwards from that. At the top of this symbol we can see a Trigram with three straight or unbroken lines. This is 'Chien' or Heaven and represents the direction of South. In Taijiquan this is represented by a Yang movement called Peng; meaning "Raise the hand/s" and equates with "Ward-off" in Taijiquan. Heaven is the source of creation and all things begin in Heaven - Tao. In more commonly found Yang Style Taijiquan, this movement requires the lifting of the hands to no higher than mouth-level with palms facing in. In Jingquanshi however we raise the hands to ward-off with palms outwards (Sun Hand), like the initial exercise of Baduanjin Qigong "Two hands Push the Sky", but not quite so high as that. A seasoned Yang stylist may ask "Why?" or may even be critical of this. It must be remembered that Yang Style originates from Old Chen Style, as mentioned before.

Similar movements to our Jingquanshitaijiquan can be found in other Taijiquan styles and is similar in some respects to Wu Yu-hsiang's Wu/Hao Style's "Grasp the Bird's Tail" posture and an opening move in Lee Family Style Form, "Gathering Celestial Energy"; not to be confused with "Ch'i Centring". This movement is a counter against the initial attack and follows on naturally into "Rolling the Boulder" and has several practical applications.

Taijiquan Forms can differ as much as Taijiquan teachers in content, depth and methods. Master Alfred Huang writes in his book 'Complete T'ai Chi' about Chen Style, Yang Style and Wu Style mainly and more or less dismisses any pre-Chen Taijiquan as being either unproven or not relevant as, he suggests, that Ch'eung San-feng only correlated a few systems that were about at the time. This is unusual insomuch as most Masters recognise a complete lineage of development rather than just a partial and more recent one that is more easily proven. Perhaps this opinion was brought about because of the information available to Shih-fu Huang at the time? In another chapter he states that he meditated before writing and was guided by the spiritual masters in his works. This is not unusual and is very common practice in Taijiquan and associated circles. This method was used in the creation of the Wellspring Form for guidance and "traditional direction" and some days it got results whilst others one would be left pondering the previous findings. It is only natural that we are likely to base any new Forms on old knowledge, or what we have been taught. Changes may or may not come later and this is what happened with Chen, Yang, Wu, Wu/Hao, Sun and latterly Lee style founders. Anyone who argues about this is pouring tea into a full cup!

'The only thing that remains constant is change" Tao Te Ching.

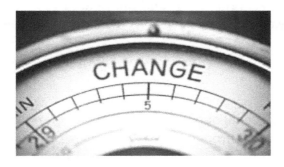

Wu Hsing - The Five Elements.

The Five Element theory is logical. In Western culture the elements would be Fire, Earth, Air and Water, in Chinese culture they are Fire, Earth, Water, Metal and Wood; it is assumed that Air is a by-product of the other elements. These elements are applied to everything from Martial Arts to Feng Shui and Traditional Chinese Medicine to every day cooking.

Wu Hsing

In T'ai Chi Ch'uan we look at the elements as a guideline towards certain principles: e.g. metal cleaves, water splashes or fire flickers. Understanding the Wu Hsing is an important part of Form and Method (Ch'uan Fa). From the Five Elements all things that we know are created and can be traced back to their roots by the same method. Your teacher will guide you by giving you insights into these aspects, but it is up to you to do the studying. Teaching in this way has a more lasting effect.

Water.

Water is the most powerful and versatile element on the planet. Think of the destructive force of the Tsunami, then the gentle trickle of a fresh mountain stream which serves all as it flows down through the valleys, to the river, then the surging river with all its currents and eddies. Water eventually flows to the sea, which supports many life forms and also is effected by the rotation of the planet and moon's pull, causing tidal flow. Water *is hard and will wear down the hardest rocks, yet it is soft and* will yield as you try to grasp it, flowing away and settling back at its own level. Water enables wood to grow.

Wood.

Think of a small seed, opening and the seemingly delicate first shoot pushing its way up through the earth, moving stones aside as it reaches for the light. Wood is flexible, it can bend and change direction, yet it can also remain rooted at the same time. Look at the trees and plants that grow on craggy rocks, the roots delving into the cracks and crannies so that the plant can hold on and not topple. Wood is a fuel for fire.

Fire.

Scorching high flames and burning embers, flames that flicker and dance. The flames can leap into the air and dance around in a seemingly random fashion or fire can be subtle like a smouldering ember. Where wood grows fire can feed though water can dampen the flames. Wood when burned leaves ash which soon returns to soil forming earth.

Earth.

The earth is a source of nutrients and these, combined with sunlight and water, are a perfect base for growing many things in. Earth is Yin, and is represented in natural laws as being "down" and "below our feet", ground and gravitational. Mother Earth holds us close to her so that we do not float away into space. Rocks, clay and minerals are also "earth" and all part of the basic sub-structure. We like to keep our feet on the ground and feel secure when closest to her beating heart. The Earth gives rise to metal.

Metal.

Think of veins of metal, cleaving through the soil, embedded in the rocks like hardened arteries of the earth. Metal is hard, yet can be melted by fire. Metal can be moulded to make use of its essence to hold water or an axe to cut trees, dig the soil in farming toil, or act as tokens for trading. Metal is quite versatile too, like other elements here. It is said, in Taoist philosophical terms, that metal attracts water because of its coldness; like condensation, so metal leads us back to water in the creative cycle.

The Pa Kua.

The Bagua (Chinese: 八卦; literally "eight symbols") are eight diagrams used in Taoist cosmology to represent the fundamental principles of reality and also equate to the four primary and four sub-directions of the compass. The symbols are Trigrams which are treated as a range of eight interrelated concepts. Each Trigram, as the name suggests, consists of three lines, each line either "broken" (Yin) or "unbroken," (Yang).

Seen here in their arrangement representing the Eight main directions, the Trigrams also have a Yang point, being South (at top of image). The Trigram representing South is Ch'ien - Heaven - Creative - Strength and Ward-off, and consists of three unbroken lines. This is because South represents Heaven (Yang), Sun (Yang) and "Creative", also Yang. At the opposite pole is K'un: Earth - Receptive - Yielding, all Yin qualities.

(Moving anti-clockwise around the circular Bagua: Yang goes leftwards and down while Yin goes upwards and to the right, progressively changing.)

The other Trigrams are:

East - K'an - Water - The Abysmal, Dangerous and Press.

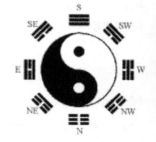

West - L'i - Fire - Clinging - Light Transmission and Push. The four sub-directions are: South-west - Chen - Thunder Arousing - Inciting Movement - Splitting.

North-east - Sun - Wood - Gentle - Penetrating - Large Roll-back.

North-west - Tui - Lake - Joy - Attraction and Elbow Strike.

South-east - K'en - Mountain - Centring - Stillness - Rest and Shoulder Press.

The Trigrams (three line representations) are taken from the book called the I-Ching (pronounced like "Yee-jing"), meaning roughly "Book of Changes". There are sixty-four in total and these can be used in combinations of two, forming six lines called a Hexagram. In the basics of Taijiquan only eight Trigrams are used at first to describe the Eight Basic Techniques and Eight Directions; Pa Kua ("Bagua"). At the South we have Fire. This represents the Sun (Yang) at its highest pinnacle in our sky as well as Heaven and all creation. The Trigram is composed of three solid lines. Solid lines are Yang, broken lines are Yin. In the North we have K'un, Earth which is formed of three broken lines (Yin). In the Hexagram seen above left we have "Harmony", when the Yin is kept above the Yang. Harmony is a state whereby nothing radical is happening and it is like the Yin and Yang of Tao working together.

There are other Taoist Arts which concentrate more on the Eight Trigrams, like Pa Kua Ch'ang or Pa Kua Chang or Ch'uan and of course the Chinese Art of Divination known as Feng Shui. These are all practised in the same vein as T'ai Chi Ch'uan, to harmonise with Tao or Nature. You do not have to understand, contemplate or even briefly ponder on these unless you intend to make a full study of T'ai Chi and T'ai Chi Ch'uan. In the aspect of T'ai Chi for Health, for example, it is important that the practitioner develops his or her strength and health; indeed this is the same for anyone beginning the full T'ai Chi Ch'uan practice too.

The Table of Bagua Trigrams and Relation to Taijiquan.

From the Eight Directions stems the Wu Hsing. These are Fire, Earth, Metal, Water and Wood. From these all things that we know are created; this is called "Ten Thousand Things" as it was a big number many years ago.

In terms of Taijiquan the Ten Thousand Things can represent permutations of movements that can occur as a result of mastering the basics. The actual number or permutations has never been calculated, to my knowledge, but could be far more than ten-thousand or even more than Ten-zillion; the actual number is unimportant, the *concept* that Tao creates all things is the only value here but you could work out *every single thing* in life, if you wished, and ascertain its Yin/Yang and Wu Hsing value; if you want to drive yourself mad and waste time!

The Table below details each of the Eight Directions, their corresponding Pa Kua (Bagua) and the T'ai Chi posture, TCM reference and opposites. This should help serious students get a deeper understanding of the Form.

Trigram	Compass	Image	Posture	Faults	Skills	Cavity	Meridian
Chien	South	Heaven (Supreme Yang)	Ward-off	Opposing	Evade	Pai Hui	Tu Mo
T'ui	South-East	Valley (Young Yang)	Elbowing	Bending Downward	Advancing	Kuan Hsuan	Yang Wei Mo
Li	East	Fire /Thunder (Mid-Yang)	Pushing	Resisting	Clearing	Chiang Kung	Tai Mo
Chen	North-East	Thunder (Old Yang)	Splitting	Splicing	Change	Ch'i Hai	Yin Chia Mo
K'un	North	Earth (Supreme Yin)	Roll Back	Leaning	Return	Hui Yin	Jen Mo
Ken	North-West	Mountain (Young Yin)	Shoulder Butt	Looking upwards	Withdraw ing	Ching Men	Yang Chia Mo
K'an	West	Water (Middle Yin)	Pressing	Discarding	Adhering	Shuang Kuan	Chuang Mo
SUN	South-West	Wind (Old Yin)	Pulling	Detaching	Circling	Yu Chen	Yin Wei Mo

Earth is sometimes depicted in the centre. This is because in the Form Earth represents being centred and rooted. For the purposes of the illustration above the order has been placed in the Creative Cycle which may help the beginner to understand their relationships easier. Each Element, yin or yang aspect and all of the "ten thousand things" have a linked relationship. There is a way that these can be used alongside T'ai Chi Ch'uan practice and study, but that is another story. There is a book by Stuart Alve Olson called "T'ai Chi According to The I Ching" which goes into the very comprehensive detail of this subject, linked to the Yang Style and a Form created for that method. This strict and finely detailed practice is not necessary in your Wellspring T'ai Chi Ch'uan as this is a more modern development, but very interesting nevertheless. Traditionally this may be chosen as a parallel study.

The basic principles have always been associated with T'ai Chi Ch'uan, to varying degrees of use and conceived importance. More details on the above aspects follows but this serves well enough as a concise guide to the essential elements of T'ai Chi Ch'uan.

The basic principles of the Wellspring style are:

• Five Steps
• Eight Methods
• Unification
• Harmony
• Non-being.

These methods, without too much need for "brain strain" for the overwhelmed novice, will naturally split into more sub-categories whilst the Form is being executed.

The main movements are based upon the Snake and Crane with a few hints of historic folklore and legends of the founders built in.

Mix these ingredients with a liquid blend of, Silk Reeling Technique, "Song" (Feng Zho) and set them in a dish of correct alignments. Let them settle for around fifteen to twenty years and "Hey presto!" A Form should appear that is very satisfying and nourishing.

Why twenty years? It is said in China that "It takes ten years to make a T'ai Chi instructor. Twenty years to make a good one!" There are other details that go into training but these are not suitable for publication in a book as trying to explain the detail would end up in a state of ambiguity; as said previously, an instructor is needed.

T'ai Chi Ch'uan Basics.

There are set basics, governed by the study of Universal principles and restrictions of human physiology. These at first seem vague or even illusive to those who do not know the true skills of T'ai Chi Ch'uan, but for those who are taught they will all become clear and essential as well as making perfect sense. On the next pages we will take a closer look at these basics but rather than being read through at speed, they should be studied until they become natural to do.

Posture.

The posture or correct physical approach is essential to Taijiquan as without it you would never achieve anything worthwhile. Your mission is to remember these postures and apply them to your everyday practice.

The common analogy of having an invisible string holding your head aloft is just one part of the postural practice. Various parts of the body need to be sunk, stretched out, relaxed or aligned. Your Instructor will explain to you the posture principles within the first few sessions that you begin. Posture also includes correct alignments and placement of feet, etcetera.

Attitude.

Your attitude is the backbone of your life. If your attitude is not strong then your learning will be weakened. By "attitude" we do not mean the subject of modern colloquialisms when speaking of people with "an attitude problem"; bad attitude, in other words. Attitude refers to the will to learn, the will to succeed, the will to do good and the will to survive and live a longer, healthier happier life. If you do not have the best attitude it must be developed.

The Main Energies.

Yee.

The Mind's intention is to develop, to do well, to perform correctly and efficiently. This will be done in harmony with nature and in line with the principles of Taijiquan. If you do not develop "I" ("Yee") within two years then you need to practice harder, more often and listen to advice more carefully. Without the "I" your T'ai Chi Ch'uan Form will be nothing more than ballroom dancing!

Jin Energy.

There are many types of Jin. Tianjin is "listening energy", not listening with the ears but listening with the body; this we become familiar with in I Fou-shou practice. Jin can be defined as the energy which controls the muscles or an energy which is produced within the body, helping health. Jin is one of the many Chinese words which has many meanings depending upon the context of the sentence or subject in which it is mentioned. External Jin is usually referred to as the power to use muscles, but this relies also on Qi and Yee. Internal Jin is the build-up and circulation of energy or

206

ability to move it to the right place at the right time. Fa Jin is when the energies are concentrated and executed in a Form. Do not worry too deeply about Jin.

Li Energy.

The Li energy is like the energy you would find in an arrow that has been shot into the air. The Bow has been pulled, so building up and storing energy. On release the stored energy is transferred to the arrow. The arrow's shaft then stores that transferred energy until the tip hits and penetrates a target when the energy is transferred to the target via the arrow shaft which had stored the energy. Li energy, in human terms, is not just muscle power but a combined energy of the body which is controlled by the mind so linking I, Qi and Li with Jin.

LI energy reminds me of the old Chinese Taijiquan Master who was being quizzed by a Karate Master, one who had never seen the once secretive internal skills before. He asked "How can you fight someone with no muscles?" The old Taijiquan player smiled and replied "A bullet has no muscles"!

Qi Energy.

The mind controls the body and develops Li energy; the most efficient form of "physical power". With correct breathing the Qi or Ch'i is developed. The mind's intent, "I" (pronounced "Yee"), drives the qi to its destination. The brain creates electrical signals that are sent through the nervous system. These signals are what make us react to different stimuli, like sneezing to clear the nose of dust; a natural energy movement. The mind controls the qi and the qi controls the muscles and governs the internal organs. Through a combination of the other training elements and correct breathing you will develop your body's ability to use a more relaxed and natural power, yet one which is more powerful than just muscle-power alone.

Shen.
Just a note here about 'Shen' (Spirit). This is something which is already present but is refined, bolstered and boosted by practice. The Spirit's job is as an overseer or operator. The disharmonies before practice are unified and the Shen controls each movement or action without the need for present consciousness.

It may be said that Shen is an accumulation of energies which, after years of practice, transform one's way of doing things. To use a simple analogy, the Spirit operates the body in much the same way as the human operates as a driver of a car. After many years of driving many tasks become "sub-conscious" and performed without thinking. Reactions may also be on this sub-conscious level. In Taijiquan we become somewhat automated through practice and understanding. This is not the only goal though. As Shen is purified and boosted, there may be more spiritual experiences, connections and "unexplained" events. Because we are "driving" a human or animal body, we may be limited to the capabilities of that body and brain (Chemicals are limited individually) to what may seem like frustratingly reduced abilities: compared to "out of body" activities of the less restricted Spiritual Form.

Summary of Shen Energy.

Shen, loosely translated is Spirit. By the gradual process of training in the Taijiquan principles you will build up Shen. These stages are like overlapping steps, like an escalator; slow, subtle and ever increasing upwards to a higher level. The more Shen is developed the more it will take over; in other words the Spirit is linked via the mind, brain and nervous system which is also utilising the higher levels of Qi and Jin generated through regular practice.

Supportive Exercises.

Depending upon the style and the instructor, or the way that he or she was taught, you may start off training with a supplemental exercise first, like Zhanzhuang (Standing as though holding a post), for example. These "multi-purpose" exercises are often good grounding methods which may be used in conjunction with specific exercises to enhance or correct conditions. Some people use no extra exercises.

Shisanqi.

The original information regarding the Thirteen Principles, which, in addition to Yin and Yang and other elements, became the mainstay of most Taijiquan styles.

Shi San Shi ("Xisanxi") means "Thirteen Postures", though these are not just postures but also techniques (named postures after drawn illustrations of each). Behind the number thirteen is the complete basic principle of Taijiquan or Taoist Boxing. This principle is respected and has been followed by all generations of Taiji groups for more than two hundred years. The 13 Postures lead to developing 37 Forms, made well known by Yang Style's original Set. These were said to create all the basics of Taijiquan and combine to build up to 250 or more techniques of self-defence in "cross-combination" or permutation. Without understanding these 13 principles well, it is said that one cannot reach high level Taiji Quan skills.

The Five Skills.

Students must learn the basic five skills before they can accomplish any level of satisfactory practice. This depends on the ability of the teacher, not the student.

Life's a long Song!

Relaxation is the first priority, all else follows when that is learned. In terms of T'ai Chi Ch'uan relaxation is not floppy, as though one has fainted. Relaxation is often likened to "steel wrapped in cotton" as the practitioner's hands may look relaxed or "soft" externally but still contain strength within. Attaining the correct posture is the key to relaxation in Taijiquan.

No book can ever do justice to the five key skills, only personal tuition can help translate and teach these elements.

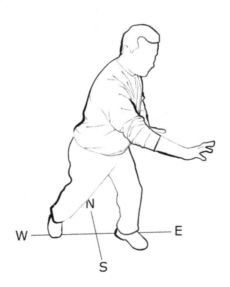

Eight "Gates" or Directions
(八門 Bā Mén)

(1) P'eng (掤, "Pung") or "Ward off" is usually an upward circular movement, in any direction, whilst "yielding" to an attack. Performed more frequently with the arms this will upset the opponent's centre of gravity (CoG) and assist in "uprooting" him. P'eng is also part of the concept of "song" (鬆), relaxation; without tension. Attention must be paid to the shoulders, elbows and waist when studying P'eng. It is also described as being an "outward and expanding energy".

Kuo, Lien-Ying, in his book 'The T'ai Chi Boxing Chronicle' wrote, "When moving, receiving, collecting, and striking, P'eng ching (energy) is always used. It is not easy to complete consecutive movements and string them together without flexibility. P'eng ching is T'ai Chi boxing's essential energy. The body becomes like a spring; when pressed it recoils immediately." This description gives more light to the common expression "Pung is like a large beach-ball that, when hit, absorbs and bounces back an opponent's attacking energy."

(2) Lü (挒 "Lo"), or "Roll Back". This is a sideways and circular yielding movement, usually sinking naturally to avoid creating tension whilst deflecting and gathering the attacker's energy. Lu is the movement which to me most typifies the statement made by my Old Master, Shih-fu Soo, when he said "In T'ai Chi Ch'uan one's waist is relaxed and turns freely like a turntable. Imagine a gramophone turntable [record deck] that is spinning. If you try to throw a hard dried-pea onto it as it spins the pea will be thrown off at an angle." This is P'eng Lu.

In using Lu ching it is the attacker who dictates the movement and its results are then created from the combined actions. The harder and faster an attacker throws himself forwards then the more detrimental it is to them as they will be redirected "into the void". The greater the force the attacker uses then the greater the loss of balance results.

(3) Chi (擠 "Chee"), "Pressing" or "Sticky". Chi is usually done with the back of the hand or outside edge of the palm or forearm. The Chinese word "pressing" can easily be misinterpreted for "push", but that is totally wrong. To Press is to "listen", also to "follow". By using Chi after Ward-off and Roll-back you can listen to the attacker and determine if or where "An" may be possible.

(4) An (按 "An") To "push" or "uproot" usually with the hand and performed with a slight "dip" with the fingers then a push down-and-up of the palm, which can appear falsely as a palm-heel strike. The pushing power comes from the downwards movement. It is somewhat like compressing a spring that is then released. This can be done with the whole body if one is subtle enough. This is a delicate movement that follows Chi more often than not.

Uprooting can be done in many directions and must always travel through the centre and outwards at one of the 256 or more directions. An is not really a "push" but an extension of Chi or pressing where the culmination of energy transfer may be completed.

(5) Tsai (採 "Tai") - To "pluck or pick or grasp" downwards with the hand, especially with the fingertips or palm. This is like the movement of the Leopard's Jaw in T'ien Ti Tao. The word "tsai" is part of the compound that means to gather, collect or pluck a tea leaf from a branch (採茶, cǎi chá): "Cha" being Chinese for tea, an infusion made with plucked leaves.

In using Tsai one does a short, sharp plucking and pulling action, usually by taking the wrist to your backward direction and downwards. Tsai is not a clumsy grab but an accelerated movement that comes from an existing action and uses the weight and momentum of the body's current "jing" to accomplish what may be described as another type of "An". Do not denigrate the technique by employing muscles alone and study it within the other key principles of T'ai Chi Ch'uan.

(6) Lieh (挒 "Li-eh") This means "separate" or "split" and in Lieh is to twist or to offset with a spiral motion, often while making immobile another part of his body (such as a hand, leg or foot) thereby destroying posture and balance. In movements like "Comb the Wild Horse's Tail" or "Cat Grasps the Bird" we use the action differently but with the same principle. The whole body moves and the resulting spiraling action is used to both neutralise the attacker and apply the counter action of "splitting". Splitting can be deemed to be like "An" in its spiraling or spinning effect but should not be confused.

(7) Chou (肘 "Chow-oo") Chou is to "strike or push" with the elbow. It can be translated as "Elbow Strike" or "Elbow Stroke" or just plain "Elbow" or even "Pork"! Chou can be direct or subtle. If used instead of the shoulder in our version of "Single Whip" and be obvious. In another situation it can be applied in close form, perhaps in I Fou Shou. The study of Chou can yield some interesting facts and some surprising techniques.

(8) K'ao (靠 "Kao") - To "strike or push with the shoulder or upper back". The word K'ao implies leaning or inclining but that does not mean translation should be literal. Shoulder Kao Ching is a full body striking energy. The P'eng energy is mobilized throughout the whole body and is then used as one unit and the force is delivered with the shoulder or back. This and some other of the "Eight" is where we learn subtle energy and Small Gate.

The Five Steps
(Wu bu).

(9) Chin Pu (步 "Chin-pu") - Forward step.

(Metal) or "Advancement". One of the key steps if not the key step
of T'ai Chi Ch'uan, Chin Pu should not be taken too literally though.
Advancing steps coordinate with the rest of the body actions and
stepping should be by correct heel-and-toe method.

Sometimes this technique is referred to as "advance and look" which
implies that care should be taken in choosing one's moment, but
also in being aware of the yin and the yang and being prepared for
withdrawal too.

(10) T'ui Pu (進步 "To-ey bu") - Backward step or "leeway", "room to
manoeuvre" (Wood). In most styles of T'ai Chi Ch'uan the player is
taught to step back on the ball-of-foot and toes. In T'ien Ti Tao we
encourage heel first, if possible. Stability is essential when moving
backwards and the "room to manoeuvre" should always be
remembered.

(11) Tsuo Ku (左顧 "Tsuar Ku") - Step Left (Water). Although this is
usually associated with "Single Whip" it is more accurately almost
any technique performed to the left or with the left leg.

 (12) You p'an (右盼 "You pan") - Step Right (Fire). There is a
similarity to Step Left, but here is the "Song of Look-Right" from the
"Yang Family Manuscripts," Edited by Li Ying-ang ('T'ai-chi
Touchstones: Yang Family Secret Transmissions.' 1983, p. 37.)
"Feigning to the left, we attack to the right with perfect Steps.
Sticking left and attacking right, we follow the opportunities. We
avoid the frontal and advance from the side, seizing changing

214

conditions. Left and right, full and empty, our technique must be faultless."

(13) Chung Ting (中定 "Zhong Ding" also like "John Ding";) - The central position, middle (Earth). Seen clearly in the technique of "Turn the Great Wheel", Chung Ting is to become like a post that is deeply rooted into the ground. It is also more than that. In "Golden Cock" it is essential that this principle is understood, otherwise the method as well as the moment may be lost. Chung Ting, represents not just the physical centre, but a condition which is expected to be present at all times in the first four steps as well, associated with the concept of "earthing" or "rooting" and is symbolic of the correct posture gained from correct T'ai Chi Ch'uan training)

T'ai Chi Ch'uan Stances.

Ma Bu ("Mabu" Riding Horse)

Mabu is often used as a transitional stance or for stability and lowering the Tan T'ien. The knees should always be over the feet to avoid injuries or weakness. The name, Riding Horse, comes from the way that you lower your weight, with feet wide apart, as though sitting on horseback. There can also be some rising and falling motion, as there might be when riding a horse which is trotting; of more use in training but in combat the weight needs to be controlled and stable.

Zou Pan Bu (Crossed-leg Stance)

Different to Scissor Stance, this step enables you to either make space - sideways - or do an 1800 turn by pivoting.

Miao Bu (Cat Stance)

Sometimes called "False Leg Stance", the Cat step enables you to make space or avoid by withdrawing the weight onto the rear leg, or by stepping, and leave the front leg empty for kicking or trapping.

Si Liu Bu (Sixty-Forty Stance)

This is common in all styles of Taijiquan but is one that needs careful monitoring by one's instructor, otherwise injury could occur. In Yang Style this is used in 'Repulse Monkey' whereas in Jingquanshi it is in 'Comb the Wild Hose's Maine'.

Gong Jian Bu (Bow and Arrow Stance.

Another version of this is Mountain Climbing Stance or Dragon Stance. They are all very similar and used for a similar purpose. Be aware of the positions of the lead foot and knee. Correct guidance is necessary.

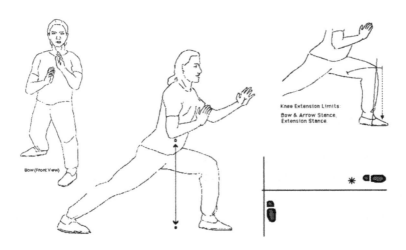

Knee Extension Limits:
Bow & Arrow Stance.
Extension Stance

Bow (Front View)

Jin Gi Du Li Bu (Golden Rooster Stance)

Also known as Golden Cockerel or Golden Cock Stands on One Leg, this is a useful stance but must done correctly or used in the right context. In Jingquanshi it is found early in the Form as an end to one technique and prelude to another.

Jian Dao (Scissor Stance)

It is important that you understand the use of stances and this one is no exception. Scissor Stance is no good if done incorrectly, so pay attention to what your teacher says and shows you. This is a useful stance and can be subtle and powerful in effect.

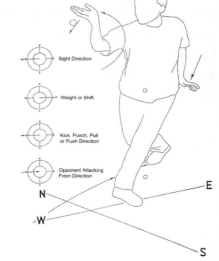

Other stances that may be used are Snake Stance, Crane Stance, Monkey Stance and Dog Stance and of course Eagle Stance, to name a few. There are many "stances" in Kung Fu but their meanings and uses may seem obscure unless you have good instruction. Their names may seem to be misleading, but this is again because of the difficulty of translating Chinese into English; for example, Alligator Stance may actually be a technique rather than a stance or posture; the "stance" is only representative of one position in a sequence or Form. The use of stances in Taijiquan is synonymous with Form, if we think of "shape" as being the appearance.

Your teacher will show you how the stances work both physically and in coordination with other principles. Do not be in a hurry to get past these in order to learn the whole Form, just for the sake of feeling good or looking as though you have completed it; you never will complete anything! Spend as much time on stances as anything else and some of the secrets will be revealed to you. Remember, there is no substitute for a well-grounded teacher who knows his or her subject.

Another very important aspect is that of weight transfer and foot pivoting. Unless the student correctly pivots on the heel, ball-of-foot or even the whole foot, then he or she may suffer twisted or sprained ligaments. Paying attention to the Yin and Yang again is crucial. Listen to your feet!

Follow the advice below to gain more from your practice:

- head and body should mostly be held upright and relaxed.
- bend your knees, not your back, generally.
- seriously enjoy your study, do not compete; abandon ego.
- the mouth should be closed with the tongue touching upper palate, breathing through the nose.
- when you breath in expand your lower abdomen, not your chest. Breath in for Yin movements (gathering in) and out for Yang movements (pushing out).
- do not push your chest out but keep it relaxed.
- Shoulders and elbows should relax and sink downwards.
- elbows and knees become weak if fully bent, never fully straighten them either.
- hands should be relaxed with small spaces between the fingers, palm cupped slightly.
- avoid a stiff body (Song). Body movements spring from a flexible waist (Song) (Song means to relax and open the joints, loosen the waist, etc.)
- your body movements are preceded by, and reflect directly your mental confidence, will, and intention. Train your

218

imagination for positive will power and confidence rather than your external physical strength.

- seek calmness in movement and do not let your attention wander.
- practice the Forms in a relaxed and unhurried manner with continuous flowing movements originating as responses to your mental images.

What you practice is what you will become. Taoist Kung fu and Taijiquan help to improve confidence as well as gaining better health, longer life and better ability in self- defence. The more you put in, the more you get out. Nothing comes easy or free in life except illness, decay and troubles.

The Treatise of T'ai Chi Ch'uan.

The Chinese language used to be very poetic, especially when used by scholars. They saw the Universe as a flowing event and sought to write in such a way as to echo the flows and rhythms of life. Hence, when it came to writing about the most intellectual and favoured pastime of many scholars, they would use verse or song to get the message across.

SONGS OF THE THIRTEEN POSTURES

(Originally Attributed to T'an Meng-hsien)

The thirteen postures should not be taken too lightly; the source of the postures lies in the waist.

Be mindful of the insubstantial and substantial changes; the ch'i spreads throughout without hindrance.

Being still, when attacked by the opponent, be tranquil and move in stillness; changes caused by the opponent fill him with wonder.

Study the function of each posture carefully and with deliberation; to achieve the goal is very easy.

Pay attention to the waist at all times;
Completely relax the abdomen and the qi (breath) will raise up.

When the coccyx is straight, the Shen (spirit) goes through the crown of the head.

To make the whole body light and agile suspend the head as though from above.

Carefully study.

Expansion and contraction, opening and closing, should be natural. To enter the door and be shown the way, you must be orally taught.

The practice is uninterrupted, and the technique is achieved by self-study. Speaking of the body and its function, what is the standard?

The I (mind) and ch'i (energy) are king, and the bones and muscles are the court.

Think over carefully what the final purpose is: to lengthen life and maintain youth.

The Song consists of 140 Chinese characters; each character is true and the meaning is complete so all you need to do is study. If you do not study in this manner, then you will waste your time. T'ai Chi Ch'uan students should think about the meanings of these verses and always keep them in mind when practising.

Pa Kua in Practice.

The Pa Kua or Bagua are an important part of Chinese philosophy and play a key role in Feng Shui, the Art of Divination. In Chinese philosophy there is a belief that no relationship can exist between two elements without the existence of a third element which then neutralizes the two elements. The third element not only comes under the influences of the two linked elements, but is also essential to the maintenance of the relationship between the two elements. This is seen in TCM where we have the body, the mind and the qi and one cannot exist without the other.

Tiandidao Taijiquan includes Sung Style *variation* for health routine; T'ai Chi for Health.

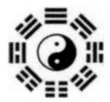 SOUTH: Heaven (Qian or Tian), P'eng; Energy like the bounce off of a beach ball. Ward Off, Roll Back, Embrace the Tiger and Return to Mountain, Roll The Boulder, Too Lazy to Tie the Coat.

Southwest: (Chai or Cai), Wood; Energy like plucking an apple. Wind/Sun. Pull down, Needle at Sea Bottom, Yin-Yang Palms, Temple Dragon (Pt.1), Sweep The Leaves off Mount Hua (Pt.2), Binding The Ox.

West (Jai or Ji). Water. Energy to adhere, deflect and counter as one. Press forwards, Brush Knee, Repulse Monkey, Elbow-lock and throw, Single Whip, Press-punch, Press and Push.

Northwest: (Kau or Kao), Mountain; Energy of look right, fake left and using the whole body to store and deliver. Shoulder Press, Deflect, parry and punch, Old Ch'eung Packs and Leaves for Wudang, Single Whip (end).

North: (Lu or Lei), Earth and Centre; Energy is sideways force, off-balancing, Roll-back, Pull, Search Clouds, Turn The Great Wheel, Cloud Hands, Play The Lute, Hsing-I Punch & Block, Black Crow.

Northeast: (Lit or Lie) Thunder; Energy of Splitting. Sit Back, Bend Back, Brush Wild Horse's Tail, Slantwise Flying, White Crane Flaps Wings, Sweep Leaves off Mt. Hua (Pt.1), Cat Grasps Bird's Tail.

East: (On or An) Fire; Downwards pressing energy. Push to Uproot, Deflect and Punch

Down, Tiger Mouth or Sleepy Tiger, Sweep Leaves (press), Repulse Monkey (low).

Southeast: (Jau or Zhou), Lake, Water; Energy chopping fist, elbow, rolling-back fist. Gather Universal Energies, Fold The Cloth, Step Back and Separate.

The above list is by no means comprehensive, not even for Jingquanshitaijiquan or Sun Style Variation for health. Some techniques contain more than one element and may even contain more than three, so to name individual parts is left to the discerning student in his or her studies. It is useful to understand the Bagua in relation to Taijiquan and it can come into one's training at various stages.

Tui Shou

Utilising the various elements of T'ai Chi Ch'uan is more of an essential principle rather than a luxury or extension. The detailed training is so complex to teach that a book cannot do it justice; hence another reason why not everything is covered in this humble

222

book. One aspect that we like to concentrate on in both Jingquanshitaijiquan and T'ai Chi for Health is I Fou Shou.

The basics have to be learned first; not necessarily explained in depth or great detail, but "experienced" by the beginner so that they can begin to build their knowledge and skill base. The concepts of P'eng, Lu, Chi and An form the foundations of Tui Shou and the teacher will explain how these link and function. Once this is done then the practice can be taken from solo to duel format and the student will experience a whole new level of perception.

There are four things you must remember when practising this technique:

1. Proper placement of the foot so as to aid balance and allow correct use of the waist.

2. Relaxing the waist and mind so as to enable "listening".

3. Learning to "feel" your partner's energy and differentiate between substantial, insubstantial, withdraw or attack, empty and full, etcetera.

4. Learning to control your own energy and refine it.

Generally the exercise is done by stepping out with the lead foot at a 45° angle to your centre line and base line. We say 45° but in reality the foot is likely to be between 45° and 65° marks. The toes are essentially pointed "inwards" so as to give maximum stability to the stance; often known as Dragon Stance (Loong Pu). There are variations to the Tui Shou theme, but we use the same as my Old Master taught us when learning Lee/Li Style T'ai Chi Ch'uan. This is 'I Fou Shou' and uses much more sensitivity.

In the first stage of this exercise you will be in a single stance and remain in it, save for changing from left to right occasionally, or vice-versa. In later variations more difficult tasks are added and you will experience feelings of "being like a beginner again" until you settle into it. Pass the first few levels though and you will see your practice open up like a Peony, with many beautiful folds and petals!

Amongst the general things to be aware of are keeping the ch'i centred at the Tan T'ien, staying calm and centred at all times, breathing naturally but in rhythm, learning to distinguish between empty and full, not locking the knees, maintaining your level, using circular movements which at times might intercept balance points, use hand or elbow and not both at once, and remember that the waist moves the arms, not the other way around! These are just a few pointers that your instructor will explain along the way.

Higher Level.

In higher levels the student may go on to learn how to use the body more effectively, like in Adhering Hands, but striking with various body parts, advanced control of the ch'i using Taijiquan weapons fluently and much more. This is one of the things that I truly love about T'ai Chi Ch'uan, it is as deep as the deepest ocean and as wide as all the oceans combined with a rich source of vast discoveries that go on and on and on throughout your life (lives?)

The Psychology of T'ai Chi Ch'uan.

In Taijiquan we use the image of Wuji, Taiji and Dao throughout the Forms. Not just the drawn image but the mental image and what it means. The philosophy of Dao uses these symbols to teach basic principles of Nature and Nature's "laws" as if by magic. Years of study help to channel thinking and within time life, like the Form, can become clearer and more "easy to do"; again this relies upon your surroundings and other people, it is impossible to avoid the negative aspects of human culture all the time. The law of the Universe is the only law. These laws are governed by the Supreme

Ultimate (Tao) and cannot be changed or excluded. In using these symbols to understand we learn and become more in tune with Nature.

Any person who has practised T'ai chi Ch'uan for ten to twenty years will tell you that it has an effect on the mind, a good effect. It can calm the mind that's troubled by anxieties, improve clarity of thought, help thoughts to flow by taking on the likeness of Wu Wei and allowing relaxed mind, just like the Form is relaxed and flows naturally. The many side-effects of health, both mentally and physically are too many to be discussed in detail.

T'ai Chi Ch'uan is the most popular exercise in the world, bar none. There is a very good reason for this. Many people have dabbled with T'ai Chi Ch'uan in some way or another, whether in a T'ai Chi for Health class, some off-shoot like Shibashi, or starting to learn a traditional Form. Sadly a large percentage of Westerners drop out at an early stage and fail to see the real benefits. Lack of patience, lack of ability to see ahead or "project" their lives; ironically some of these people can create a Business Projection but cannot create a Life Projection for themselves! T'ai Chi Ch'uan is a long term study and achievement. Some people may be put off by this. Why? There is no reason there to put anyone off, nothing at all. It is a folly of the imagination, fear, lack of perception and more. Why worry about how long the future training takes when you can enjoy it now? Yes, T'ai Chi Ch'uan is something that from day one you can enjoy and benefit from, so why worry about that which you do not know and cannot see? It is the "here and now" that is important and taking up T'ai Chi Ch'uan is dealing with the here and now. The future will unravel year by year, month by month, week by week, day by day, hour by hour, but all you need to do is carry on enjoying your T'ai Chi Ch'uan for it too will unravel day by day and improvements will come surely and slowly; the way that benefits most positively.

The TAO of T'ai Chi Ch'uan

The philosophy of Tao is expressed in many ways throughout life, Martial Arts, Traditional Chinese Medicine and more besides.

Most people have either seen a Yin/Yang symbol or at least heard of the basic Yin and Yang theory. Many may take this as being the core of the philosophy. It is not, it is the outcome. The physical and mental practices of T'ai Chi Ch'uan are the living embodiment of the Taoist philosophy and we can understand more about life, the Universe and everything from the practice of this wonderful Taoist Boxing Art; I use the term "wonderful" as it is meant and as T'ai Chi Ch'uan is, "full of wonder"! As mighty as the pen is it is not capable of describing the feelings and experiences of long term practice of T'ai Chi Ch'uan, not even in a large book. T'ai Chi Ch'uan is personal, like the feelings extreme grief and extreme joy, they have an extra effect on the body as well as the mind, you can feel it, and others cannot.

Wellspring T'ai Chi Ch'uan attempts to communicate with the original concepts and principles (Tao). It does not attempt to emulate or copy any other style or system, even the movements that honour Li and Sun are performed in a natural way and do not attempt to emulate closely. The principles within the 24 Forms are basic, yet they reflect all of the "essential" principles of T'ai Chi Ch'uan. The 24 Form is performed in a completely natural manner, expressing the essential elements of Tao as one would in a fighting situation. For example, Turning the Great Wheel is an Earth Element (Centre or North) technique, yet it is performed to the East (Li - Fire). It is still "centred" as there is no movement other than from the Tan T'ien upwards, absorbing the attack through loose arms (a Yin condition). While most styles of Taoist Boxing follow a linear footwork pattern Ching-chuan follows a Compass pattern; eight directions leading out from a central point, like an Asterisk or a ship's wheel (☼). Ching-chuan Forms, like life, are not predictable if taken from the perspective of a flowing Form, or Linked Forms, as it is usually known.

The only thing in life (Tao) which is predictable is change. If all Taoist Boxing Forms or Styles were to follow a pattern true to Tao, then they would all look virtually the same*, following the patterns of the Pa Kua and the I-Ching; elbow to south-east, or performing "splitting" to the north-east, shoulder press to the north-west, et cetera. The Ching- chuan Forms use change as a key factor, there are no intellectualised changes, just natural changes which may reflect also the patterns of attack and defence; e.g. if one is facing east using a Crane Kick and an attacker comes in from the south-east, he may see that the sides of the defender's body are unprotected and attack the right flank, thus a right-handed ward-off and roll back to the north may be appropriate. There is also a predilection for the movements of the Snake and Crane in Wellspring T'ai Chi Ch'uan, the two creatures which purportedly spurred Ch'eung Sam Feng into the creation of his new style of T'ai Chi Ch'uan, or whatever it was called at that time. Wellspring is only a short Form but contains much of the Snake and Crane's movements and essence. It attempts, like much of T'ien Ti Tao's outlook, to return to the original source and reflect the Great Principle. It is unique in this respect.

*This is Nature's Way, just as trees look different, animals look different and people are different shapes, colours and sizes.

'Snake winds around a branch'

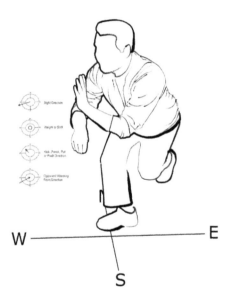

228

Chapter Eight

WELLSPRING T'AI CHI CH'UAN:
The ('40 Step') 24 Forms illustrated

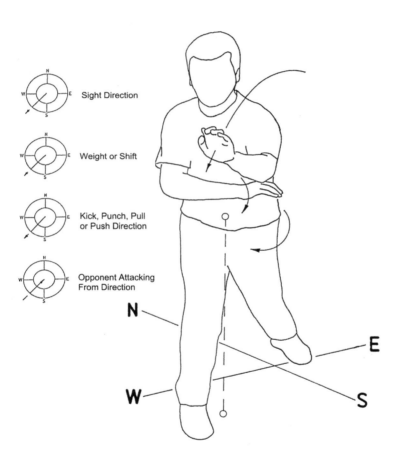

POEM OF T'AI CHI CH'UAN

Like a piston the diaphragm moves,
The breath below the waistline goes.
Ch'i will sink like mud in a pool,
To form the lining of the soul.
With spine erect like young bamboo;
To flex, support, give health to you
Slowly move both body and mind,
Aware of space but not of time.
Never lock the elbows or knees,
Float like down upon the breeze,
Plant your roots sure and deep;
Above the pelvis your head must keep.
Exercise hard and practice soft,
Remember, keep your crown aloft
Flow like water from mountain stream,
The Yin and Yang remain Supreme.

Readers Note:

Some of the foot positions or angles may not look entirely accurate due to the "flat" nature of 1D line art illustrations. This illustrated guide serves as a rough guide and reminder for new students but can never be relied upon as a replacement for an instructor. Anyone attempting to learn from the book alone will make mistakes that will not be easily repaired and does so at their own risk of injury through attempting to learn without proper personal supervision and instruction.

DO NOT ATTEMPT TO LEARN THIS OR ANY COMPLEX FORM WITHOUT PROPER PERSONAL INSTRUCTION AS ERRORS CAN CAUSE HEALTH PROBLEMS OR INJURIES AS WELL AS LOOKING A FOOL IF YOU GET IT TOTALLY WRONG;

YOU CANNOT LEARN T'AI CHI CH'UAN FROM A BOOK OR VIDEO! Why? Because you need to be corrected and have reasons, postures and techniques explained.

T'ai Chi exercises are loosely based on three concepts; those that prepare the body for more exercise, those that prepare you for the Form, and those that develop a healthier body. In most of the exercises the same attitude and posture is required.

GENERAL GUIDELINES:

* Always maintain correct posture, walking or sitting.

* When standing and moving follow the "heel & Toe" principle.

* Develop Tan T'ien (Dantian) breathing as a natural way, but never force it.

* Perform all the movements as though "swimming in air".

* Centre your thoughts at the beginning and end of every session.

* Sink the elbows, shoulders and waist, tuck-in the pelvis and pullback your chin/raise top of head.

* Do not tightly clench the fists, keep the arms relaxed but firm.

* Concentrate on every movement, what it is and what it does.

* Aim to join every movement together to make one fluid Form.

* NEVER do ch'i Kung or T'ai Chi when you have a HIGH TEMPERATURE.

BEFORE YOU BEGIN EXERCISING:

There are at least three things that your instructor should know. For instance,

Have you any knee, spine or joint problems?

Have you any muscle, tendon or ligament injuries? Have you any Angina or other Heart problems?

Do you have any other health conditions?

If you are unsure, then a visit to your GP/Doctor should resolve the doubts. Tell him/her that you intend to take up T'ai Chi Ch'uan and affiliated health exercises. Most spine or back-muscle problems can be helped with T'ai Chi Ch'uan exercises. As the head is not twisted and the spine is held erect then this develops better posture and healthier muscles, etc.

Knees can be strengthened and tendons, muscles, arteries and nerves will become healthier and stronger. T'ai Chi Ch'uan also adjusts the cardiovascular rate to a better level, thus it is said that with all these beneficial side-effects and many more, T'ai Chi Ch'uan can prolong life.

Some have claimed that cancers and tumours or cancer growths have also been cleared by the frequent, daily practice of T'ai Chi Ch'uan and Chi Kung Breathing Therapy. The author himself would attest to this. These may sound like high claims but it has been documented and witnessed. Some Doctors of modern medicine n the western world, of course, may not be too hasty to accept anything else which they do not understand or cannot legally recommend. Many scientific and medical tests have been carried out throughout the eastern world though and there is little doubt that both T'ai Chi Ch'uan and Chi Kung are powerful medicines. The multi-million pound/dollar drug companies are likely to be most opposed to "free treatments" though.

There are many facets to the ancient Arts of this world that are invaluable to you and me. The only wisdom and method that we can trust is that which is tried and tested by the course of time - T'ai Chi Ch'uan is one of these, Ch'i Kung is another.

Pa Tuan Chin or Baduanjin is a wonderful complimentary exercise set for T'ai Chi Ch'uan. The "New (safer) Standardised Set" in particular has no movements which would conflict with the general principles of T'ai Chi Ch'uan, such as bending backwards. Used by itself it is a simple yet effective way of helping daily fitness and health. Used in combination with T'ai Chi Ch'uan it becomes a tremendous duo with ch'i building powers and glowing health attributes. You can find out more about this popular exercise in the accompanying linked series book "Qigong & Baduanjin" - ISBN-10:

0954293223 or ISBN-13: 978-0954293222. This book also details the very rare Seated Set which Shih-fu Symonds has revived and made more popular after extensive research and study.

Always wear comfortable COTTON clothing, nothing restrictive.

Choose an airy, light, dust and fume free place.

A garden, park or by a stream or seashore is ideal. Failing that a nice dust- free and uncluttered room would do. An open window and/or an Ioniser' will help to improve the atmosphere; most buildings absorb negative ions that are good for your health so an Ioniser will help replace them and make you feel better.

Early morning, midday and late evening are the best times, when the air is both clear and traffic fume free. Regular daily practice pays off. So be determined to continue once started.

Do not hurry or be hurried. Should you be outside, then concentrate on your movements, not those of others. If you are inside and you are disturbed by important callers (telephone/door), then cease SLOWLY and smile. Say to yourself, "I am unruffled, calm and receptive. I shall continue later, as though nothing had happened." Smile from your heart.

Follow these basic guidelines and you can benefit from Wellspring T'ai Chi Ch'uan and Pa T'uan Chin for the rest of your life.

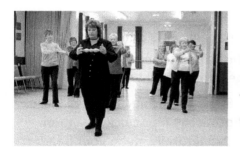

Pictured here are some of our "T'ai Chi for Health" group learning the T'ai Chi Ruler. This is a powerful exercise and one which is complimentary also for practice as it is in actual fact an "extension" exercise for developing the ch'i, concentration and strengthening the body in the same manner as T'ai Chi Ch'uan.

Ching-chuan T'ai Chi Ch'uan Form by itself is a good exercise, but it is not a complete exercise system. T'ai Chi's exercise values are more 'internal', that is to say they have beneficial effects on the internal organs, circulation, nerves and energy (ch'i). The majority of people taking up this type of exercise need their bodies 'tuned-up' a bit before they can 'feel comfortable' in their 'Form' practice. The following set of very simple exercises plus the Eight Strands of Silk Brocade (Pa T'uan Chin) are included to help you and your loved ones to the first two steps on the ladder to better health. Thus the head-to-toe warm-up exercises have been included to benefit everyone from the unfit to the fit (even the impatient!).

Head-to-Toe Warm-up.
Please do these exercises under the supervision of a competent instructor if you are fit enough to do them. Always start gently.

Fingers: Hold your hands out a little way in front of your chest. Wiggle your fingers powerfully, as though 'clawing'. (1 minute.)

Wrists: From the same position. Flex your wrists from side to side in

a large 'infinity' ∞ pattern. (1 minute.)

Shoulders: Rotate the shoulders forwards-up-and-back, then the other way. Breathe naturally. Repeat ten times each direction.

Neck: Gently turn the head left, centre, and then right. Exhale as you turn and inhale as you centre. Look down, and then look up. Two to three times each way.

Torso: Inhale. Relax and bend slowly to the side as you exhale. Inhale as you straighten. Repeat this five times each side. Do five slow forward bends, keep the spine straight and knees bent.

Hip Region: (Hip/Leg Joints, Lower Spine and Sciatic Nerves). Place the hands either side of the hips. Rotate the hips clockwise then anti-clockwise in large circles. Breathe naturally. Keep your head still. Ten times each way.

Upper Legs: (and balance) Stand on one foot and raise the other behind you, hold the raised foot and pull it up towards your buttocks. Keep a straight spine. Two to five times each leg.

Place the feet together, toes pointing out at 45°. Bend the knees and slowly exhale and stretch forwards as far as possible. Inhale as you straighten. Repeat two to five times.

Knees: Lower your weight and bend the knees, placing the hands upon them to keep the knees together. Rotate the knees clockwise then anti-clockwise, not too vigorously. Keep the back straight. Five to ten times each way.

Calf Muscles & Achilles: Stand on tip-toe, then lower. Rock back onto the heels, keeping the knees bent, then lower. Repeat ten times each way.

Ankles: Standing firmly on one foot with the knee flexed, then raise the free foot off the ground. Rotate the toes in a large circle, ten times clockwise, ten times anti- clockwise. Repeat with the other foot. This stretches and strengthens ankle ligaments.

Shake out: Shake the arms, then each leg, really loosely to finish.

Stand quietly for a moment.

Centre your ch'i at the Tan T'ien.

Form Guides.

The author has developed special symbols to help the student remember the important points of each posture (Form). These are in the simple shape of a circle, which represents a compass face (see diagram below). The first or upper image shows which way you should be looking, but not necessarily turning the head; the direction of sight is generally the same direction we face.

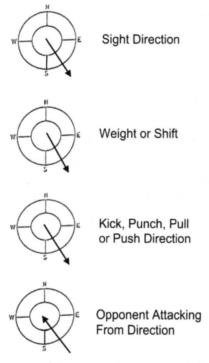

Sight Direction

Weight or Shift

Kick, Punch, Pull or Push Direction

Opponent Attacking From Direction

The second image down tells you which direction the body weight is shifting to.

The third image down tells you which way you are operating, a kick, punch, elbow or pull, for example.

Finally we have the direction from which the opponent would be attacking us from.

Together these symbols give you some of the most important information regarding each posture or Form.

Just in case you are confused about the term "Form" and how it is used herein, the word can mean an individual posture or it can refer to the whole "set" as a Form. This derives from original Chinese meanings as in Traditional Chinese one calligraphic character might mean various things according to the context of the sentence in which it appears.

The Form.
(Illustrated)

Preparation and Gentle Breeze: Stand in 'Eagle Stance', heels together, toes pointing out naturally. The eyes are "gazing at the horizon", Qi centred at the Tan T'ien/Dantian and the body "rooted". This is the "Wuji" posture and is an important first step in getting the Form right and attaining the right results.

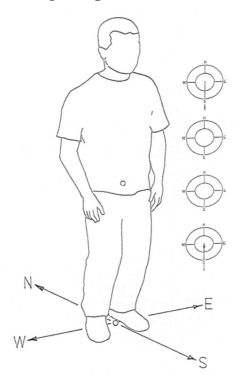

The posture should be correct. Make sure that your shoulders are relaxed so that there is a slight "hollow" just above and in front of the armpits. The Ba Hui is held aloft without pulling in the chin unnaturally. Relax the neck, jaw and tongue as well as the arms and shoulders.

Bend the knees slightly, as though someone has just poked the back of your knee, letting you "Earth". Allow the body to be balanced will alleviate any stress and help calm the mind. There should be a small space beneath the armpits. The Qi will settle and you can then attain Wuji. As said before, this preparation is important so take your time and practice it as much as possible before moving off to the next posture. All postures should be natural and relaxed; not floppy.

Form 1:

Transfer your weight to the right foot, step out a small pace to the East (Bear Stance). Raise your palms up to belt-level, fingertips touching, as you settle your weight down 50% - 50%.Turn the hands over.

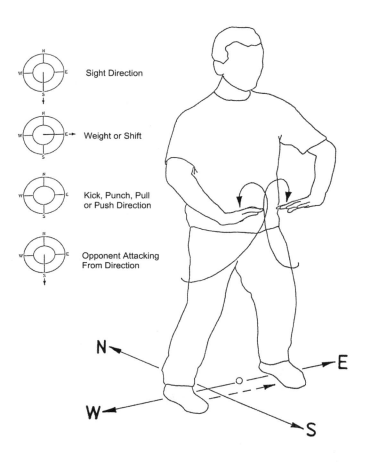

Sight Direction

Weight or Shift

Kick, Punch, Pull or Push Direction

Opponent Attacking From Direction

Form 2: Gathering the Energies:

Slowly scoop both hands out-and-upwards until at head height.
Then bring the elbows in towards the waist. Do not crease the neck.
Gaze ahead.

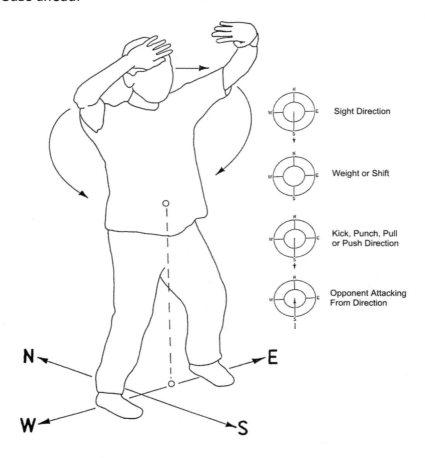

Sight Direction

Weight or Shift

Kick, Punch, Pull
or Push Direction

Opponent Attacking
From Direction

The dotted line and small circles show where the Centre of Gravity
(CoG) should be.

Form 3: Roll The Ball:

Transfer the weight to the right foot and step straight ahead with the left foot. As you sink your weight to your left foot, extend the fingertips forwards at shoulder level (Tongue). Look between the finger-tips of the left and right hand.

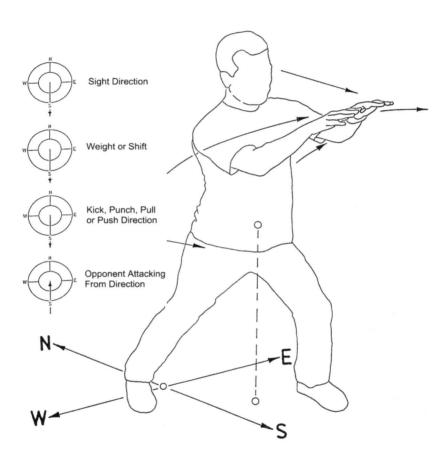

4: Cloud-hand West & Kick:

Lower the elbows. Transfer the weight to the left foot. Step up and right to form an "L" shaped stance. As you transfer weight to the right leg, perform a Right Cloud-hand deflection. Allow the hips to "sink" and keep the waist relaxed.

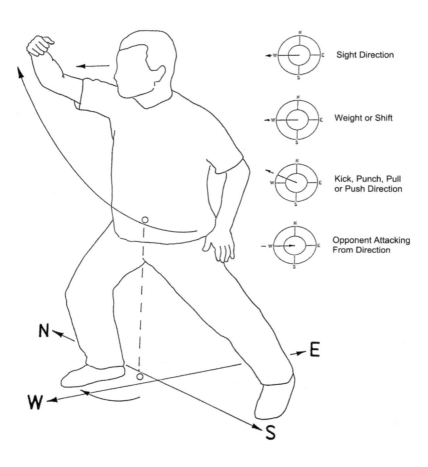

Sight Direction

Weight or Shift

Kick, Punch, Pull or Push Direction

Opponent Attacking From Direction

Golden Cock:

Raise the left leg and perform a right-footed kick; this completes Cloud Hand West & Kick. Then fold the right leg into 'Golden Cock Stands on One Leg' style. Root the weight down your right leg as you sweep the left knee back to the South.

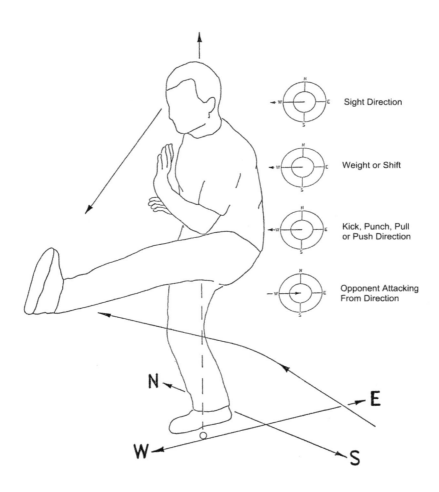

Sight Direction

Weight or Shift

Kick, Punch, Pull
or Push Direction

Opponent Attacking
From Direction

Yin-Yang Palm 1:

Step the foot down and slightly outwards (South-East) to where it came from, to replace it to its original position during 'Rolling the Boulder'. Raise the left arm in Cloud-hand and perform left Yin-Yang Palm.

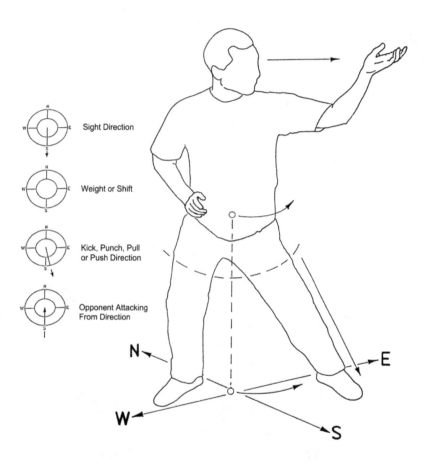

Sight Direction

Weight or Shift

Kick, Punch, Pull or Push Direction

Opponent Attacking From Direction

Yin - Yang Palms 2:

Sink the left palm to the left hip as you transfer weight and step through to face East. As you pull to the left hip, the right hand follows through with a 'Sun Palm' to shoulder height. Continue to turn fully to the left then begin to transfer your weight to the right leg for the next technique.

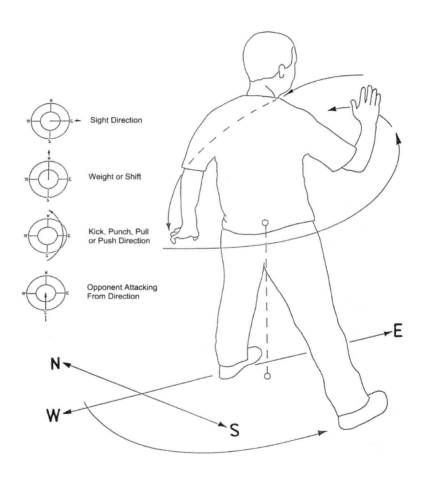

Sight Direction

Weight or Shift

Kick, Punch, Pull or Push Direction

Opponent Attacking From Direction

N

W

S

E

Sun Palm & Dog Kick:

Perform Yin-Yang Palm with the left hand, bringing it down to left hip-level as you transfer the weight back to the left leg. The right hand performs the shortened version of this, as the right leg is primed. Execute a right Heaven Palm and a right Dog Kick simultaneously.

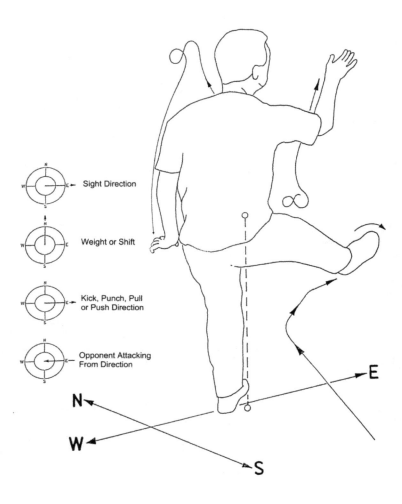

Sight Direction

Weight or Shift

Kick, Punch, Pull
or Push Direction

Opponent Attacking
From Direction

N

W

S

E

Step Down Knock-kneed with High Guard:

Step down with the right toes pointing to your left. Raise the right arm in High Guard and bring the left arm around in a Cloud Hand, as this is happening, sink and turn naturally to face north. The weight transfers to the right leg.

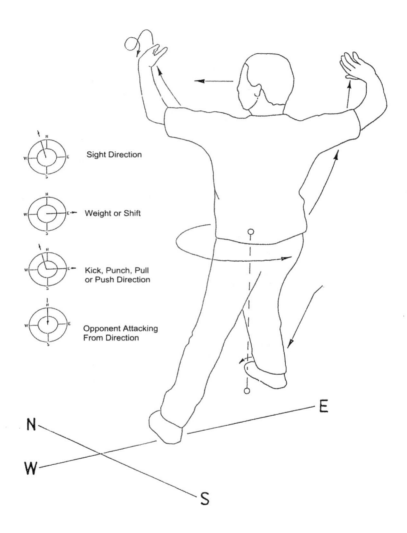

Sight Direction

Weight or Shift

Kick, Punch, Pull or Push Direction

Opponent Attacking From Direction

N

W

E

S

懶豹 - Lazy Leopard:

Perform Lazy Leopard. Keep the trunk upright (although inclined slightly in illustration) and look down nose. Weight is on the right leg. Note: illustration misrepresents posture!

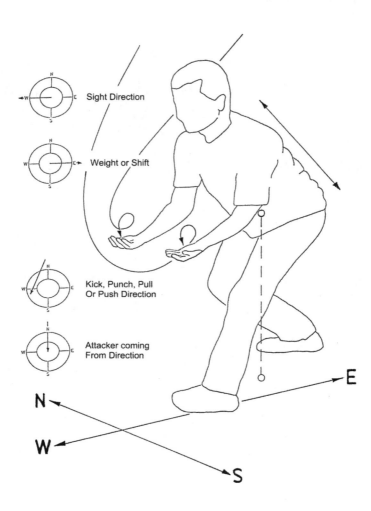

Turn The Wheel 1:

Move weight to the left leg whilst turning the torso clockwise to face east. The right hand rises to forehead level and the left stays by the abdomen. Perform the first rotation, clockwise, of Turn the Wheel. Your right foot forms Monkey Stance.

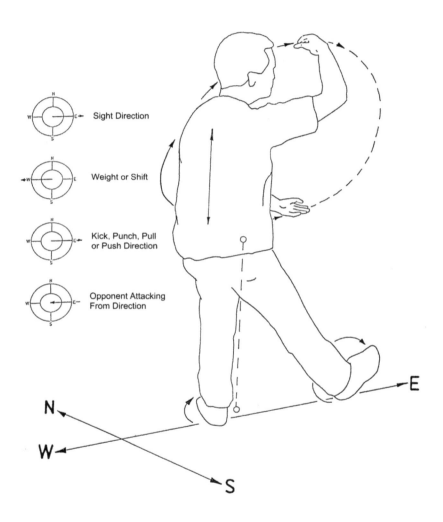

Sight Direction

Weight or Shift

Kick, Punch, Pull or Push Direction

Opponent Attacking From Direction

Turn The Wheel 2:

Turn 'the wheel' anti-clockwise. The arms must remain a constant distance from each other, as though turning a large wheel by the rim. The hands should be level with the forehead (Upper Dantian) and Lower Dantian forming a large circle.

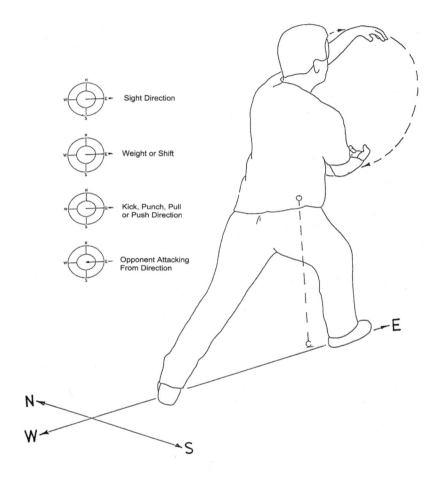

Sight Direction

Weight or Shift

Kick, Punch, Pull or Push Direction

Opponent Attacking From Direction

Once more, turn the arms clockwise. As you do so, step forwards and ESE into right Dragon Stance. Note: Illustration should depict space between feet!

White Crane Flaps Its Wings:

Raise the right hand up to form "folded wings". Spread the fingertips as you swing both hands down, outwards and up into, White Crane Spreads its Wings. As you do this, transfer your weight to the right leg, raise the left leg into a forward pointing Crane Kick.

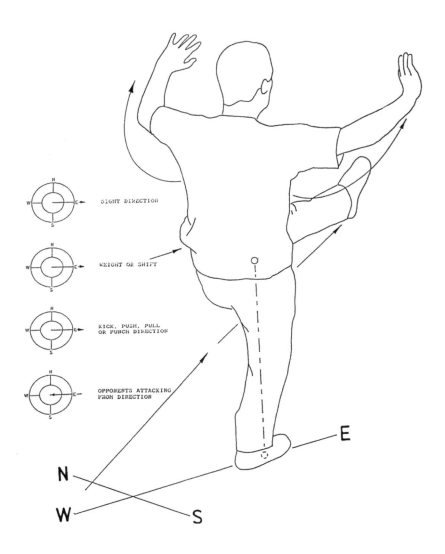

SIGHT DIRECTION

WEIGHT OR SHIFT

KICK, PUSH, PULL OR PUNCH DIRECTION

OPPONENTS ATTACKING FROM DIRECTION

Ward-Off: (15 to 17)

Eyes look right. Step down and left with the left foot. Swing the right palm down and in, lower the left elbow and let the right palm rest below it. Transfer your weight to Left Leopard Stance. (Illustration now viewed from the East)

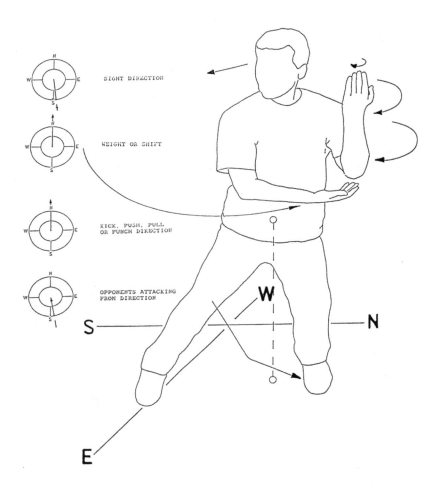

Roll Back, Ward Off: Step the right foot backwards through a quarter-circle. Transfer the weight to Right Leopard Stance as you swing your left hand down, right and in front of your right. Bring both hands up until the fingertips rest on the sides of the neck. (Viewed from South West)

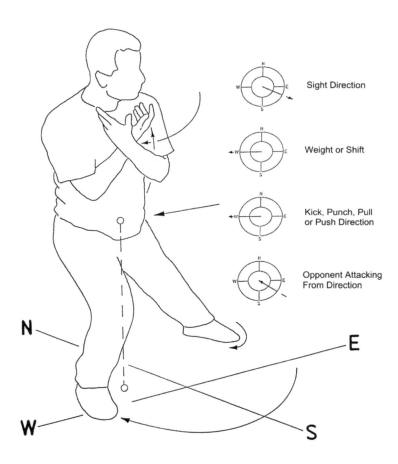

Sight Direction

Weight or Shift

Kick, Punch, Pull or Push Direction

Opponent Attacking From Direction

Continue through "Mud Wading Step" as you Press & Push.

Press & Push: Step forwards to the South-East into a Left Dragon Stance. As you do, bring the left forearm forwards and the fingers of the right forearm lightly to touch the inside-left forearm's surface. Follow through with a "Press". Sink into "Push" – shown here half-way between the two.

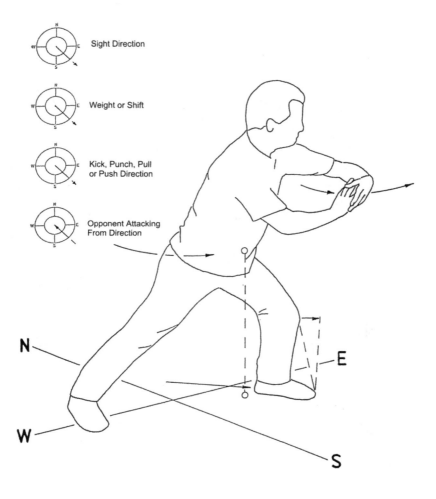

Sight Direction

Weight or Shift

Kick, Punch, Pull or Push Direction

Opponent Attacking From Direction

Note: Illustration exaggerates posture! Hips should be down and forwards and balance, harmony and triangulation achieved.

Cat Grasps the Bird:

Eyes look right. Drop back to 'Left Cat Stance'. Swing your left hand up as though beckoning someone. Swing your right hand up the opposite way, as though waving on someone to pass.

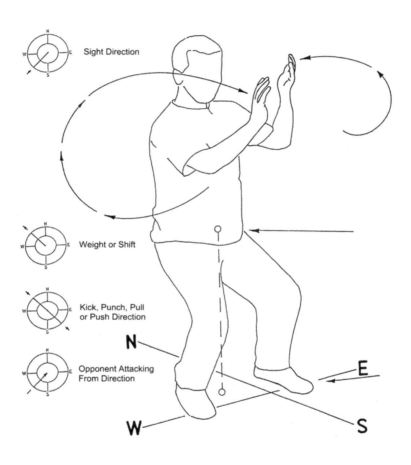

Sight Direction

Weight or Shift

Kick, Punch, Pull or Push Direction

Opponent Attacking From Direction

裁縫褶皺布 - Tailor Folds the Cloth 1:

Transfer your weight to your left foot. Step through South-West into Dragon Stance. Slightly lower the right palm. Bring the left palm over and down to chest height. Direction is south-west.

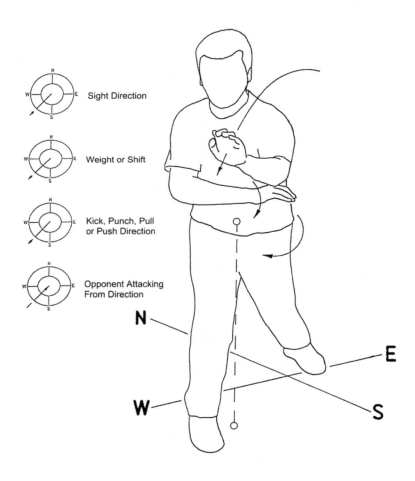

Sight Direction

Weight or Shift

Kick, Punch, Pull or Push Direction

Opponent Attacking From Direction

The weight is transferred mainly to the right foot as the technique is completed. Keep the shoulders and elbows down at all times.

Fold The Cloth 2:

Swing the weight towards the left foot. Pull the left elbow back. Make a 'Monkey Hook' with the right hand. Hook it from left side to right as you push off rear leg and swing-punch with left fist.

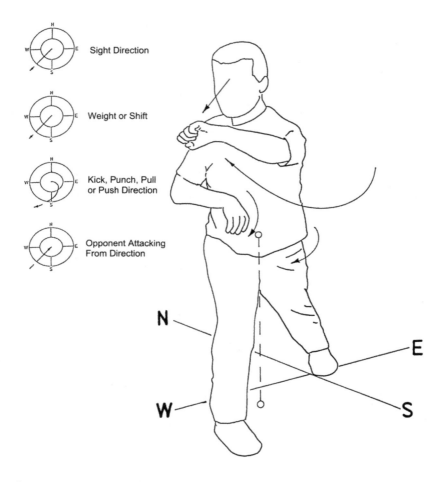

Sight Direction

Weight or Shift

Kick, Punch, Pull or Push Direction

Opponent Attacking From Direction

The arms are moved with the body, the body by the legs; initiate the movement from the roots and Dantian.

Step Back & Separate:

Transfer the weight back to the left foot and swing the right foot back to the East. Torso facing west, swing both hands up, over and inwards, backs of hands together and then down, as illustrated here.

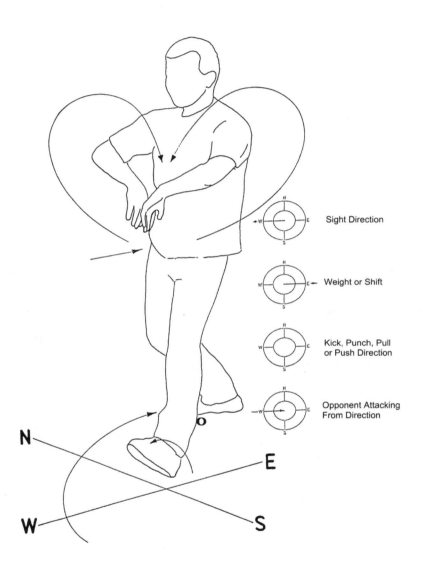

Sight Direction

Weight or Shift

Kick, Punch, Pull or Push Direction

Opponent Attacking From Direction

Push To Uproot:

Circle both hands outwards to shoulder height. Stepping forward with the left foot (Tongue), drive off the rear leg, sink and push.

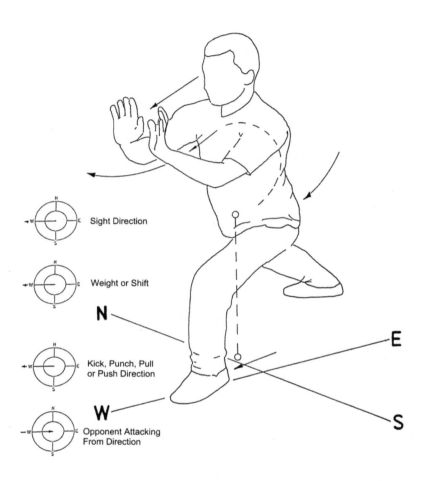

Sight Direction

Weight or Shift

Kick, Punch, Pull or Push Direction

Opponent Attacking From Direction

黑烏鴉 開翅膀 - Black Crow Spreads its Wings 1:

Bring the right foot up alongside the left (Sink & Root), rest the toes on the floor. Keep your weight low and balance the torso above the feet. Cross the arms, left in front of right, fingertips by the throat.

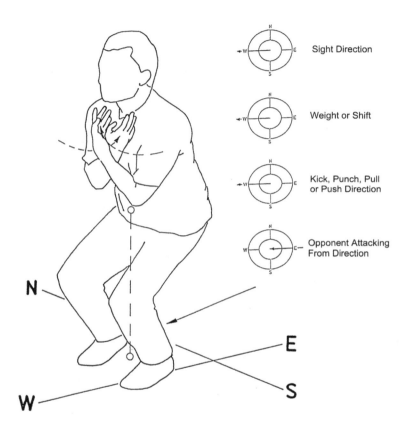

Sight Direction

Weight or Shift

Kick, Punch, Pull or Push Direction

Opponent Attacking From Direction

Black Crow Spreads its Wings 2:

Step right into Leopard Stance and look over the left shoulder at the floor behind you. Form a "twisted left Cat Stance", still keeping balanced and low. The heels should not be too close together (see below).

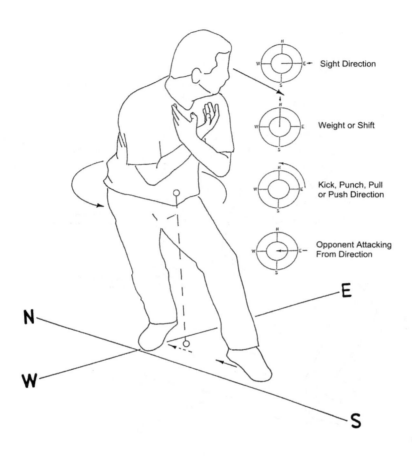

Sight Direction

Weight or Shift

Kick, Punch, Pull or Push Direction

Opponent Attacking From Direction

Black Crow Spreads its Wings 3:

Step the left foot through to the rear into 'Riding Horse Stance'. As you do so, crouch down. When your left foot is placed, then raise up strongly pushing out the elbows. This is 'Black Crow Spreads Its Wings'. Do not lean backwards. Look at left elbow.

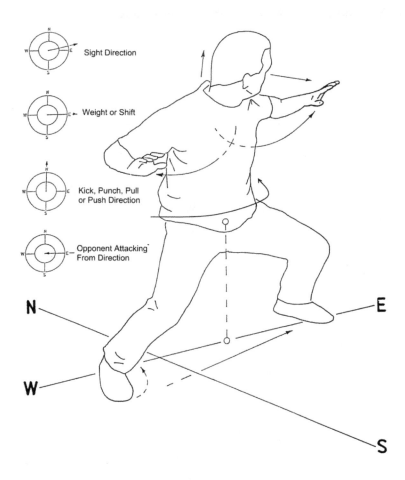

Sight Direction

Weight or Shift

Kick, Punch, Pull or Push Direction

Opponent Attacking From Direction

N

E

W

S

Again the reader is reminded that a two-dimensional graphic illustration is no comparison to having a three-dimensional instructor.

Temple Dragon Shows its Claws 1:

Look right. Transfer your weight to your left leg and step behind with the right foot into 'Scissor Stance'. At the same time perform a right Yin-Yang Palm. As you sink the right hand to your hip level...

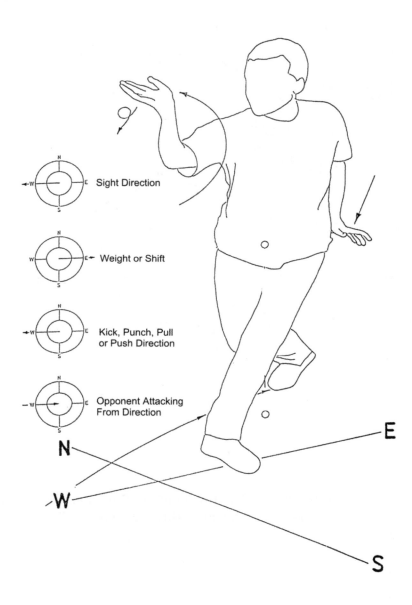

Sight Direction

Weight or Shift

Kick, Punch, Pull or Push Direction

Opponent Attacking From Direction

Pivot in your stance, clockwise, through Riding Horse Stance and continue to take your weight to the right. The left hand follows through naturally.

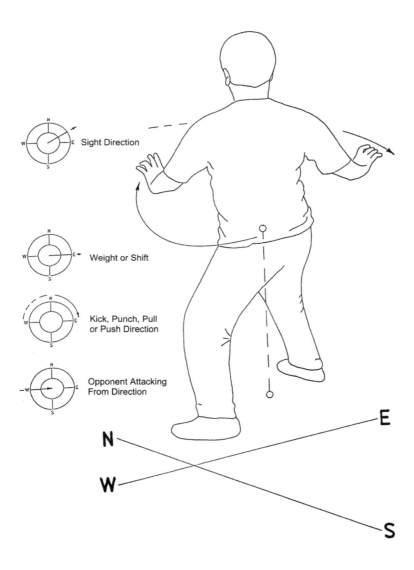

Sight Direction

Weight or Shift

Kick, Punch, Pull or Push Direction

Opponent Attacking From Direction

N

E

W

S

Temple Dragon 2:

Turn out the toes of the left foot anti-clockwise. Transfer your weight to the left leg and step the right foot through towards West into Riding Horse Stance. As you step, perform a wide 'Monkey Hook' with the left hand...

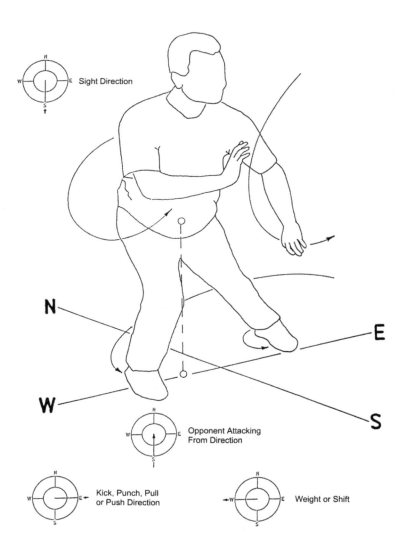

Sight Direction

N

E

W

S

Opponent Attacking From Direction

Kick, Punch, Pull or Push Direction

Weight or Shift

... Kick relaxed, but controlled, with the left toes at abdomen height, direction South-South-East. Do not lock-out the knee either in stance or as kicking.

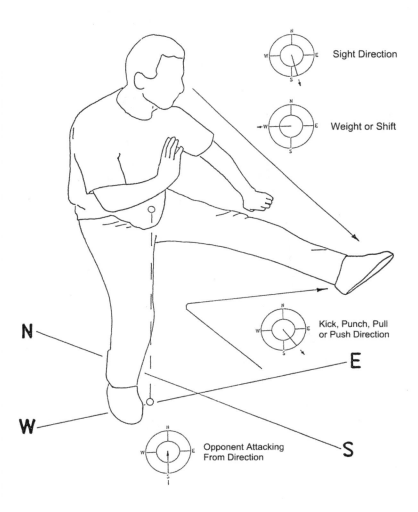

Sight Direction

Weight or Shift

Kick, Punch, Pull or Push Direction

N

E

W

S

Opponent Attacking From Direction

Note: There is a transition in graphic style on the next page due to a later batch by the artist who used a different technique.

Brush the Horses Maine: Step your left foot down and forward as you execute a double 'Metal Palm' Press.

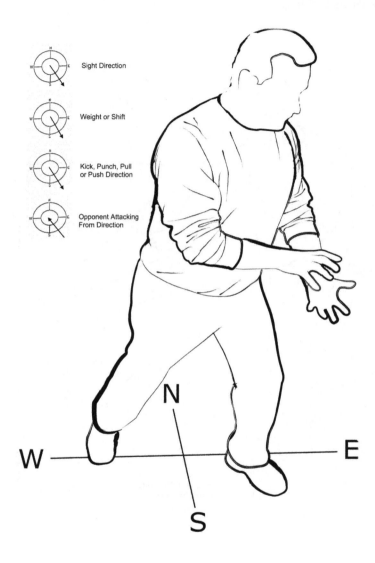

Sight Direction

Weight or Shift

Kick, Punch, Pull or Push Direction

Opponent Attacking From Direction

N

W —— E

S

Push from the front foot as you complete the move....

....and then step-up and step forwards with the right foot to complete the movement.

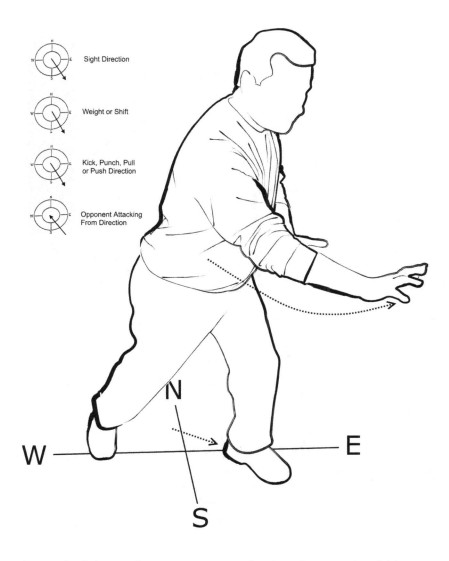

Sight Direction

Weight or Shift

Kick, Punch, Pull or Push Direction

Opponent Attacking From Direction

At the end of this technique your weight distribution should be approximately 60/40 towards the rear foot. Remember the transitory phases of Yin and Yang here and to allow foot movement and "gearing the force".

Triangle Stance: Pivot leftwards to face N.W. as you raise your left hand to neck height and settle into a three point posture.

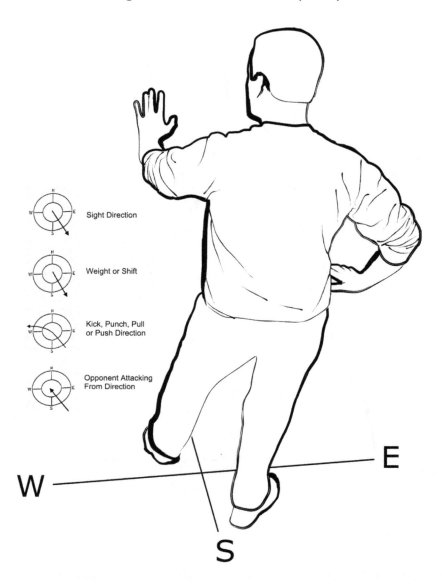

Sight Direction

Weight or Shift

Kick, Punch, Pull
or Push Direction

Opponent Attacking
From Direction

E

W

S

Step up with High Guard: Step up with the right foot and keep your left hand 'on the spot' as you thread your right arm through between left and body shooting the right hand up to head height with palm facing out at forehead level.

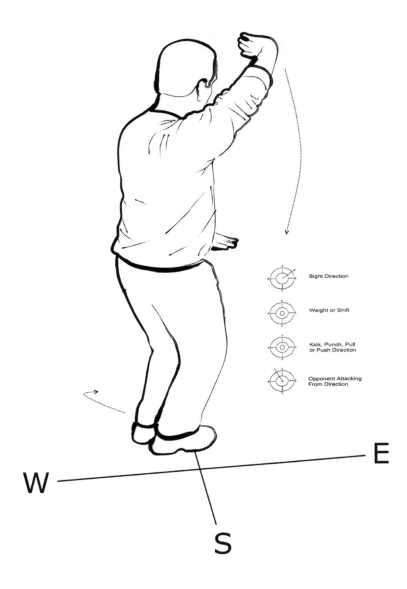

Sight Direction

Weight or Shift

Kick, Punch, Pull
or Push Direction

Opponent Attacking
From Direction

E

W

S

Single Whip: Bring your left foot forwards in a small clockwise arc and place it firmly down. Bring your right arm to the right as you execute a Single Whip.

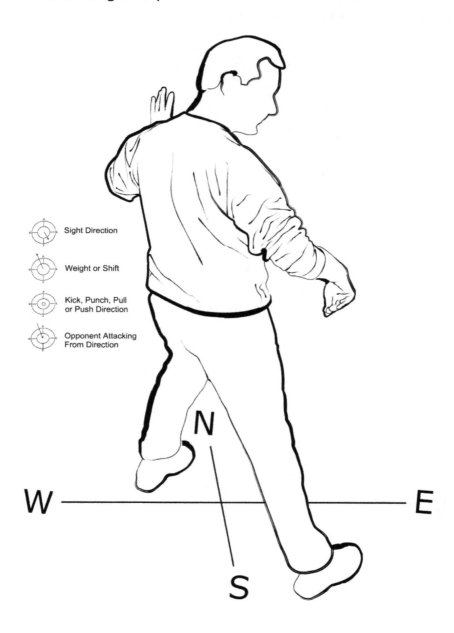

Sight Direction

Weight or Shift

Kick, Punch, Pull or Push Direction

Opponent Attacking From Direction

N

W —————————————————— E

S

(The "looking" has been emphasised here in this illustration. Keep neck as straight as possible in practice!)

Turn to S. West: Pivot your left foot leftwards and step around in a small anti-clockwise circle with your right. Bring your left hand up in a high block as you pivot your right foot anti-clockwise and transfer your weight to the right. Step out S.W. with your left foot as bring your weight forwards on to it and perform a Palm Strike at chest height.

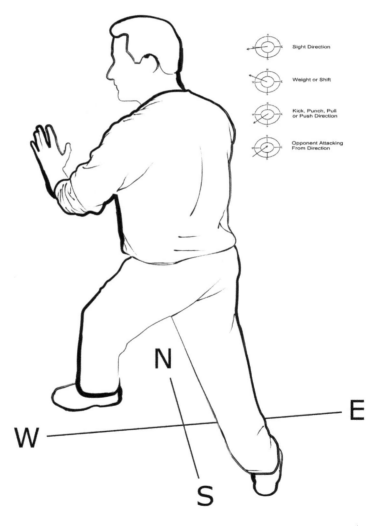

Continue to turn towards the SW and prepare for...

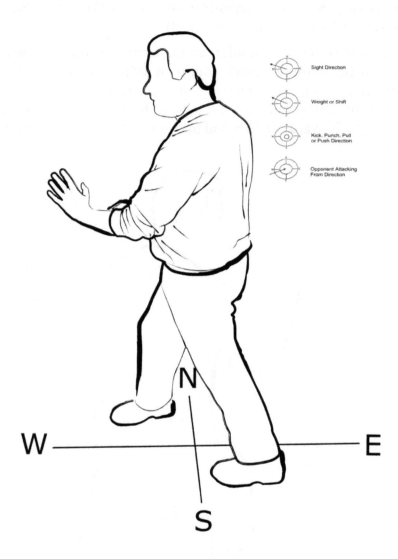

Sight Direction

Weight or Shift

Kick, Punch, Pull
or Push Direction

Opponent Attacking
From Direction

... Working the Shuttle. Remember the posture pointers that your Shih-fu has given you in this technique as well as the eye focus and internal aspects. Remember to keep your weight down and to focus correctly as you execute this technique. The artist's drawing is deceptive; do not raise the left hand too high and make sure that you also sink the shoulder.

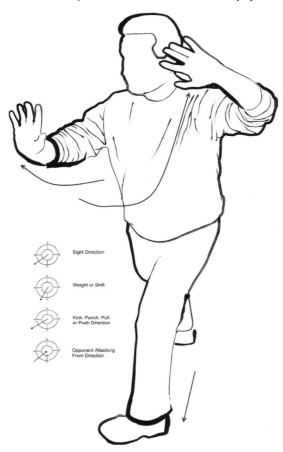

Sight Direction

Weight or Shift

Kick, Punch, Pull or Push Direction

Opponent Attacking From Direction

To those of you who have studied other styles of T'ai Chi Ch'uan, you may find this name somewhat familiar. In Yang Style, for example, there is a movement named Fair Lady Works the Shuttle. Our name is non-sexist but represents the same principle, one which is common in T'ai Chi Ch'uan in all of its many styles and forms.

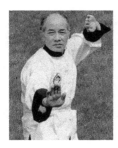

Here you can see Great-grandmaster C. C. Soo, my revered Taoist Arts Master, performing a technique called 'The Archer', which is very similar to 'Working the Shuttle' with a slight variation of lead-hand strike.

Play The Lute: Step back into Left Cat as you extend right palm. Step 45 degrees to the left-rear with your left foot, twisting to face east as you block with left hand. Step down and perform a Half-step as you deliver a right palm to chest height.

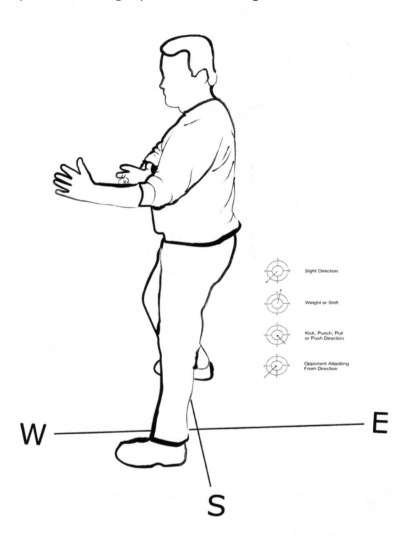

Sight Direction

Weight or Shift

Kick, Punch, Pull or Push Direction

Opponent Attacking From Direction

W ——————————————— E

S

Continue with Play the Lute Right style, including full Song and subtle waist movements.

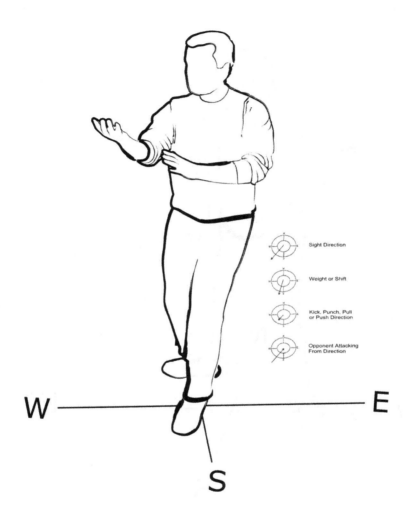

Sight Direction

Weight or Shift

Kick, Punch, Pull
or Push Direction

Opponent Attacking
From Direction

W —————————————— E

S

Brush Knee & Twisting Step:

Begin with your turning step and raise the right open palm to shoulder height, and then continue with the twisting step and "push".

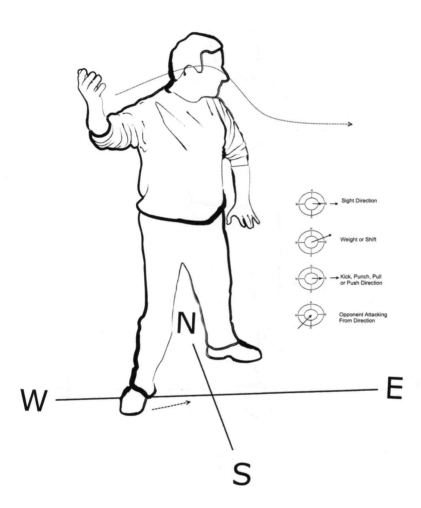

Sight Direction

Weight or Shift

Kick, Punch, Pull
or Push Direction

Opponent Attacking
From Direction

Continue the "push" as you prepare to shift weight forwards (image on left) and use "follow step" (illustration on right).

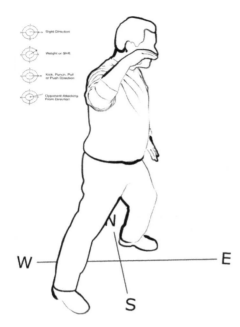

2: Move your left hand forward to cover palm-heel. Swing your right arm leftwards in a large clockwise circle and pull it back to the right waist.

Swinging the clasped hands from left to right as you move position, prepare to step towards the South-South-East.

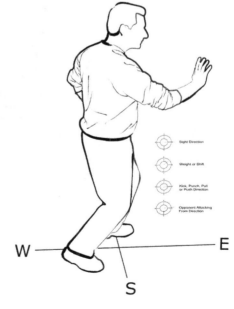

Block & Close Step:

Step back into Left Cat as you "Play the Lute". Step forwards with left foot as you perform this technique.

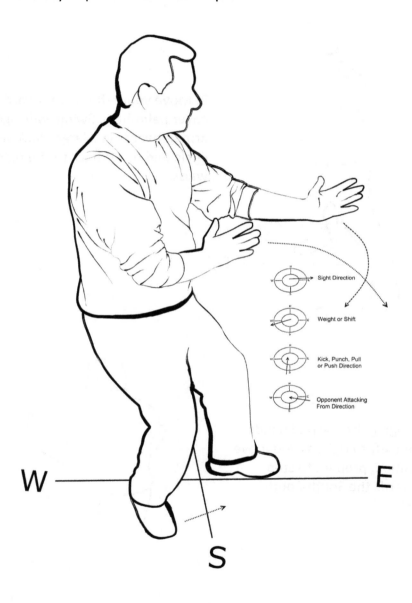

Sight Direction

Weight or Shift

Kick, Punch, Pull or Push Direction

Opponent Attacking From Direction

W ———————————— E

S

Parry & Punch.
Step up to close and simultaneously punch downwards with right fist in crouching stance.

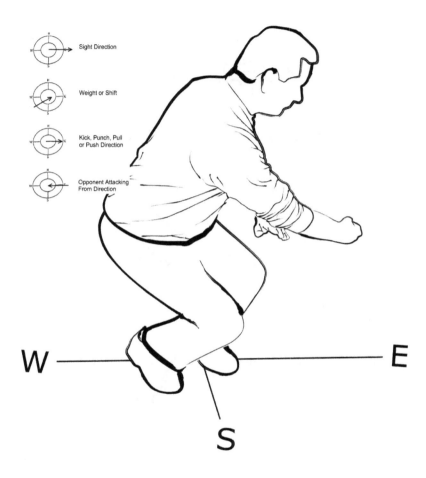

Please adhere to your teacher's advice about crouching or kneeling stances, step sizes and foot/knee/hip/shoulder/elbow positions.

秋 掃葉華山 - Sweep Autumn Leaves off Mount Hua 1:

From Left stance, pivot to your right to face S.E. and bring right hand around at waist level with left hand following to join elbow.

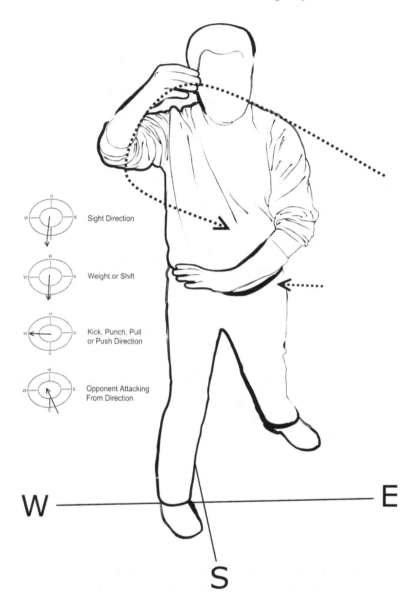

Sight Direction

Weight or Shift

Kick, Punch, Pull
or Push Direction

Opponent Attacking
From Direction

W ——————————————— E

S

Sweep Autumn Leaves off Mount Hua 2:

Use the "spiral power" o generate the next part of the movement as you "swing" into action, your right arm continuing the clockwise circling movement.

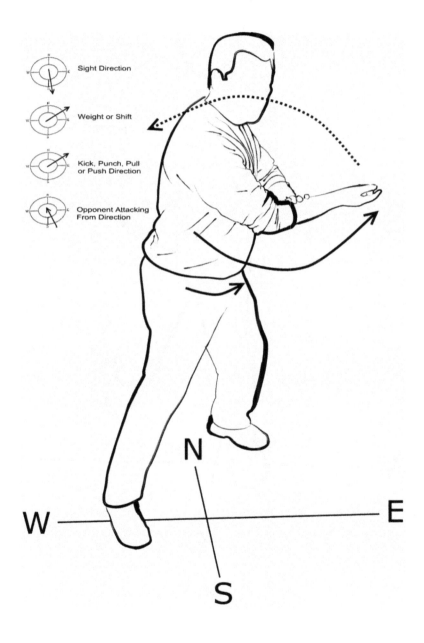

Sight Direction

Weight or Shift

Kick, Punch, Pull or Push Direction

Opponent Attacking From Direction

N

W ——————————————— E

S

(2: continued)

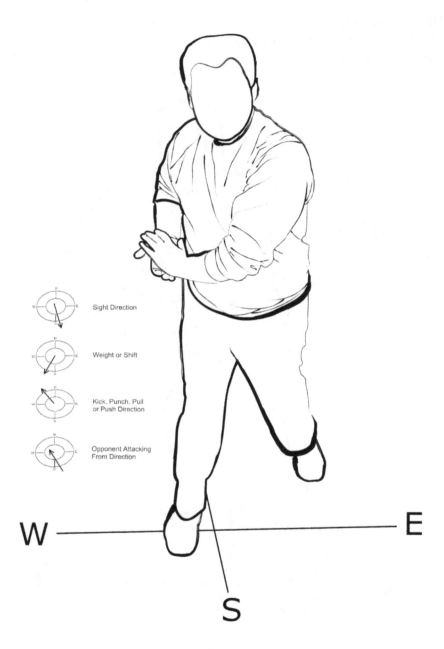

Sight Direction

Weight or Shift

Kick, Punch, Pull
or Push Direction

Opponent Attacking
From Direction

W

E

S

284

3: Step forwards with your left foot as you 'sweep the leaves'. Be careful of the knees as you bend them.

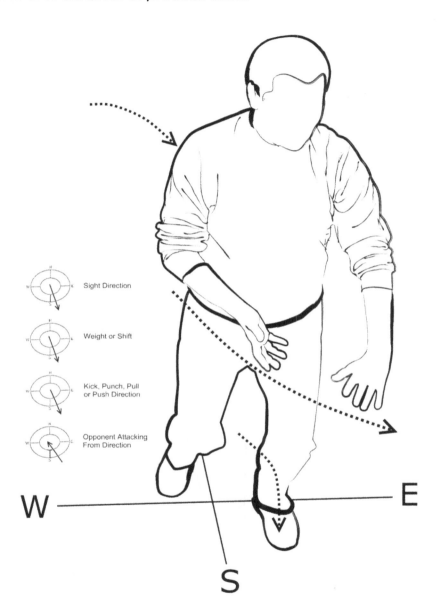

Sight Direction

Weight or Shift

Kick, Punch, Pull or Push Direction

Opponent Attacking From Direction

W ——————————————— E

S

4: Step back with your right foot, then left as you take 'the gathered leaves'

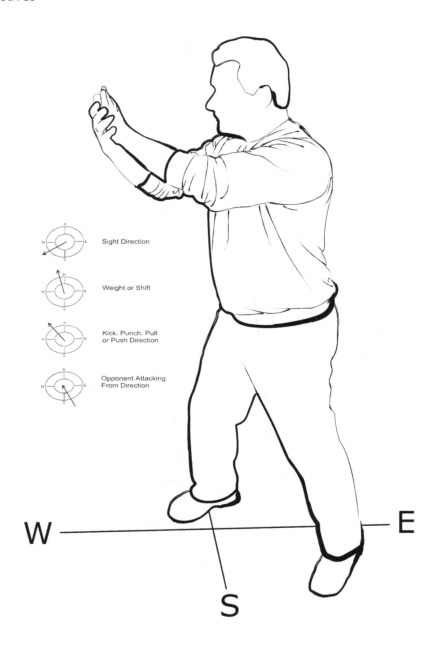

Sight Direction

Weight or Shift

Kick, Punch, Pull or Push Direction

Opponent Attacking From Direction

W ———————————— E

S

Sweep Autumn Leaves off Mount Hua 5:

... and drop them into the barrow (N.E.) culminating in Crouch Stance. Stand up to finish.

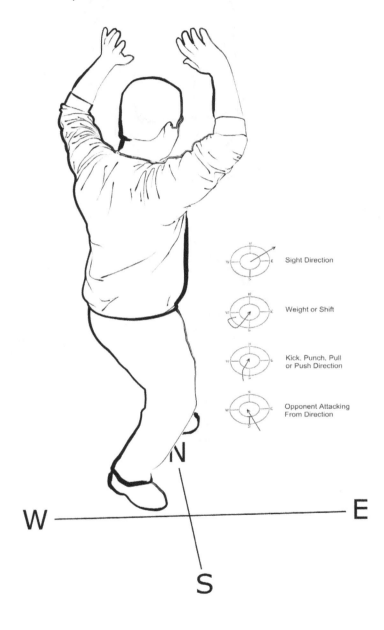

Sight Direction

Weight or Shift

Kick, Punch, Pull or Push Direction

Opponent Attacking From Direction

N

W ——————————— E

S

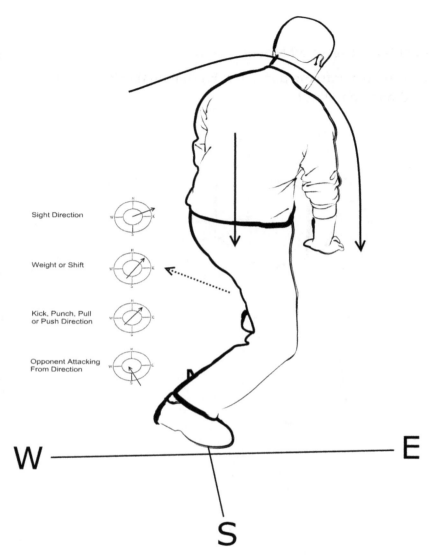

Sight Direction

Weight or Shift

Kick, Punch, Pull
or Push Direction

Opponent Attacking
From Direction

W ——————————— E

S

(Stand up to finish.)

雲手 - Cloud Clearing Hands: Perform Left Cloud Hand, step through to right stance and perform Right Cloud Hand, step through to left stance and perform Left Cloud Hand.

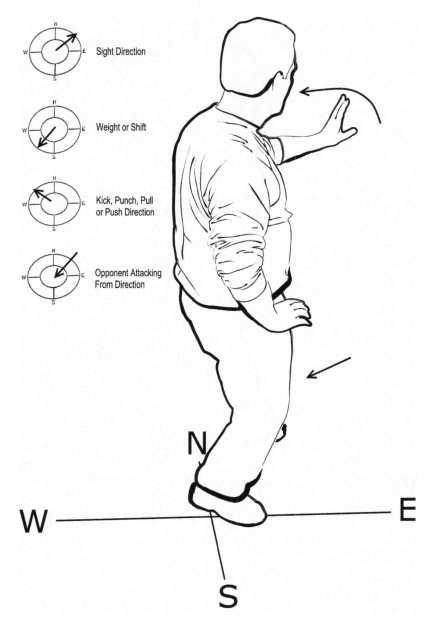

Sight Direction

Weight or Shift

Kick, Punch, Pull or Push Direction

Opponent Attacking From Direction

N

W ———— E

S

(continued)

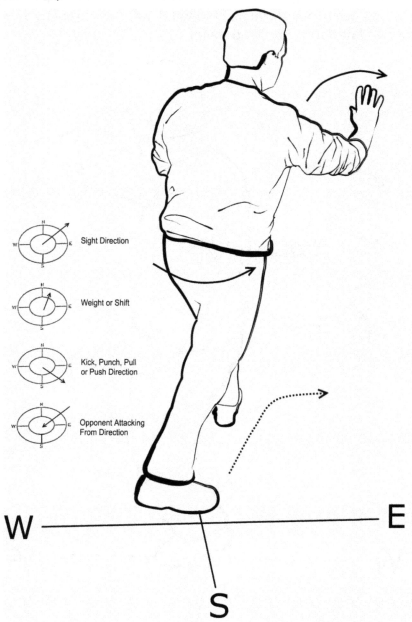

Sight Direction

Weight or Shift

Kick, Punch, Pull
or Push Direction

Opponent Attacking
From Direction

W

E

S

(continued)

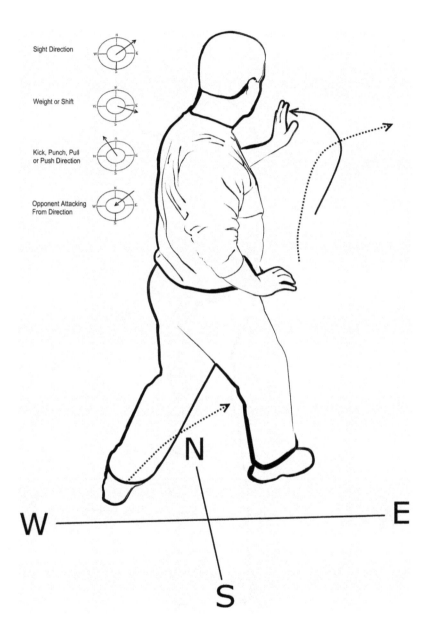

Sight Direction

Weight or Shift

Kick, Punch, Pull
or Push Direction

Opponent Attacking
From Direction

N

W ———————————— E

S

Cloud Hands (Continued)

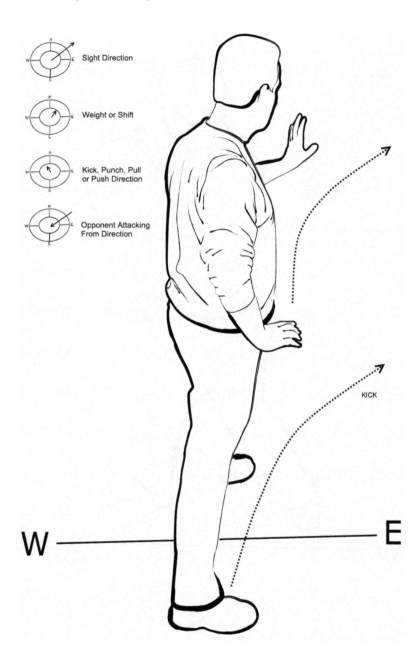

Sight Direction

Weight or Shift

Kick, Punch, Pull or Push Direction

Opponent Attacking From Direction

KICK

W ——————————————— E

2: Continue with "Cloud Hands" as you step forwards: avoid double weighting.

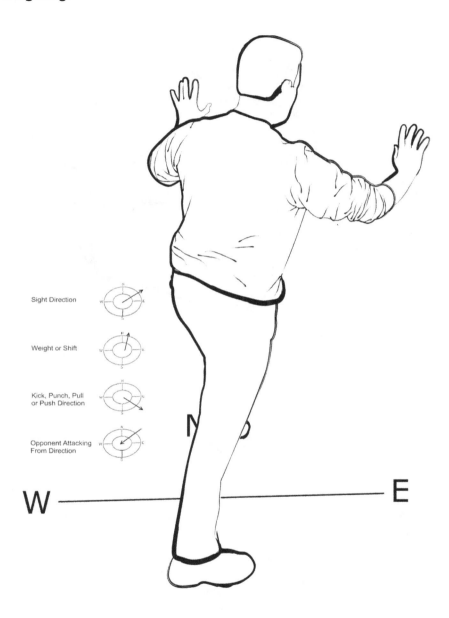

Sight Direction

Weight or Shift

Kick, Punch, Pull or Push Direction

Opponent Attacking From Direction

W —————————————— E

White Crane: Separate and kick.

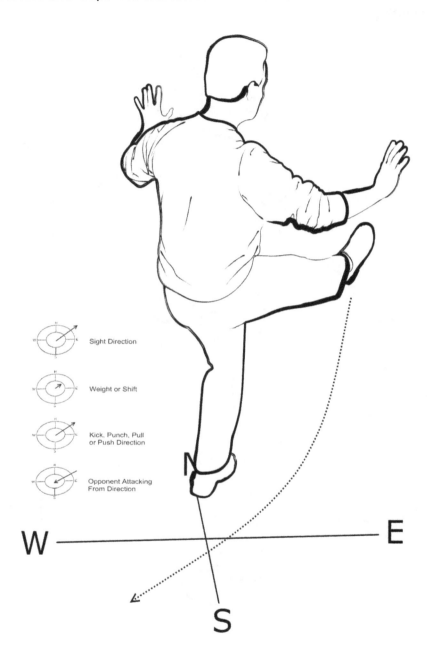

Sight Direction

Weight or Shift

Kick, Punch, Pull
or Push Direction

Opponent Attacking
From Direction

N

W —————————— E

S

Snake Winds around a Branch: Toe-out and continue to pivot as you perform a right-handed Snake technique.

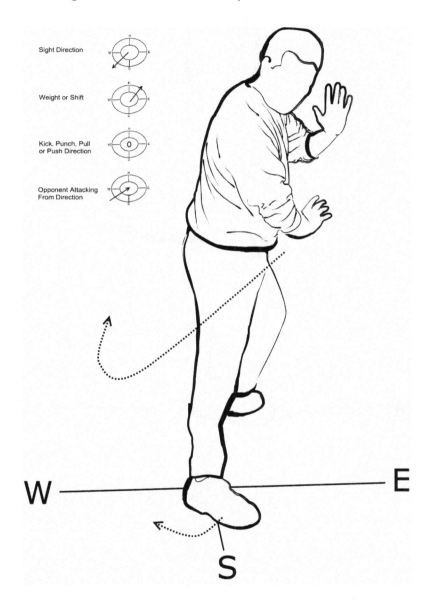

Crouch low and "wind around the branch".

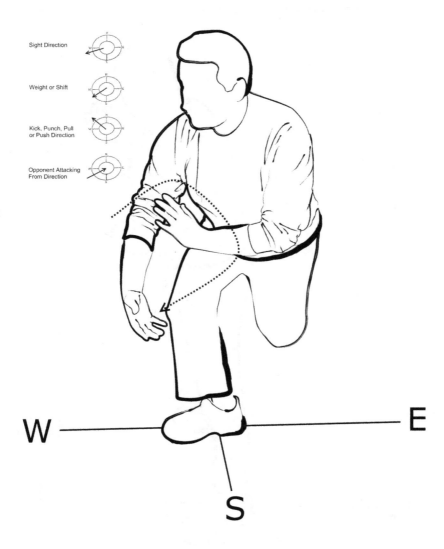

Sight Direction

Weight or Shift

Kick, Punch, Pull
or Push Direction

Opponent Attacking
From Direction

W —————————— E

S

(continued)

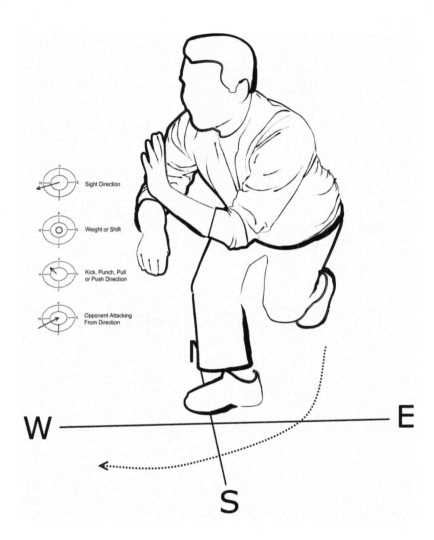

Sight Direction

Weight or Shift

Kick, Punch, Pull
or Push Direction

Opponent Attacking
From Direction

W

E

S

4: Apply the "snake's tail trap" and move into the next posture.

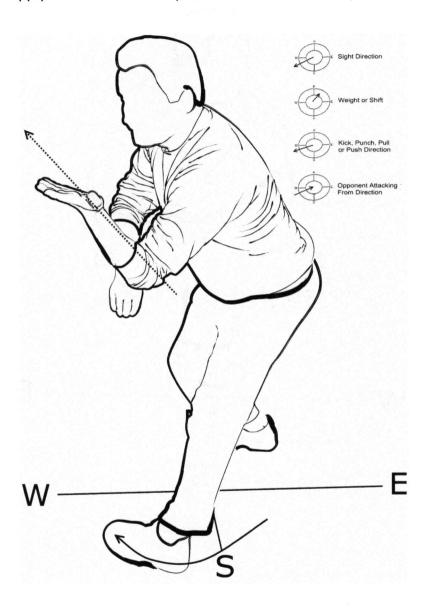

Sight Direction

Weight or Shift

Kick, Punch, Pull
or Push Direction

Opponent Attacking
From Direction

W ——————————— E

S

三豐葉片慎食 - Ch'eung San-feng Packs and Leaves Shensi - 1:

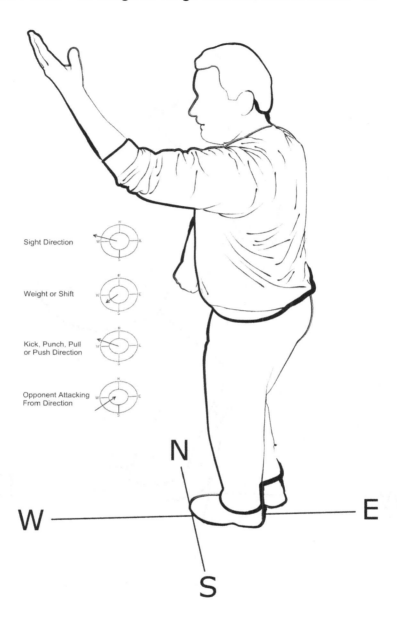

Sight Direction

Weight or Shift

Kick, Punch, Pull
or Push Direction

Opponent Attacking
From Direction

N

W ——— E

S

Execute the "stamp foot and bear weight" technique to finish.

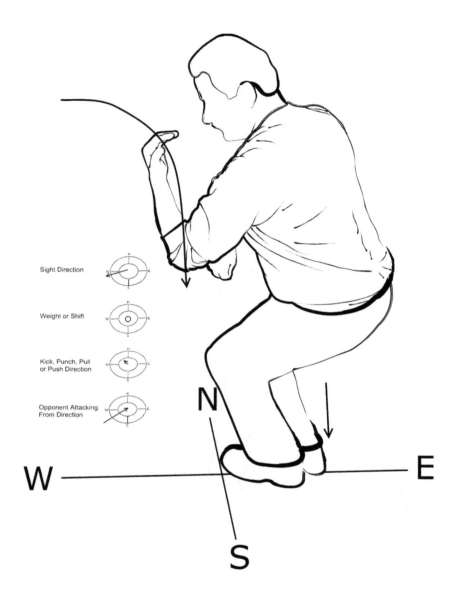

Sight Direction

Weight or Shift

Kick, Punch, Pull or Push Direction

Opponent Attacking From Direction

N

W ——————————— E

S

Single Whip: Step left in a small hooked step and plant your weight down firmly, drop your weight as you perform a Single Whip taking your hook-hand out to the right.

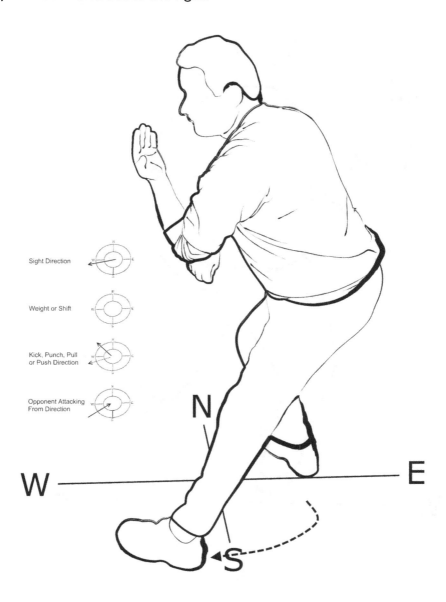

Sight Direction

Weight or Shift

Kick, Punch, Pull
or Push Direction

Opponent Attacking
From Direction

N

W ——————————————— E

S

Tip: Remember to avoid double-weighting.

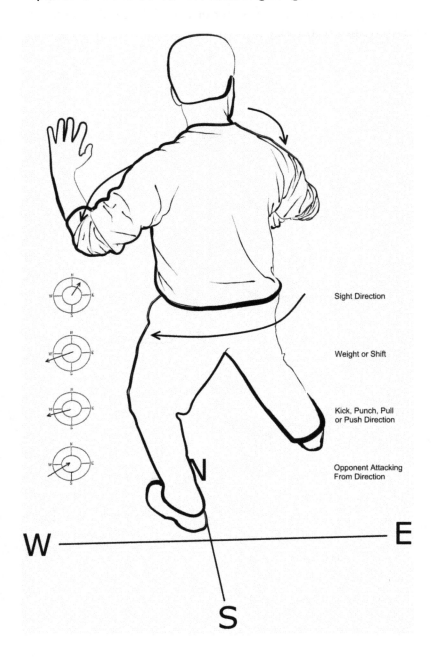

Sight Direction

Weight or Shift

Kick, Punch, Pull
or Push Direction

Opponent Attacking
From Direction

綁定牛I Binding the Ox - 1:
Shift weight leftwards as you prepare to bind a rope around the ox's neck.

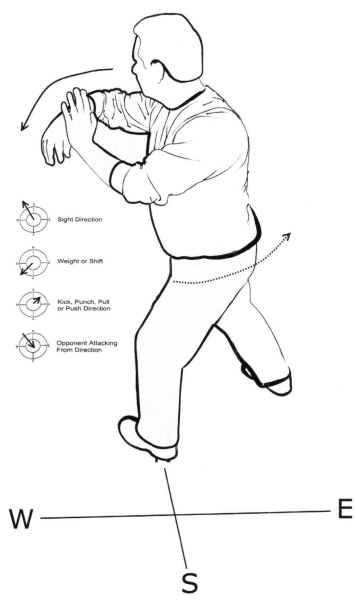

Sight Direction

Weight or Shift

Kick, Punch, Pull
or Push Direction

Opponent Attacking
From Direction

W ———————————————— E

S

When you have performed the first section, do the same again
(images on next page)

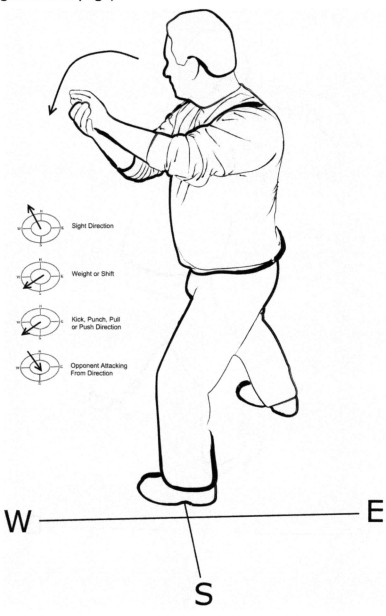

Sight Direction

Weight or Shift

Kick, Punch, Pull
or Push Direction

Opponent Attacking
From Direction

W ——————————————————————— E

S

Ox 2: Perform Yin-Yang weight shifts as you continue.

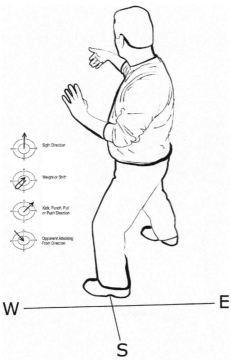

Bind the Ox and then shift
your weight to the left leg to
finish, ready to begin 'Sleepy
Tiger'.

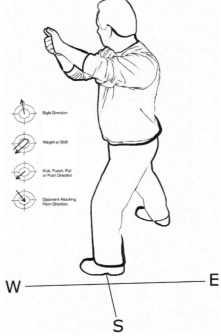

累老虎打哈欠I Sleepy Tiger - 1:
Having performed a "wrapping" technique, shift your weight to your right foot.

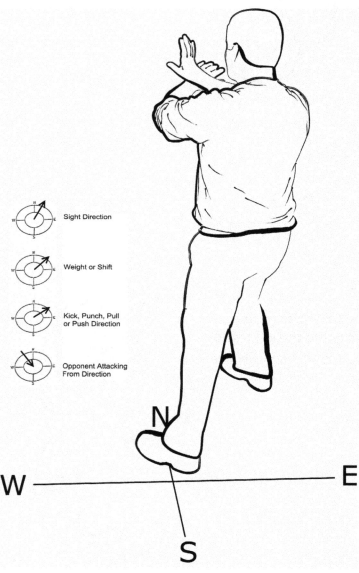

Sight Direction

Weight or Shift

Kick, Punch, Pull
or Push Direction

Opponent Attacking
From Direction

Sleepy Tiger – 2.

(Seen from back view) Continue the movement in a wide arc. Prepare to step you're your empty left foot.

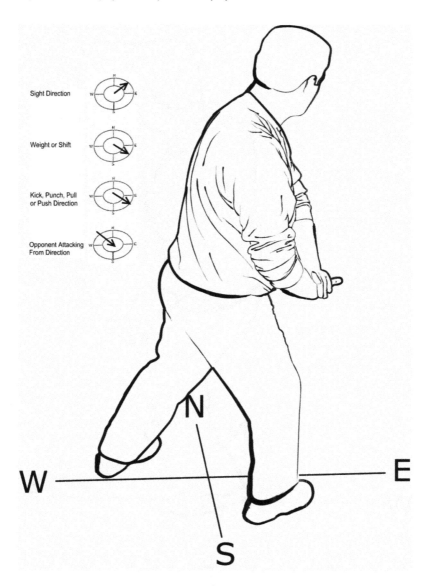

Sight Direction

Weight or Shift

Kick, Punch, Pull
or Push Direction

Opponent Attacking
From Direction

N

W —————————————— E

S

累老虎打哈欠 2: Bring your weight fully to your right leg and using the Tan T'ien to lead.

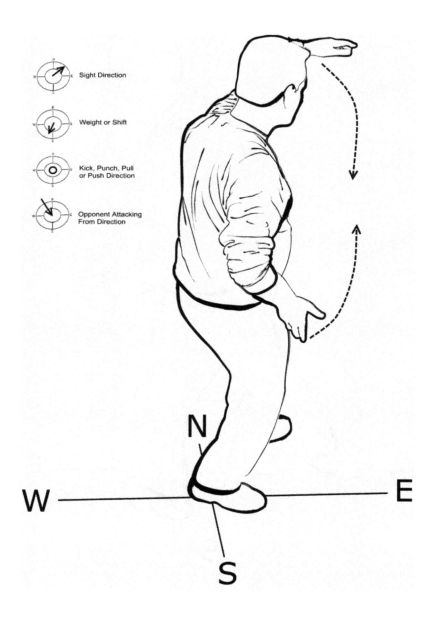

Sight Direction

Weight or Shift

Kick, Punch, Pull or Push Direction

Opponent Attacking From Direction

Sleepy Tiger 3: Perform "Yawning Tiger" as you prepare to transfer your weight to the North East.

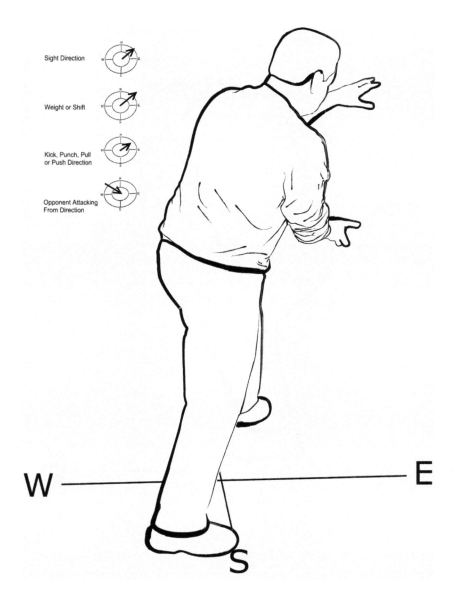

累老虎打哈欠 4: "Press" as you step forwards to the north-East then half-step up with the rear foot.

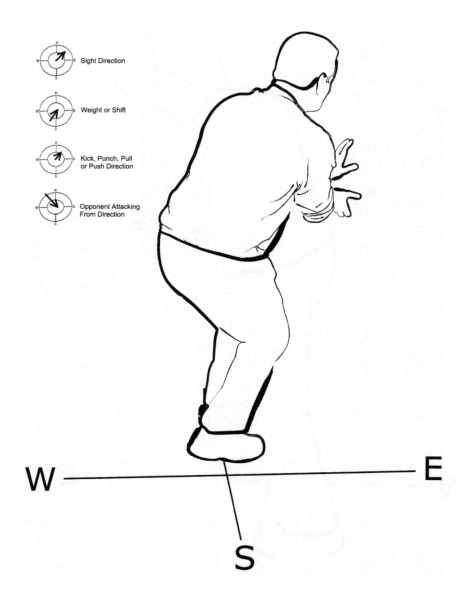

Sight Direction

Weight or Shift

Kick, Punch, Pull or Push Direction

Opponent Attacking From Direction

W ——————————————————— E

S

尋找精神 - Spirit Searching 1:

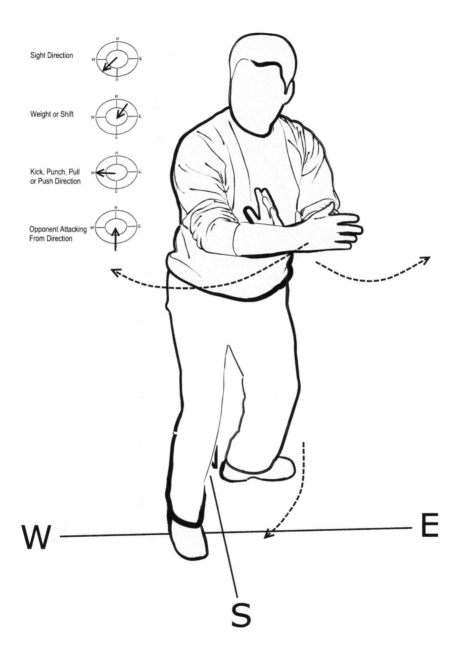

Sight Direction

Weight or Shift

Kick, Punch, Pull
or Push Direction

Opponent Attacking
From Direction

W

E

S

(Continued) Look over your shoulder as you begin the actions of ch'i centring.

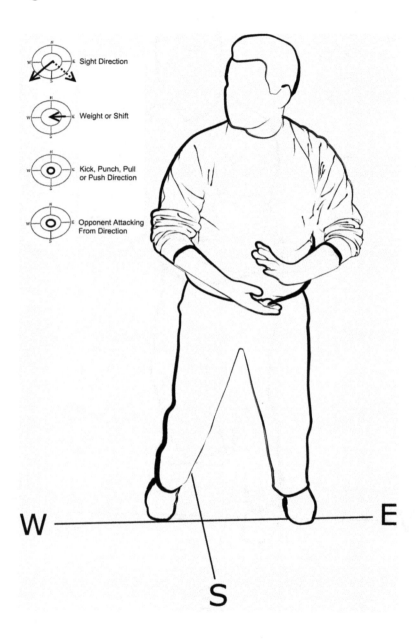

Sight Direction

Weight or Shift

Kick, Punch, Pull or Push Direction

Opponent Attacking From Direction

W ———————— E

S

Turn to the South as you show "beauteous palms to the sun" to offer peace. Using the "sensing" technique your Shih-fu has explained, continue to Ch'i Centring.

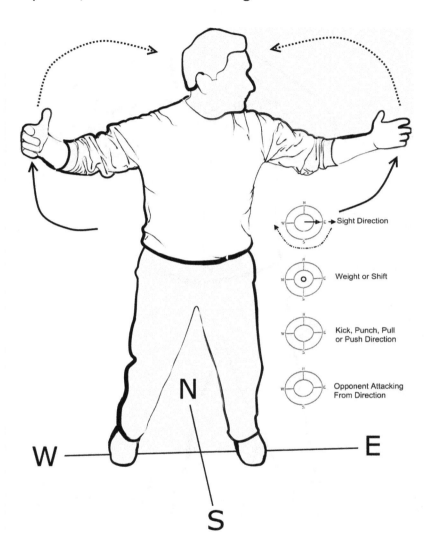

Sight Direction

Weight or Shift

Kick, Punch, Pull or Push Direction

Opponent Attacking From Direction

尋找精神 2: Bring your left foot forwards into Bear Stance as you glance to the right then prepare for Ch'i Centring.

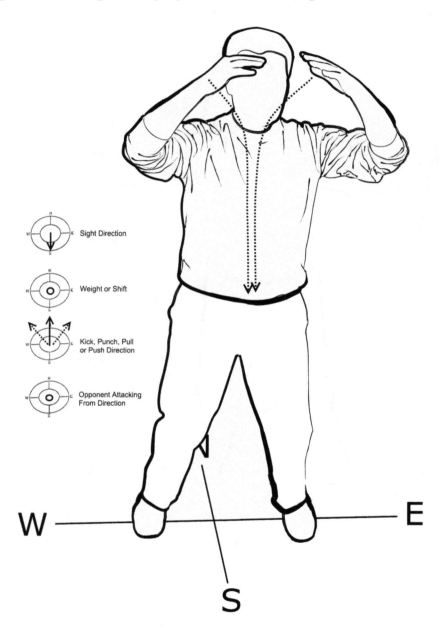

Sight Direction

Weight or Shift

Kick, Punch, Pull or Push Direction

Opponent Attacking From Direction

W ——————— E

S

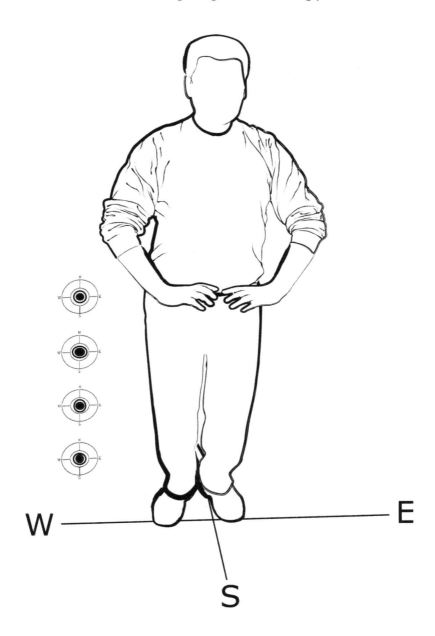

Return to Wu Chi:

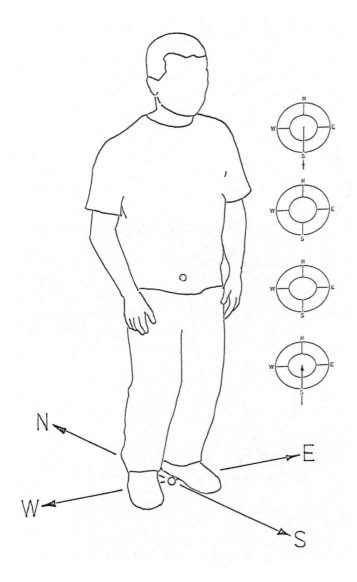

之前宇宙的狀態: Close.

Note: It is advised that many years of practice are spent in order to fully appreciate this Form before teaching. A 'Teacher Training Course', just learning the Form and supporting exercises, may only last two to three years; however, to become a proficient teacher will take at least ten years of dedicated learning and practice after this.

SHI-FU'S PRACTICE ADVICE:

If you are new to Taijiquan and wish to do the whole thing:

First spend up to 2 years practicing Qigong; absolute minimum time required is six-to-twelve months. This time will be useful in making the body stronger, the ch'i circulation better and the mind more clear as well as relaxing the body. This is the best preparation for Taijiquan.

If you are not new to Taijiquan:

Begin as usual with Qigong. Study the stances and basic principles for at least two months. To the western beginner this may seem "boring" and one might want to get onto the Form in more detail, but progress will not be made so well this way. Remember the old Chinese saying, "Quickly learned, easily forgotten!" And the other one that says "A house built on sand will soon subside and collapse. Build your house on a thick and solid foundation, then you can make it taller and more lasting!"

Practice each posture, holding - with correct postures only - for up to two hours, allowing the qi to open the energy channels and "shape" the mind's mould. Practice the Metal Element of meditation with each posture.

Before doing the Linked Form or Flowing Form, practice the applications after each posture. This will reinforce "I and Ch'i".

(Continued)

When doing the linked form remember the advice that you are given in class. Remember it well as it will serve you well if you do. T'ai Chi Ch'uan is a beautifully simple Art but at the same time it is complex, with many, many small points to remember. Without these details your Form/s will never amount to anything worthwhile, even if you do feel more relaxed or healthier for doing them; just as there are many levels to practice there are also many levels of benefits and achievements too. What you get out of it is equal to what you put in.

See also the advice at the beginning of this chapter.

Chapter Nine

T'ai Chi Kun

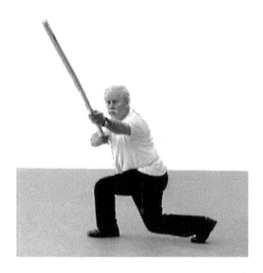

Taiji Gun

The Staff of Supreme Ultimate Boxing

Taiji Staff

(Simplified Chinese: 太极棍; Traditional Chinese: 太極棍; Pinyin: Taiji Gun)

All styles of T'ai Chi Ch'uan, (pinyin, which I shall use here) or Taijiquan have a Staff or Kun, pronounced "Gun" training method. Tiandidao is no exception. It is commonly believed that after learning the main Form or Quan that practising the Gun will help to develop more power, greater coordination and the ability to "extend", which is useful in expressing. There are mainly three types of staff, the "Gun" being the most common. Its length should be roughly the height of the practitioner. In the west we may have problems finding any other length than the near "six-foot pole" or Bo (Japanese) length poles; as it seems to be called by most suppliers. As far as I am aware, the Northern schools pronounce it more like "Gan" but sometimes "gan-er" as well.

Materials differ for staves now but the most common traditional material was thought to be "Waxwood", a smoothed white wood which has a waxed finish; it is also very tough and inflexible but durable. Waxwood or other hard wood is preferred by Weigong schools. Rattan Cane, white oak and red oak are also quite widely found nowadays but the correct materials and being a well-made staff is necessary for good practice. Rattan is preferred for Taijiquan as the characteristics fit in with the principles of practice. Rattan Cane is a vine that usually grows around trees and can be straightened, skinned or left unskinned. The skinned canes are far better for Taijigun.

In the earliest times farmers may have used a stout wooden pole to balance heavy loads across the shoulders. This is thought to be originated in China, like many, many other inventions that we take for granted today. However, being a "stick" various methods may have started in Europe or other countries at or around the same time. It seems to follow that something like this being to hand when attacked by bandits or robbers would become a common weapon of defence. Easy to cut, straighten and smooth, the wooden branch or stem is a world-wide resource that is available to all.

Once developed for Martial Arts and Self-defence purposes it was thought that a length of "one hand's with" taller than the wielder was the best. This obviously causes disparity when we are faced with the standard length staves that we buy from suppliers nowadays. This can be overcome, I found, but takes a bit of research and then some travel, followed by home-spun straightening or smoothing techniques. This is time consuming and challenges you to find new skills and techniques of handy crafting that you may never have tried before, but satisfying.

After development within the various schools of Chinese Boxing the Gun was shaped to be thicker at the base end, thinner at the "business end". A short stick is generally called a Bang; fitting in the West as we may naturally think that a "bang" comes from one end of a Gun! The stick that comes up to eyebrow height, or thereabouts, is called Gun. Some systems, like Wing Chun, use a longer pole, often referred to as a "six point pole", this is called Ch'ang Gun. The name Gun probably originates from the first cannon or rifle invented. The Chinese, who invented gunpowder, used a hollowed out bamboo to fire projectiles out of with gunpowder charges, hence the name.

In Taijiquan it is important that the correct principles are applied throughout and one should follow the advice of a good instructor closely, otherwise it will be nothing more than "waving a dead stick." In Taiji Gun the stick should be "alive", not dead. There will also be some additional method teaching and pairs practice, but this will vary according to the level of the students and their abilities. Your instructor should be able to link all practices throughout the various Forms or Methods and can show you how the essential principles apply to each Quan. Your teacher should be able to demonstrate how the staff is used and by this demonstration you should be able to see the correct techniques and energies involved. It should not look dull or lifeless, even when done slowly. Practice diligently and as often as possible to get the best results.

In Europe the use of a wooden staff is not recorded until around the mediaeval times. This was usually a hard wood, such as Blackthorn, a very strong and resilient wood. In these times in Europe it was generally known as the Quarterstaff. The reason for this is simply because the hands are positioned a quarter ways up from each end. The rather flamboyant illustration below, taken from an old European Sports book, shows something quite different and more like the Chinese grip – figure on right.

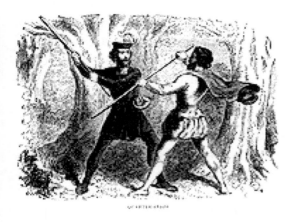

In the more familiar tale of Robin Hood, a character said to have lived around the 11th century, he famously used a Quarterstaff in a fight with John Little when he confronted him on a "ligger"; a fallen tree used to cross a stream. According to legend, Robin was outlawed for killing a "King's deer" and had to live life as an outcast in the forest. One day he approached a steam and wanted to cross by the fallen tree-trunk. A large man carrying a heavy staff also was crossing from the other side Robin, being young and allegedly cocky and hot-headed, told the man to get off and let him pass. The big man laughed at the lad's insolence. After a brief exchange, Robin said "Why if I had a staff I'd beat you off!" The big man laughed all the more. John Little looked around and said, "Tell you what lad, there's a blackthorn tree over yonder. Go cut yourself a staff and we'll see what stuff you're made of!" This he did. When read they fought on the log and eventually John Little knocked the cheeky lad off into the stream, giving him a good drubbing. After the big man had stopped laughing, they introduced themselves. When Little told Robin his name, Robin laughed, looking at the size of the man who was around six-foot seven, "Ha! John *Little*? I think I'll call you Little John!" They became good friends and colleagues.

In old China, the most famous accounts of Staff fighting must surely be from early Shaolin days. Just a few monks held a strategic bridge against cavalry charges and defeated the attackers.

Another famous Chinese legend was born from a novel. A fictional character called 'Nine Dragons'; he had nine dragons tattooed over his body. According to legend he could defeat many attackers and was never scathed in battle. There have been throughout history many accounts of fighting with a wooden pole. Being the easiest material to source, in most places on Earth, it is not only convenient but can be made to fit many purposes; e.g. cut to fit the fighter, made tapered at one end to hold a blade, or even used in sections, joined by a chain or rope, as in the Chinese weapon called simply "Three Section Staff".

The Taijigun method is, even to the uninitiated, different to the Shaolin Staff Method, which often uses the harder Waxwood Kun; although nowadays Oak and other materials may be substituted. In either school, the dexterity and technique is quite astounding compared to the very basic techniques seen in old western films, like those about Knights, for example. Films made in the twenty-first century, like those featuring Jackie Chan and Jet Li, tend to show more and more of the deft skills developed within Chinese Martial Arts.

Tiandidao Divine Staff
(地 道 神 棍; pinyin: Shen Gun)

The Staff is considered to be the grandfather of all weapons. This is because it is the basic and also essential weapon that can be owned easily by all people in many formats; e.g. cut from a tree, made from bamboo or even a metal pole. It teaches the necessary skills in "extension" and coordination; something which most beginners find difficult with a long weapon and often either drop it or hit their selves with it. The staff acts an extension of the arms and while it might be comparatively simple to use arms and fists in combat, wielding a six-foot long staff can prove awkward at first. Basics should always be taught first and the student must get used to holding the staff as well as moving smoothly from one technique to another without mishap.

In any proper Quan-shu schools the staff will be taught before any other weapon, always. It forms the foundational training, awareness and handling skills required of students before they can go on to learn anything else. Mastery of the staff is more than just waving it around, you must also be familiar with it as though it was an extra arm, or leg, and in dealing with its theoretical use against all other weapons. Finally, as a requirement of Tiandidao, you should be able to disarm a person with a staff.

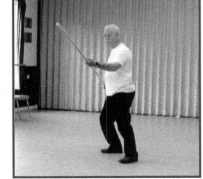

In Tiandidao our Divine Staff Form is not only an extension of the Taiji Quan Form but also a prelude to learning other weapons. It must be remembered that all weapons are an extension of the body and arms.

As the Taijigun falls into the Neigong category of training it must be practiced with correct values.

Chapter Ten

TAIJIQUAN DAO & JIAN SWORDS

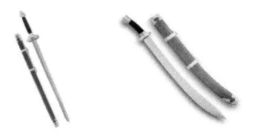

Legends of China

T'ai Chi Sword.

Jian.

The Jian is a sword of almost mythical powers, especially in Taoist legends. It has been featured in films such as Crouching Tiger, Hidden Dragon, Dragon Inn, Heaven Sword and Dragon Sabre. It is nicknamed "the gentleman's and lady's sword" as it requires refined techniques to play it properly. The Jian feels more like a precision tool rather than a weapon, and for good reasons. A well-crafted Jian has superb balance and therefore feels light, even though it can weigh from one-and-a-half to two pounds; depending on the correct length for user. The balance point is about four to five inches in front of the guard.

Some Jian produced seem to have a hand guard that has "wings" facing forwards. While this allows the maker to apply a "clip" action to it for locking it into the scabbard, it may not be the best item for advanced T'ai Chi Jian practice as it allows an opponent to "lock" or control your sword. This is a feature which depends upon the age or era of sword being copied. Shih-fu Adam Hsu, the internationally renowned and respected author, practitioner and authority on Traditional Chinese Arts, has developed sword which is now produced by Paul Chen called "The Adam Hsu Jian". This comes in one-handed or two- handed variety. This is a highly crafted piece and suitable for someone advanced in their practice. Normally students will start with a wooden straight sword. These again should be one piece blade and hilt with a good hand guard. Many students in China often keep and use the wooden swords for life; and in this day and age where people no longer have need to carry swords on the street, a real sword is only suitable for private practice so as to get an enhanced feeling and understanding of the Form.

The name Jian has different meanings to many people. It can mean "three sharps", as Shih-fu Hsu alludes to in his book "Lone Sword Against the Cold Sky" (Plum Publications). It has also referred to a steel rod in the past, one which is tapered and has "knots" along the length of the non-sharp blade that look somewhat similar to the pattern of bamboo; a strong material. This Jian was used to smash an enemy sword and maybe strike the enemy or poke them with it too. There are two very similar types of straight sword, one having a very slight flexibility at the tip end (Jian) and the other no flexibility but a thicker blade for cutting power (Gim).

Generally, for T'ai Chi Ch'uan practice, the sword should be lighter, around 1.2 to 2.0 lbs. in weight and the balance point just two fingers width or 4 cm away from the front of the guard. These swords are not used for "hacking" or chopping, so lightness is required for the major principle techniques of the style to be applied with deftness and agility. The heavier Gim would still allow this but because of the weight some people may find it more "unwieldy" than the lighter version.

Sword Forms and Styles.

There are many Forms or sets about these days, all variable in content, origin and style. Some may look "flowery", as the Chinese say, whilst others may look extremely practical. There is a great deal of difference between the two. I am no expert on these but there are experts out there that have travelled afar and wide and seen almost all there is to see regarding these Forms and "Kung Fu" in general. According to these opinions expressed by trustworthy and revered practitioners there are very few "practical" Forms around, so finding one of these in the West may be more difficult than finding someone who teaches genuine skills for no profit; there are many Traditional Martial Arts Instructors around who do not seek profit from their teachings of authentic Martial arts, but what I am saying here is that such things as a genuine, practical Jian Form may be more rare than rocking horse pool You would find one in China, if you looked hard enough and was "recommended" or introduced; and they liked your attitude, of course. You can find one in Taiwan and maybe somewhere in the USA, but that is a big plot of land. It all depends upon you and what you are content to settle with. Personally, whilst I am familiar with some Jian basics I am still looking for a genuinely good teacher after around fifty something years of dedicated study to the practice and development of Traditional Chinese Arts. I am not content to learn the variations of modern Competition Style. So far I have only discovered two possible Masters of Jian that I would wish to learn from, one is in Taiwan and the other mainland China; both unaffordable and unreachable for me!

The style depends upon the school or system that the swords "Sets" emanate from. For example, Pa Kua Ch'uan may incorporate the "walking in circles" methods whilst another, say Yang, may use slightly bolder techniques, and another more stepping, jumping and snake stances. It stands to reason though that if you are studying Pa Kua Ch'uan (The Eight Diagrams Boxing) then you would continue to learn that method of Dao and Jian. Usually the style fits the school's curriculum.

There are two major sword forms in T'ai Chi Ch'uan, as there are in most Chung-Kuo Ch'uan styles generally. These are Dao (Broadsword) and Jian (Straight double-edged sword). The Jian is a straight sword that is tapered and sharp on two edges.

History.

In terms of legends, the Jian tends to get more airing than does the Dao, but both are indeed stuff of great battle legends. In ancient China there were stories of Ten Famous Swords; The sword of delicate elegance: Cheng Ying, The sword of majesty: Chun Jun, The sword of bravery: Yu Chang, The swords of love: Gan Jiang and Mo Ye, The sword of integrity: Qi Xing Long Yuan, The sword of prestige: Tai E, The sword of sovereignty: Chi Xiao, The sword of kindness: Zhan Lu, The sword of divinity: Xuan Yuan – made for the Yellow Emperor.

Here I shall be happy to bring you the legendary account of the 'sword of integrity'.

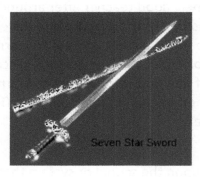

Seven Star Sword

Qi Xing Long Yuan.

Chinese legend has it that this sword was the joint work of two revered Chinese sword makers, Gan Jiang and Ou Yezi. In order to make this sword they brought stream water from Cishan Mountain (During the Japanese colonized times, in consideration of the ungraceful old name, Cishan was renamed according to the highest mountain "Mt. Chiwei" in the area) to the seven ponds around the sword-making fireplace. Because the seven ponds were shaped like the seven stars of the Big Dipper, the sword was named Qi Xing (seven stars). If you look down the sword, it looks ethereal and profound, as if you are in a high position overlooking a valley where a huge dragon lives, which is why the sword was also named Long Yuan (an abyss with a dragon).

To this day the Chinese make Seven Star Swords; although most are not so well made as they are meant as cheap tourist decorations, not practical swords; be warned! A more practical solution, but not a Seven Star sword, is made available by Scot Rodell, based in USA.

According to the Annals of Wu and Yue, another version or story that made this sword famous was based upon a fisherman, whose name is unknown. He saved Wu Zixu's life. In order to express his gratitude to the fisherman, who refused to tell his name, Wu sent him the sword, Qi Xing Long Yuan. The fisherman sighed and said, "I saved your life because you are a loyal official of the country, not because I wanted your reward. Now that you think I am a man longing for profits, I have to show my nobleness with this sword." With these words, he committed suicide with the sword. Therefore, Qi Xing Long Yuan was a sword of integrity.

Long means 'Dragon'. Chuan means 'Well'. Together this makes Dragon Well; Longquan. There is a region in Southern China where the water coming down from the mountains is rich in minerals that make swords extra strong. There are many factories based in the area these days making what they call Dragon Well Swords, based on the legend. As said above, many people are of the opinion that most are unsuitable for sword practice, as they could break or fall apart with vigorous use, so endangering not only the user but bystanders too.

Dao.

Dao means "Big Knife" in literal translation and it is believed that the shape and style was taken from a cookery knife; as in Chef's knife. A popular misnomer in the West is to call it a "broadsword". This sword has a thick end to the blade and is used in much the same way as a large kitchen knife when chopping vegetables. The

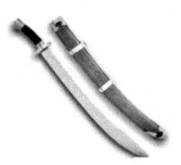

difference being here that the Dao is several times larger and therefore more difficult to wield. It used to be used in the military and to good effect. It was said that when the Japanese invaded China and used their Katana swords that the Chinese Broadsword soldiers outmatched them. Although I have seen no historical evidence of this personally it seems feasible. The Dao has a heavy blade with a thick, blunt edge on top. In theory it is possible that a blade with such dimensions could smash a thinner blade if used correctly.

There is a saying that it takes "six months to learn the Dao". This might seem reasonable in a militaristic scenario, when troops have to be trained quickly, but in T'ai Chi Ch'uan it can and should take a lot longer so as to learn the subtleties that are normally hidden from plain view. In T'ai Chi Ch'uan the object of learning to use the Dao is not for war or violent purposes but for the development of mind, spirit and energies. Each weapon trained with will have a different effect on the mind, body and ch'i.

For practice purposes most people use the wooden Dao. This is more than adequate for learning. There are other alternatives though and the reader should be aware of quality and purpose. Flimsy swords or those with two-piece blades and handles are not suitable. Only those with a strong construction should be used. During the Cultural Revolution all Martial Arts were banned, as mentioned earlier in the history section. The making, owning and using of real weapons was also banned. The governments did not want another revolution, like the Boxer Rebellion (1898-1900), and we all saw the Chinese Communist Government's brutal reactions to the peaceful demonstrations of Tiananmen Square, using brute force against *unarmed* protestors. The Chinese Communist Government (CCG) of the time did not want people to have arms with which to defend them, so swords had to go as far as they were concerned. This also suited their intent to banish real Martial Arts and replace them with a more stage-like performing art they called Competition Wu Shu. This featured "flowery hand" sets and theatrical weapons that were of anything but "combat quality" and more like toys. Only in recent years when new members of the CCG made changes, restored battered buildings (like Wu Tang) and damaged graves of Chinese heroes, did they reinstate the traditional Martial Arts, to a degree, then in the late 1990's plans were made to allow the making of real swords once more. However, sadly, many cheap and nasty products of the earlier regime were already being churned out of factories in their thousands and exported across the world in their attempt at capitalising on culture and trading.

Nowadays it is still changing and makers such as Hanwei (Paul Chen) are producing reasonable steel swords for practice that are similar to traditional swords. Traditionally though, going back a few hundred years, there were not very well made swords in China.

Ironically the Japanese took a Miao Dao; meaning "leaf-sprout knife" because of the shape being likened to a new wheat sprout, or similar. The Japanese are said to have taken this sword as a base shape and then manufactured the "Samurai Sword" from this shape, but the grip following the same curve as the blade instead of counter-curving like the Miao Dao or being straight. These Katana were made by Japanese blacksmiths who folded and beat the blades to make them sharper and stronger. This technique may have been available in China but from my studies it seems that most swords used then were made of alloys, such as bronze. These would last a short while but were really not up to serious use.

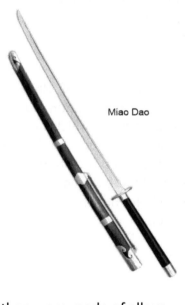

Miao Dao

For practice I would recommend the wooden Dao that is made from red oak or similar. The ones traded as "Wooden Chinese Broadsword" from well-known Martial Arts wholesalers in the UK are usually superb. They are made in China to the correct specifications (pictured below right). Even the balance is quite fair, for a wooden sword, thought it will be far lighter than steel or even alloy sword.

Aluminium or "alloy" practice swords are also available and these are much heavier, almost similar in weight to a steel sword. The grips are "bound" to make them safer and more comfortable, but beware of the weight pulling it out of a beginner's hand on a big sweeping movement! Some come with two coloured "scarves" or red and yellow cloths that are attached to the pommel and these may be wrapped around the hand or wrist to help beginners keep a hold of the sword; although they are not made for this purpose.

As mentions earlier, Hanwei make steel swords to a reproduction standard based upon old swords of China. In recent years this range of "practical" swords has been added to by a range of "historic swords of Europe" and the Practical Dao is very good value for money if you wish to own something close to "the real thing". These should not be used in class or public practice due to their edges, which are not sharpened but still capable of damage if a slip-up occurs!

338

Chapter Eleven

Taiji Qiang

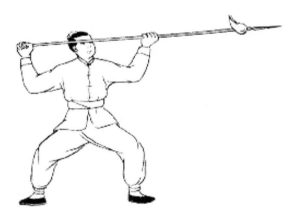

The "Qiang" Spear

Qiang - Spear

The Chinese Spear is often seen as being slightly different in use than the spears of other nations. This maybe because the Chinese Spear, Qiang or Chiang, is used with quite a bit of skills variation and specific stance work too.

Traditionally, world-wide, spears come into two broad categories, the throwing spear (includes Javelin) and the held spear. The latter was most commonly used by foot soldiers who would march forwards in a tight line, with another tight line behind them and perhaps more behind them. This formation created a formidable "wall" with long-reaching spear-points at its front onto which any charging enemy or his horses would be impaled. Should the wall of spear men be confronted with other spears, swords and shields they would use their spears to parry and then stab at any weaknesses in the defence of the enemy lines and in this way set about trying to create an opening.

The Chinese spear was used in a similar way, but also subjected to the usual Chinese thinking and development, making it an even more formidable weapon. By using stances, special parrying and deflecting techniques and rapid thrust or pulls, the spear's use was amplified. The Chinese spear was further divided by using two different shaft materials, Waxwood or other hard wood, or Rattan Cane. Rattan is very flexible and therefore offers the opportunity to use its whip-like qualities in defensive or offensive modes to great advantage. The Taiji Qian falls into the last category.

Like some other weapons Forms, the ultimate principle rests on the design of the tool, the rest is up to the bearer and methods can vary. In the case of Taijiquan though there must be at least Yin and Yang involved in the movements. Generally the waist comes into play and the feet are, I would say, of equal importance. All movements are coordinated by the mind and eye in turn.

Many people who are ignorant of the values of such practices may condemn the use of any weapon at all for training, perhaps saying that it is unnecessary violence. This is of course a ridiculous type of Un-thought-of statement to make and shows just how the ignorant may make rash statements because they do not know.

Training in "empty-hand" Forms will require you to Master yourself; mind, body and spirit. Training later with weapons requires awareness of the actual weapon, be it long, short, wood or metal. The most basic priority is awareness of space and where your limbs are, which should have been well learned during the initial Empty Hand Form.

In learning the Taiji Qiang it is soon realised that the spear is very long, has a metal point on one end, a "blood beard" and a very long, whippy shaft. It is not that heavy but nonetheless not that easy to wield and manipulate. It requires different skills to those of Taiji Dao and they again are vastly different to the skills of the Taiji Jian. By learning three, at least, such distinctively different weapons we learn a vast array of movements, all of which demand heightened awareness and specialised self-control in each Form, plus a "feel" for each distinctly different weapon. This is said to develop a more flexible qi/ch'i and mind-set, a stronger body and more focused mind.

If you are a well-polished practitioner you may be able to think of other things that I have omitted here. Otherwise for the novice reading this it will hopefully plant a seed that can be returned to later. For the intermediate or advanced student there is enough information here to perhaps give more "fuel" for the journey.

T'ai Chi Spear.

Quiang (Pinyin) or (mao 矛 in Mandarin) is the general name for Spear, one of the four classical weapons of Chinese Martial Arts. As the Pinyin version is more common these days and the Mandarin version has been all but lost in use, I shall use the modern variant here.

In T'ai Chi Ch'uan, usually, you will find the spear has a flexible shaft made of rattan, which is also quite strong. Others may be made of Waxwood and be inflexible. The flexible shaft is preferred by internal stylists as it is favourable for using ch'i and internal techniques. It has a red tassel hanging from underneath the head of the spear, this is the "Blood Beard" and is meant for distraction more than anything, but also serves to stop blood from running down the shaft onto the hands in battle and making the shaft sticky. In modern competition forms it can be seen to move correctly or incorrectly by judges awarding points for proper "form".

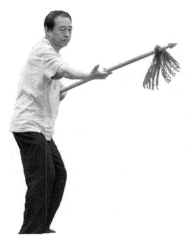

In history the Quiang was used on the battlefield, the cavalry would use it to eliminate foot soldiers, perhaps guards, while the foot soldiers would use it against horsemen, alongside such weapons as the Miaodao. It could also be used against swords, staves or chain whips. Its versatility and long reach meant that it was a very practical weapon and quite unlike the usage of Western spears it was never thrown. The Chinese philosophy, as usual, is very practical on this subject "Don't ever throw a good weapon away!"

Exercising with the Quiang is different from the staff in many respects, yet similar in others. Probably the most noticeable difference is within the footwork - stance work. In Quiang some very distinctive Ladder Steps and Side-steps may be used which can be quite tricky for newcomers to this weapon. Training, as usual, should be done only with a competent teacher, there are obvious "points" to observe and it is not for the novice or inexperienced Martial Artist as you need to be acutely aware of your surroundings. A Staff in the wrong hands can be lethal enough and being "lethal" is not the aim of practice in T'ai Chi Ch'uan; self-control and development of ch'i and spirit is though, so you would be wise to avoid anyone who seems to have the wrong character or teaches it in a way that encourages a weapon's use in violence.

So concludes this introduction of the four basic weapons that are most commonly found in the gentle Art of Taijiquan. A well-studied practitioner may come across other Chinese weapons that are used in one or another style, but these may be unique to that style or family system; there are not just five styles of Taijiquan but hundreds!

Any teacher claiming to teach Taijiquan, Tai Chi, T'ai Ch'i Ch'uan, etcetera, will be able to explain the use and practice of these weapons in Neigong; not Weigong method! Finding a teacher who is "expert in everything" is not a practical aspiration though. Each aspect of Taijiquan is something that can take years and years to "master", so trying to master five or more aspects is a high ideal for anyone to have! I suggest that students dedicate as many years as it takes to learn the "empty hand" methods first, then move on to the base weapon, the humble but demanding Taijigun. From there he or she can decide on which other aspect to learn in depth and try to master. This will be a lifetime's work.

Chapter Twelve

T'ien Ti Tao P'ai

T'ai Chi for Health (Illustrated)

A Growing Aspect in the West
Also deriving from China, but
must not be confused with the
"Real T'ai Chi Ch'uan"!

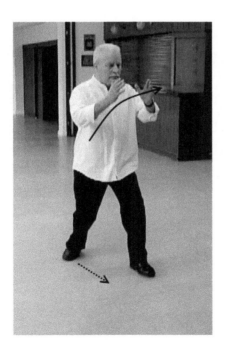

WOOD

The element of growth and art,
The roots that cleave the Earth apart,
The great Oak tree grows
With limbs so large and seeds to sow.
Those born in a Woody year
have fingers long and musical ear.
Perennial grows the carpet of grass
expanding shrubs and woods so vast.
Our bodies may be water and earth
but our growth is wood, constant from birth.
For humans multiply at alarming rate;
It's not always good to overpopulate.
Though this element is controlled by Fire
Wood stokes the flames of desire.
As ashes turn to new made earth;
from whence wood nestles to give birth.
Water nourishes the humble seeds
and from this another forest breeds.

T'ai Chi for Health?

You may well wonder why this title is used if T'ai Chi Ch'uan is supposed to be healthy for you anyway! In T'ien Ti Tao we have a variation of the Sun Family Form of T'ai Chi Ch'uan. Some may ask, "Why a variation?" Firstly, I was inspired by Dr. Paul Lam and his untiring work to better the health of his patients in his surgery in Australia, and then all around the world. Dr. Lam arrived in England for his first course on what he calls Tai Chi for Arthritis. This was in Oxford, October 2001. People arrived from all over the UK, some already practising various styles of T'ai Chi Ch'uan to varying degrees, some who had never done anything like it before. Out of the latter, some of these people were so badly stricken with arthritis that they were either in wheelchairs or using crutches. This course presented them with real hopes, they were desperate and the National Health Service had been unable to do anything for them to improve mobility; in fact many complained that all they were offered were drugs or wheelchairs!

The course began with Paul introducing himself and explaining how he came to realise the need for a programme based on T'ai Chi, as he calls it, that offered sufferers an exercise plan that was not so demanding as the full traditional T'ai Chi Ch'uan programme might be. Many of these sufferers would never be able to stand for such long periods and indeed, many on the course had to have a sit down after just ten minutes or so.

Everyone enjoyed the first weekend and some arthritis sufferers even felt energised and mild improvements to mobility after those two days; although also tired and aching, they were at least smiling and some proclaiming "It's not as painful as it was after doing that!" I studied the programme with interest and have great admiration for Dr. Paul Lam, Shih-fu. The follow up course just two years later, not far from Heathrow Airport, was a pleasant surprise indeed. Some of the arthritis sufferers who had turned up using crutches or in wheelchairs walked into the hall, unaided! The results that I witnessed were testimony to the need for an abbreviated Form of

T'ai Chi Ch'uan that was specifically aimed at people with health problems who possibly could not otherwise enjoy the benefits of the "full" system, especially if it had tight turning kicks and moves which might make them trip or fall.

After running a Tai Chi for Arthritis class for around five or six years I noticed that we had a variety of people with illnesses, disabilities and mobility problems. Further observations revealed that the results were indeed positive but also that the Form was lacking any strength building moves beyond "mild". Using my (then) 30+ years of experience in teaching I began to experiment with Ch'i Kung movements that pushed out the envelope. One Qigong exercise that I had already introduced was our "new and safer" variation of Baduanjin, the Eight Strands of Silk Brocade; this in itself offers strengthening movements, as well as opening up the meridians, toning the muscles, enhancing the nervous system, moving bile and fluids, increasing the body's ability to protect and promoting a healthier blood flow, to name but a few! Further improvements in the students were noted. Eventually, to cut a long story short, I began to meditate on how I could vary the Form. As this was based on Sun Style (Competition Form), which I had already converted back to "Family Style", being much more relaxed, the main problem was making it suitable for people with injuries, long term disabilities and various balance, mobility or skeletal problems. Eventually a new part was developed, this being in keeping with Sun Lu T'ang's original ideas on using Hsing- I, Pa Kua Ch'uan and T'ai hi Ch'uan. At first this had to be integrated into the existing Part One, Two and Three of the 'Tai Chi for Arthritis' Form (which by the way Paul has changed several times in several places since 2003). The new part was inserted as Part Three and the old part three moved out to become Part Four. This new section has a focus on balance and strengthening the lower body, working on balance control and agility.

Interestingly, at the same time as this development, Shih-fu John Bennett Jones in South Wales had studied the Sun Family Style with Dave Martin (UK & European Sun Family Representative; trained by

Sun, Jian Jun) and developed a Five Element Form of T'ai Chi for Health, which is also proving popular. He has now moved to a new Teacher, one of the Chinese "Sun Style inheritors" who was trained by Madam Sun.

Our new Part Three was taught carefully and elderly or vulnerable students were told to monitor their actions for any pain or indications of joint stress, etcetera. They were also told to moderate some of the harder movements, like "High Crane Kick" or "Dive for the Needle" whilst at the same time aiming to improve; students should always be encouraged to progress, rather than stagnate or accept small changes as the ultimate. The whole Form now makes a really good work-out and has strengthened the students who are all happy with it. As a later test, a year after this alteration, they were taught T'ai Chi Chih (Rule). This is a quite demanding Form and can be very hard work on the legs. The results were very good.

The class is till of mixed ability. Most of the members who joined over six years ago are still doing it and some of the ladies meet up at one or another's house during the week to practice their Forms and socialise at the same time. A couple have been made class assistants and one is going on to learn traditional Jingquanshitaijiquan and more Ch'i Kung. This is a very good result as far as I am concerned and cannot imagine that it is far different in China; with the exception that most people their already accept T'ai Chi Ch'uan as a health giving exercise; although, as can be seen of early morning parks, not all practice T'ai Chi Ch'uan, some do dance, aerobics, Ch'i Kung and many other exercises, medical or general.

Some Western traditional Form practitioners or teachers may think that there is no place for T'ai Chi for Health. There is and it is a very valuable place, especially in the Western culture. T'ai Chi for Health is a doorway in, with "ramps", for those who cannot take the full steps. Even those confined to wheelchairs can do something, perhaps even seated Baduanjin. This concept has never been seen in

China because until now anyone with a disability was hidden away from public view; much like they were in UK up until the 1970's.

Our Form name is copyright. Our Form and our full name is "T'ai Chi for Health; T'ien Ti Tao Sun Style Variation©". Again readers are reminded for their own safety and that of others do not attempt to learn this from a book or without a competent teacher. To protect the public we qualify Instructors with recognisable and traceable certificates which we advise students everywhere to check up on; we also have a Family Tree on our official web-site with current and "retired" Instructors names on: www.tttkungfu.com

The Health Benefits

The many health benefits of T'ai Chi Ch'uan have been known for hundreds of years in China but are only now being discovered by the rest of the world. Using movements extracted from the full Sun Family style, Dr Paul Lam (originally from China but now resident in Australia) created a new wave of T'ai Chi Ch'uan practice for those who are less able with his "Tai Chi for Arthritis" brand of exercise routine. This was so successful that he further developed routines for Diabetes sufferers, older people with mobility problems and even long distance air travellers. Some traditionalists amongst us might ask "Why bother? We already have several Forms of T'ai Chi Ch'uan. Let them do that instead!" We have to remember that the culture in the west, and even other parts of Asia, is different to that of China. Whereas many Chinese people grew up with the practice of T'ai Chi Ch'uan and Ch'i Kung in the streets, parks and probably in their family homes, we did not. A few years ago in the UK if you mentioned T'ai Chi to any older people here they might say either "What's that?" Or "Isn't that that funny sort of slow dance they do in China?" Dr Paul Lam originally told people that they could go and join classes wherever they lived, but he came under pressure from people who looked at Chen Style, for example, and shy away because of the low stances and stomping actions. Older people with arthritis, or other bone diseases, being told by western medicine to take it easy and not do anything drastic, for example, thought that such exercises were not for them. Paul's clever idea about extracting the safer movements brought these people in and made a big difference.

Within a few years of tiring world travel and much hard work, Paul's "new system" of 'Tai Chi for Arthritis' not only took off around the world but caused all sorts of sudden positive interest in the medical world. The South Koreans were amongst the first to publish medical test reports stating the benefits of his programmes to arthritis sufferers. Many others followed. This has led to a small but steady surge of acceptance and involvement amongst the otherwise "unchanging" Orthodox medical practitioners in the UK and elsewhere who still appear to be behind the times and lacking any form of preventative medicine, such as T'ai Chi for Health, to date.

Being a "traditionalist" myself, I do not see T'ai Chi for Health, as I call it, being a threat to other practises. What the CCG did and called "Competition Style" was more of a threat to the traditional styles as well as the health and progress of individual members of society. Instead I see it as a positive step forwards. Paul's programmes and great efforts have introduced T'ai Chi Ch'uan to a huge number of people that would otherwise never have got involved. Personally I saw people arrive on the first course in England in wheelchairs and using Crutches. On the second course, a year later, they were walking. That can only be a good thing. Whilst more needs to be done to make new instructors aware that they do not know everything about T'ai Chi Ch'uan or Ch'i Kung, let alone healing, I would heartily recommend that anyone, knowledgeable about T'ai chi Ch'uan or not, goes on at least one of Paul's courses to learn more about the needs of the infirm or elderly; and, by the way, if you think it's going to be very easy training, think again.

Jou T'sung-hua called Sun Style "a hodgepodge of Taijiquan, Xing-I Quan and Bagua Quan." That's exactly what I love about it!

Part One:

01 - Commencement Form.

Stand in Eagle Stance facing 12 O' Clock or South. The knees should be slightly bent and you should be in a completely relaxed state; relaxed but not "floppy". Enter Wu Chi.

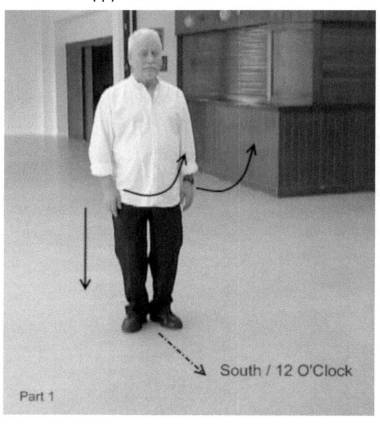

Part 1

South / 12 O'Clock

Sink the weight down when ready to commence by bending at the knees slightly more. Begin to raise your hands up in front of you as though playing basketball and about to take a shot at the hoop. As you bring your hands back towards the chest, raise height, then sink and lower again as you bring the hands down towards the hips. Transfer the weight to the right leg.

Step forward and slightly "South-East" with the left foot and as you transfer weight towards the left foot raise your hands as though passing a ball to someone.

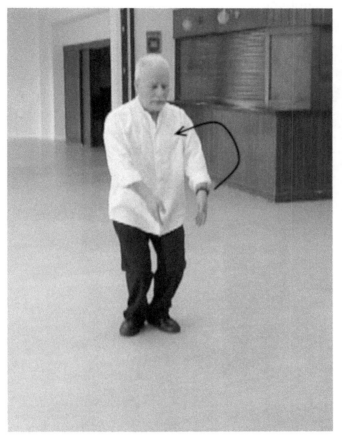

When the weight is safely balanced on the left leg, step forwards ("step up") with the right foot into Bear Stance (Feet shoulder's width apart) and then distribute the weight 50/50.

Do not forget to sink into the posture!

Opening (continued)

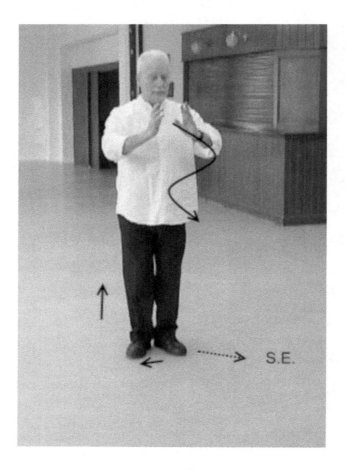

As you finish the Yin-Yang opening hand movements, sink your weight to your right leg and prepare to step slightly S.E., or towards 11 o'clock direction.

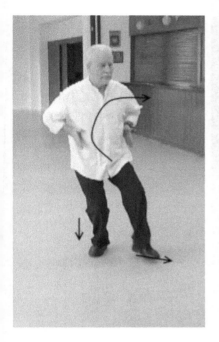

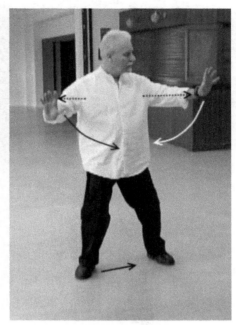

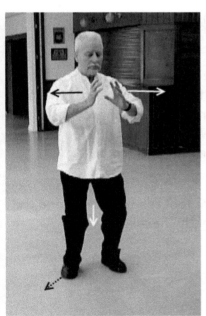

As you bring your hands back towards your waist, step forwards and perform what we call "offer the ball"; as though you are passing a basketball to someone in front of you (seen clearly in image above and right). Step up or "follow" with the right foot and transfer weight 50/50.

02 - Opening and Closing Hands

Bring both hands to upper chest height, fingertips pointing upwards to the ceiling. Gaze between the hands as you perform Open & Close; do this exactly as recommended by your instructor.

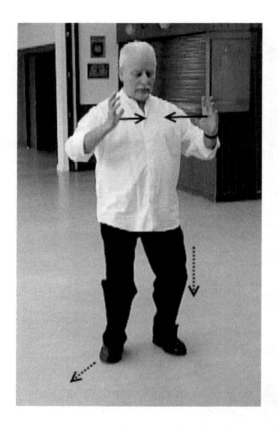

As you "close hands" sink your weight onto your left leg. You should feel that as you sink the weight onto the left leg the torso "twists" slightly clockwise and the heel of the right foot begins to lift slightly as the right leg becomes empty (non-weight bearing). Keep your back and pelvic muscles relaxed all the time!

Note: The image above shows the right foot ready to move and the dotted arrow indicates the direction of the next step.

03 - Single Whip (to right side)

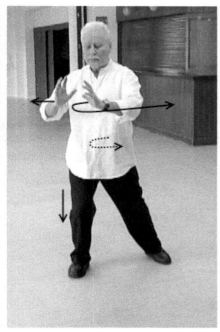

Step half-a-foot length forwards with the right foot, toes pointing directly ahead towards 12 o'clock. As you transfer the weight to the right foot, push the hands forward to a point just over the toes; the right knee should not be any further forwards than over the centre of the right foot.

The right hand then only does a short movement to the right side. The left hand does a larger movement to the left; this is done as though pasting a decorative wallpaper border strip onto a wall, on a flat plane, not in an arc! Keep the hands open and relaxed but fingers spread slightly.

As your arms part your weight should sink onto the right leg and your hips "settle" into a position just above the right leg. Let this happen naturally and do not try to force it. Keep the tailbone tucked in and do not lean forwards or stick your bottom out. The eyes should be looking at the left hand. This is the action that combines to give the "whip" like action in the name of the technique.

Feel the weight on the right leg and be aware of your knees. Never let the knees overextend; that is, do not allow it to go past your toes! For ultimate safety the knee should never go past the centre of the foot.

The illustration here is of Single Whip - Application, taken from Jingquanshitaijiquan, but the principle is the same. The feet must be firmly planted and the qi balanced so as not to be "double weighted" on the right side; you will have noticed that Shih-fu is looking at the left hand. Be aware of Yin and Yang at all times; in this instance the rights side is active.

As you finish Single Whip Right Side, centre and prepare for the next movement.

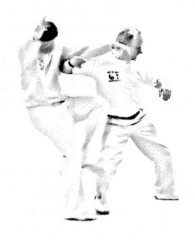

04 – Searching the Cloud

(3 steps to right side)

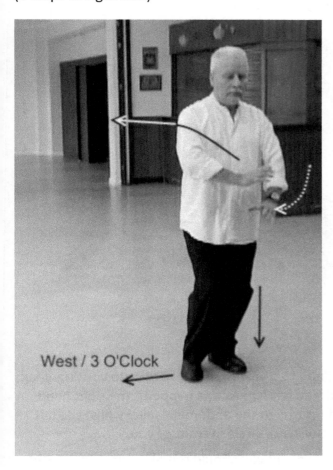

West / 3 O'Clock

After stepping in from Single Whip, transfer the weight to the left leg. Step out with the empty right leg, just one small step to the side; this is done as though edging sideways carefully along a ledge.

Bring your hands down to abdomen height, and then continue a clockwise sweep with the right hand as you step out on the right foot. It is important to remember to keep your weight on your left leg until you are sure that it is safe to place any weight upon your right leg.

Be careful not to "lean" over sideways as you move. Keep upright, as shown here. Also allow the waist to relax and turn naturally as you move from one direction to another.

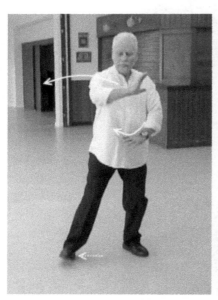 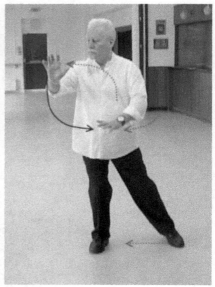

(04 Continued) Continue to transfer your weight onto your right leg and then step in with the left leg. As this happens, the right hand closes the circle and returns to the abdominal level whilst the left hand begins an anti-clockwise circle in front of you.

The eyes follow the hand and you should remain calm and relaxed throughout the whole movement.

Repeat the steps to the right so that you do three steps and six arm movements, like a Sky Dragon searching methodically for food amongst the clouds.

Allow the waist to sink and turn freely with each movement. In the lower-right illustration you can see how the head, torso and leg are "in-line" above the leading foot. Pay attention to balance. Readers will observe the background as an indication of the direction of movement. The arrows also indicate this: dotted lines may indicate the next movement.

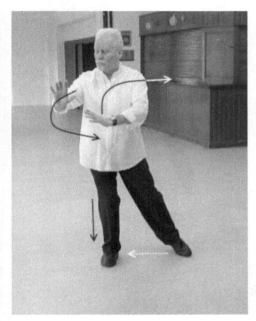 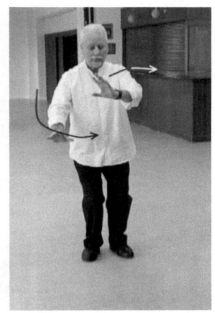

On the last step, as you bring your left foot in, you also bring your left hand around and back down and in towards the abdominal region. Allow your weight to sink in between the two feet so that you settle into Eagle Stance.

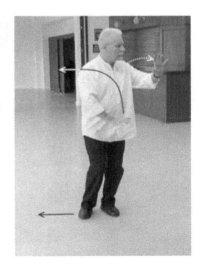

Slowly raise the hands to upper chest height as you prepare for the next movement. Continue for three "figure-of-eights".

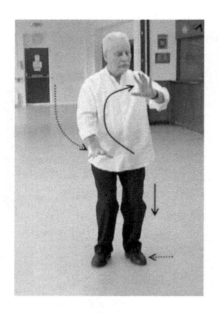

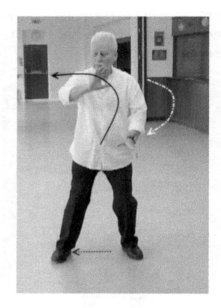

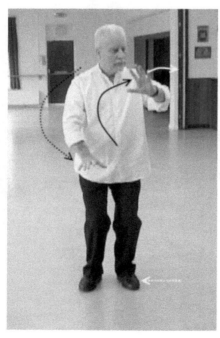

Be aware of your balance when stepping and do not drag your foot along the floor, raise it and "glide" over the floor about an inch high. Awareness should also be given to Yin and Yang plus keeping your posture relaxed and the weight sinking down.

As you finish this sequence bring in your left foot, sink the weight down 50/50 and prepare for the next Form or "technique".

05 - Opening and Closing Hands.

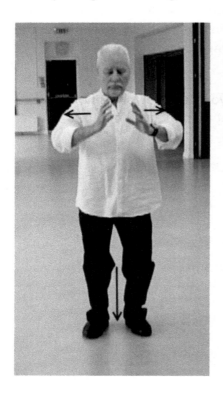 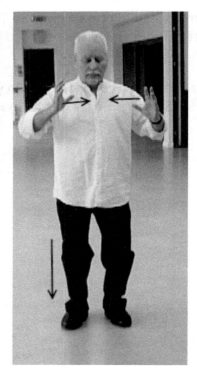

Open and Close hands was originally included by Sun Lu'tang to create more Ch'i Kung in his Form, according to one story about him. He also taught the self-defence applications to this; a sign of good mastery when someone can see applications in just about any movement! Shih-fu Sun was acknowledged as being the first public Master to teach women's self-defence too; although a system was traditionally handed down from mother to daughter, some say.

When performing Open and Close hands, keep the eyes focused between the hands. The weight, shown here by an arrow pointing downwards, should be lowered slightly through the hips, knees and feet, but do not lower the whole body; generally in T'ai Chi Ch'uan, one lowers his or her weight at the beginning of the Form and stays on that same plane, with the exception of some movements where a bend or dip is inevitable.

As you open, you should feel a slight resistance as though your hands were tied by a weak elastic band. As you close there should be a resistance again but this time like squeezing a large sponge or piece of foam. You will notice that the chest expands greatly, but not "forced", in this movement, enhancing the oxygenation of the body; itself a great health giver, as long as you are not in a dusty or fume filled atmosphere! Always exercise where there is clean air (see the book 'Qigong & Baduanjin' for further advice and more detail on this subject.)

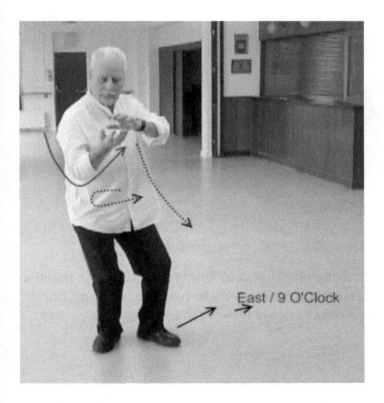

East / 9 O'Clock

06 - Brush Knee and Twist Step (leftwards)

As you "close hands" lower your weight to your right leg and when the left foot is empty and your balance good, step out with your left foot towards the 9 o'clock direction or East.

Your right hand begins to move forward as if holding a ball that you are offering to someone standing at 12 o'clock; palm upwards, arm relaxed; do not over-reach. Your left hand begins the "brush knee" movement.

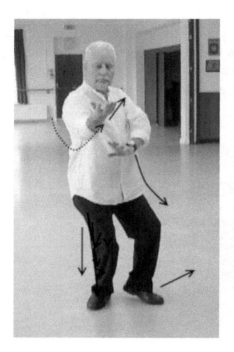 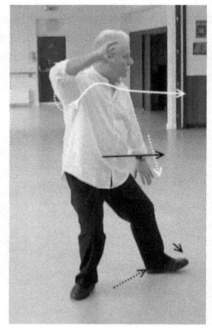

As you step left, make sure that your feet are not too close together. Shih-fu's tip: "Step as though stepping to two sides of a box, but make sure your balance is good on your supporting leg. Sink and relax!"

Bring your right hand up to the Temple as your left hand swings down to the side of the left thigh. The white arrow here shows the movement the right hand makes. The dotted arrow shows the left hand movements. The black arrow is your general direction of movement; as you move forwards to the East.

As you continue forwards to the East or 9 o'clock direction do not make the common mistake of "bobbing up and down", stay level but also stay relaxed and let the waist sink and keep the hips relaxed, letting them "settle" into place. Complete the movement with "Follow Step" (white short arrows).

You end up with your weight almost all on the leading foot and well balanced.

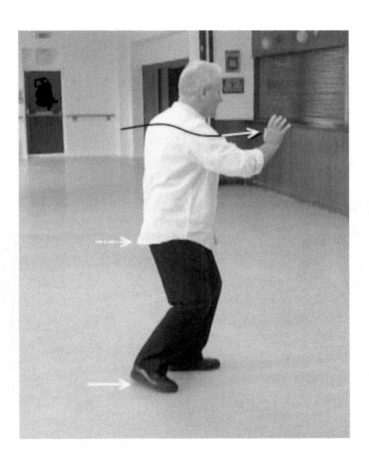

07 - Playing the Lute.

Step back with the right foot more or less to where it was previously, but with the toes pointing rightwards. Sink your weight into the right leg as you lightly withdraw the left foot - left foot forwards in Cat Stance. Your left hand comes forwards and your right hand comes back, level with left elbow, as though "strumming a lute". Shih-fu's tip: Look down with the eyes, do not tilt the head. Keep your shoulders relaxed and remain centred."

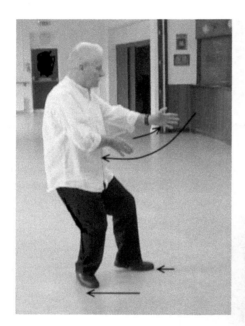

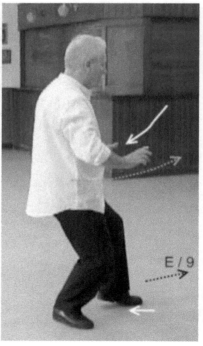

Your empty left foot goes forwards and the toes point outwards. Your weight sinks and spirals forwards as you push from the rear leg. The right hand comes forwards, as though you are holding a book out to read. The black arrows show the directions of waist, foot and hand. The dotted arrow indicates the next step.

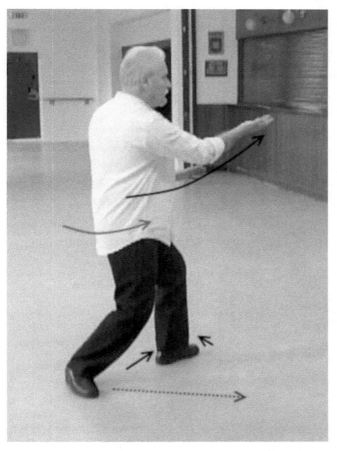

Shih-fu's comment: "The Flat Walk is a great inclusion as it enables more secure stepping, as well as other factors. The player should resist the temptation to speed up here but instead pay special attention to posture and control. "

Continue stepping forward placing the weight onto the left leg and stepping through with the right leg, toes outwards. Bring the left hand through in the same manner as the right hand in the last movement. As you can see from the illustration, the rear hand is level with the elbow of the lead hand.

The dotted arrow shows the next step.

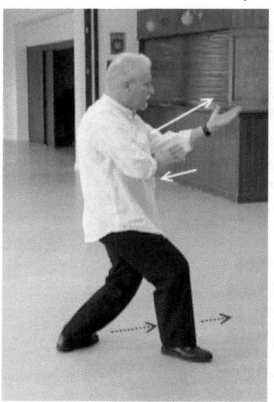

Shih-fu's Tip: "Stay upright, as usual, and do not overreach when punching. Keep the waist relaxed and lead from the Tan T'ien as you do these movements. If you are uncertain as to whether or not you are doing any movement correctly, please ask your instructor to look at you and give guidance; do not build mistakes into the Form."

Prepare for the next move by folding your right hand over left and then down, back towards your body as you prepare to step back into Cat Stance (step back towards the West).

09 - Step Forward to Deflect Downwards, Parry and Punch

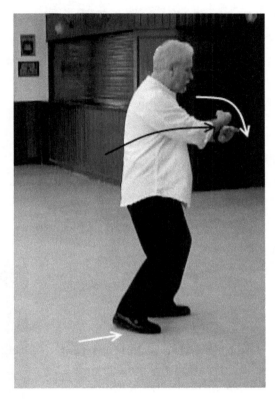

Stepping through with your left foot, into a normal stance, parry with the left hand and punch over the wrist with the right "Beauteous Fist". Step up the right foot in Follow Step as you deliver the punch.

As you can see from the picture above, you have covered some two to three yards/metres in this "advancing step" sequence.

10 - Embrace the Tiger & Pushing the Mountain. This follows the "Cover and punch" movement and, like all other movements, flows continuously from one to the other.

From the punch, wrap your top hand around the lower wrist, almost as though you were going to fold your arms. Allow the "active" hand to go around the lower wrist, all the way around, until both hands appear to be palm upwards. Spread the hands as though accepting a tray to carry.

After "wrapping" the wrists, bring your hands out as though you are going to lightly grip two handrails to pull yourself along by. This is accompanied by a withdrawal into Left Cat Stance as you step back and separate the two hands, bringing them back to just in front of the waist (as in second illustration).

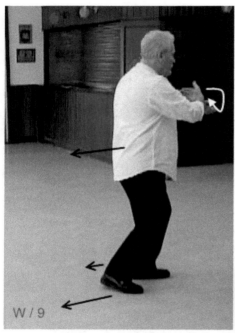

The follow step is an important consideration for elderly and those suffering from balance problems. This is why Dr. Paul Lam originally decided to use the Sun ("Soon-g") style T'ai Chi Ch'uan for his variation of the Form for health.

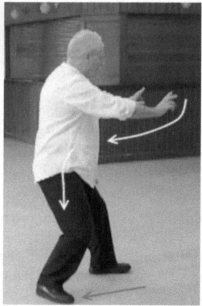

Without leaning forwards or backwards, convert the "draw back" into a push and step forwards with "follow step", as indicated in the picture on this page, and push.

In Taijiquan the push is not done with the arms, as most people instinctively think, but with the whole body moving forwards and the arms acting like a frame; like the "bumper" or "fender" on a vehicle.

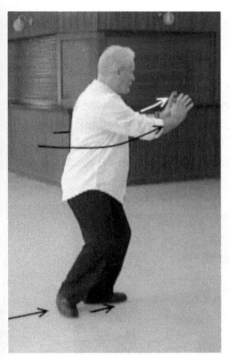

The previous illustrations above show the second part, "...return to the mountain". The "push" is done with the step, not with the arms. I always liken this to pushing a car or, as it used to be called in less reliable transport days, "Bump starting". The legs are used to deliver power whilst the arms act as the buffer or focal point for the push action.

Remember that the Dantian must be kept leading at all times, the centre of gravity low and the mind focused on the job at hand.

There are two versions of what "Embrace the Tiger and Return to the Mountain" means. In one, you are receiving an aggressive attack, like a ferocious tiger's rush, and neutralising it. In another, it is suggested, that you are embracing your own spirit and returning to Wu Tang!

After "embracing the tiger", step forwards with your left foot as though pushing at chest height. Perform a follow step (as illustrated here). At no time should you raise your head level; in other words you stay on the same plane as you go backwards and forwards.

Finishing off Section One:

11 - Opening and Closing Hands.

Bring your weight onto your left leg after the "push" and begin turning towards the starting direction or 12 o'clock. Pivot the right heel inwards, towards the left foot, and when in place sink your weight mainly to the right leg/foot. Pivot the left toes inwards, so that you face 12 o'clock in Eagle Stance and perform Open & Close Hands, slowly.

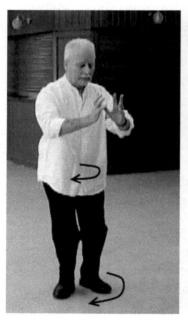 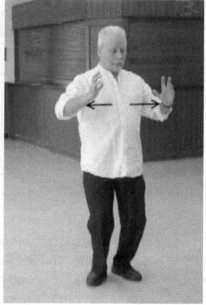

Remember to focus your eyes between the hands and "feel" the resistance as you both open and close them. Sink your weight down through the hips into the feet and bring the weight distribution back to 50/50.

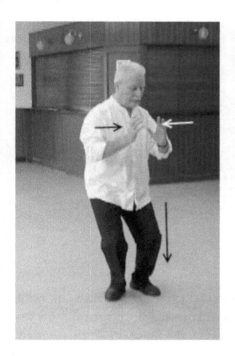 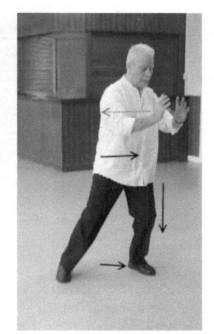

Part Two:

12 - Single Whip (to the left side)

As you close your hands, drop your weight to the right foot and prepare to step out leftwards with the left foot.

 In performing Single Whip, left style, make sure that you only place your left foot forwards just a half-length ahead of the right. The toes should point forwards. At first the eyes gaze between both hands, then as you step and separate the hands the eyes follow the right hand.

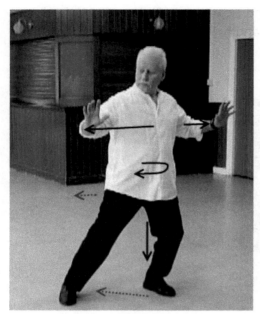

The eyes follow the right hand as you open the hands. It is important to know where to look and what to do with your ch'i/qi. Ask your Teacher for advice when you have learned the Form well enough not to worry about the movements.

Shih-fu's Tip: Do not overextend the right hand. Take it to the right in a straight line, as though fixing a decorative border to the wall with paste and smoothing it with your right palm. Keep the weight above the left leg and do not lean sideways or forwards. Allow your weight to sink and settle.

At the end of Single Whip, Withdraw the left foot after and place both your feet into Eagle Stance, but leave a small gap between them. Bring the hands together in front of your chest.

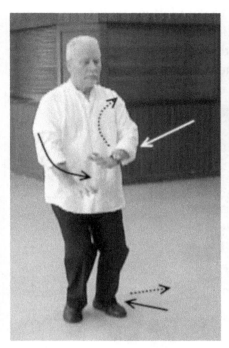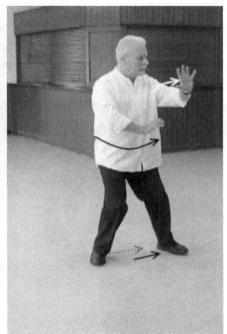

13 - Searching the Clouds (3 steps to left side)

(Above left) Prepare the left hand for a block and at the same time bring the right foot in towards the left foot, leaving a small gap, as previously stated. (Above right) Step to the left as you begin the first "Searching the Clouds" left style.

The hand movements are impossible to illustrate in full by a photograph, but the hands perform a "figure of eight" type circular returning motion; by "returning" it is meant they return to the centre after each circular sweep; as illustrated by my right hand here in the above left picture.

Continue to transfer all the weight to your left leg whilst withdrawing the right foot. In this illustration the white arrow represents the movement or direction of the left hand whilst the black arrow represents the movement and direction of the right hand.

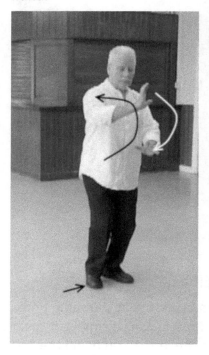 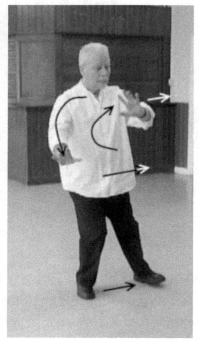

(Above left) The short black arrow, on the floor, is showing you that the right foot has just been withdrawn inwards.

(Above right) Transfer the weight to your right foot and step out leftwards, as though sliding sideways along a narrow ledge. Make a "sweep" with your left hand as you step left, then close your right in as you step your right foot inwards (close).

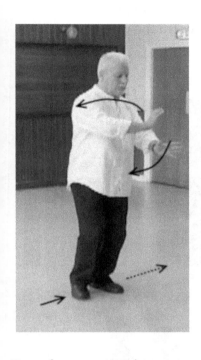

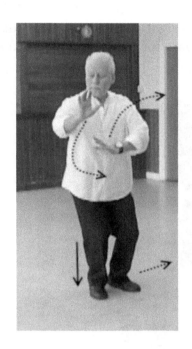

Transfer your weight to your right foot and step left again, performing the same technique. It is important that you keep your weight low and knees bent! The waist remains loose and relaxed.

Remember to keep the hands open and the palm curved with fingers lightly spread; "The beauteous palm" as the Chinese call it.

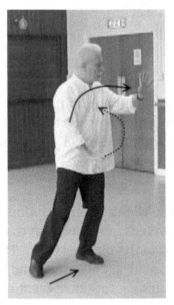

Finishing off "Search the Clouds" after three complete cycles with the weight ending on a leftwards step. Centre the weight as you prepare for "Open and Close Hands".

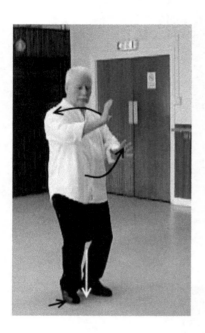 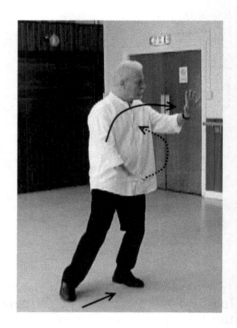

Always remember that when you move, your ch'i moves. When you centre, your ch'i centres also. The action is like moving water, it flows and then settles flows and settles. When it settles it seeks a lower level.

Just like all the other techniques in T'ai Chi Ch'uan, the Cloud Hands is "blended", meaning that there is more than one application going on within the obvious Form. This, like Nature, is one of the wonders of original T'ai Chi Ch'uan and is, like Yin/Yang and the Wu Hsing, a never ending source of creation.

14 - Opening and Closing Hands (image on right.)

Come in to "centre" from your third Search the Clouds step. Perform Open & Close hands as you have done before.

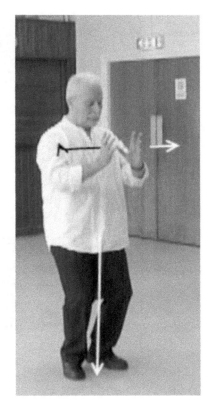

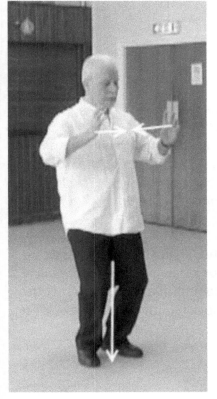

This qigong technique helps you to centre and relax, as well as generate more energy throughout the Form; Sun Lu'tang included this technique specifically for health purposes in his original Form (Sun Style 97 Forms).

15 - Brush Knee and Twist Step (1st time step to face right or West)

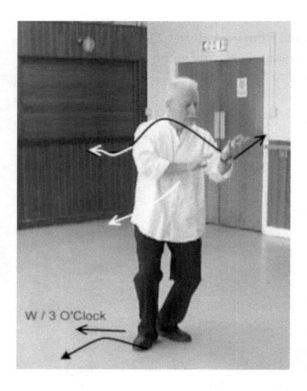

W / 3 O'Clock

From Open and Close Hands, transfer the weight to your left foot. As you close your hands, act as if rolling a ball anti-clockwise, then extend the left hand as though holding the ball out to the front. As you left arm extends, the right hand begins to move backwards and slightly down, as though stroking your left arm.

Sink your weight onto the left foot and begin stepping rightwards with the right foot. This step should be done as though stepping from one side (say, South) of a square floor tile to the other (North) and will take you to face from 12 o'clock (South) to 3 o'clock (West), body-wise.

Shih-fu's Tip: Look at the left hand as it extends.

As you lower your weight to your left leg, the hips should sink and twist or "corkscrew" as the weight transfers. Stay level and do not bob up or down.

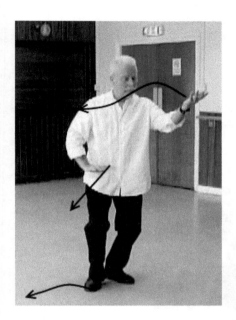

As you step to the right, bring your left hand up towards the temple are of the head. Your right hand performs "Brush Knee" and you begin shifting your weight to your right leg.

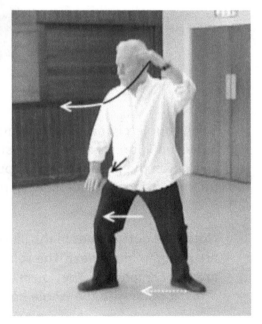

(Brush Knee and Twist Step - continued)

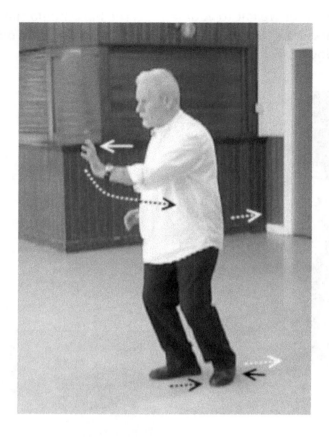

Bring your left hand forwards and down - following the illustration above until it rests at upper chest height. At no time must you fully straighten the arms when you "push". As you perform the push, step up the left foot with a follow step.

Note: The dotted lines in the illustration above show you where you are going to move next. The solid arrows indicate the movement you are just completing. The "push" in Taijiquan is never done with the arms, it done with the whole body movement.

16 - Playing the Lute (Right Cat - right foot forwards to 3 o'clock)

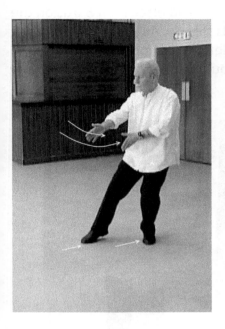 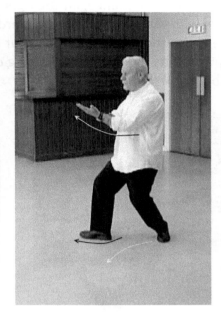

Step back to 'Play the Lute'. Place the weight onto the right foot and step backwards and slightly to the side with the left foot; more or less taking the left foot to where it was before the follow step in Brush Knee and Twist Step (previous move).

As you step back into Right Cat Stance, bring your left hand back to in front of the abdomen and your right hand back too (as in picture above left).

(Picture above right: beginning "Blocking and Closing")

Shih-fu's tip: Always make sure that you step back safely, being aware of where you put your feet and how you place them. Keep the weight above (centred) one leg, the supporting leg, and do not lean over in one direction; stay upright.

17 - Blocking & Closing (two steps).

From Right Cat Stance, lift the right foot and place it forwards on the heel with the toes pointing outwards slightly. As you transfer your weight to the right foot, bring your left fingers forwards, palm upwards, as though slowly holding out your hand to show somebody a book (picture above right).

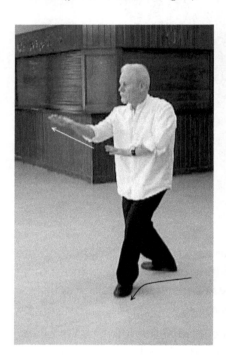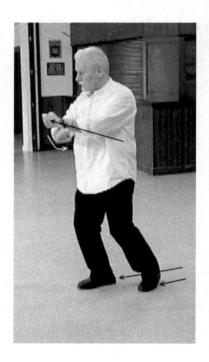

Shih-fu's Tips: Lead with the abdomen as you "slide" your weight forwards. Be calm, relax and concentrate.

Continue by stepping through with your left foot, placing it on the heel in a similar manner to the last step. As you transfer the weight forwards, onto the left foot, bring your right palm forwards as though offering a book for someone to look at; do not overextend the arm.

Do not be tempted to speed up during movements like these. The objective is to do the whole Form as slowly as possible with full concentration on each individual technique.

18 - Step Forward to Deflect Downwards, Parry and Punch (left hand punch – picture above right).

Bring your right hand over and down in front of you in an arc as you step through with your right foot; do not "toe out"! As you pat down, gently form a "beauteous fist" with the left hand and punch over the right forearm, but not too far. Your left foot steps up in a half-step or follow through step.

19 - Embrace the Tiger & Return to the Mountain.

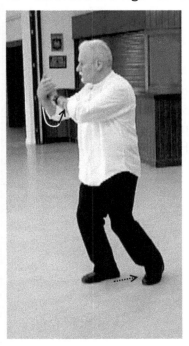 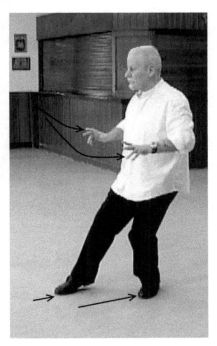

Step back into Right Cat stance and wrap your left hand around your right wrist, then bring your hands back towards you as you withdraw; palms downwards(pictured above). Make sure that you step back safely and place all your weight onto your left leg so that you are well balanced.

Lower the hands slightly before stepping the right foot forwards and then pushing forwards in an upwards arc. Do not raise your head height. Perform a follow step as you reach the forward position.

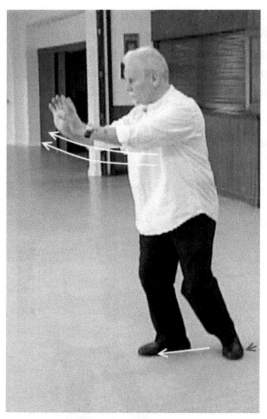

As you finish the push, prepare to turn again to the South or 12 o'clock, and perform Open and Close Hands.

20 - Open and Close Hands (facing 12 o'clock).

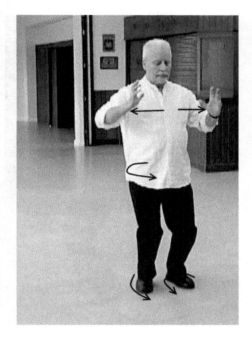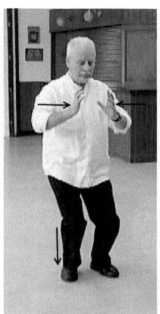

Transfer weight to left foot, pivot inward the right foot. Perform Open and Close Hands.

Drop the weight to Right Foot on Close if you are about to begin Part 3 of the Form, otherwise keep the weight central and perform the "centring" routine. This concludes Part 2 of the Form.

Shih-fu says: This is one of my favourite techniques of Sun Style. It shows part of the essence of T'ai Chi Ch'uan and is a shining example of Yin and Yang; the two equal but opposite forces. In higher levels, the use of energy in "earthing" and other methods are very clearly felt. This and "yee" (I) are very satisfying in this simple but effective technique.

Part Three:

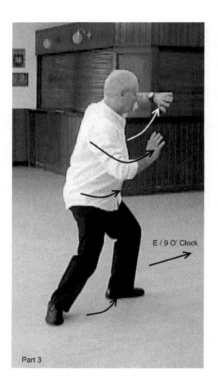 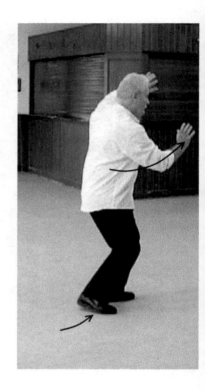

21 - Step back "East" with your empty left foot using "Diagonal Step", and as you step towards the 9 o'clock direction, swing both arms up as illustrated below. Perform Working the Shuttles (Sun Style).

When performing this technique do not raise the shoulders or swing too far or too fast. Stay at the same slow pace as before.

22- Follow through with the right foot stepping forwards as you execute the Hsing-I Double Punch/Block formation (illustrated on next page).

Anyone with a background in Hsing-I Ch'uan will automatically know this form. It is a pleasure to perform and is included here because it opens up the chest and armpit cavities. Many of the movements like this also encourage better blood flow, especially in the arms and hands; this is where many older people feel cold because of poor circulation.

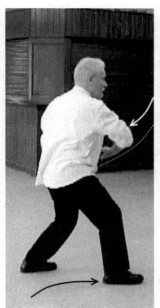 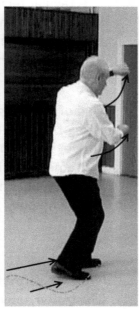 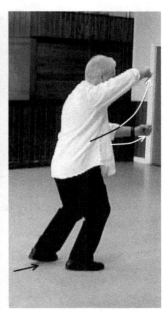

(Continued on next page)

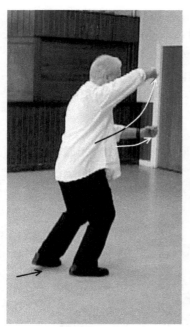

This concludes 'Hsing-I Block and Punch' double step. For better technique the steps employ "Flat walk" from the Hsing-I repertoire.

As you perform this unique and spectacular technique, keep your weight down and glide the feet forwards planting the lead foot firmly as you approach the end.

One of the things I love most about Hsing-I (Xing-yee) is the feeling of "drive" as you power through the movements. This has similarities with most T'ai Chi Ch'uan Forms where the power can be clearly felt in each technique.

23 - Snake Darts Out:

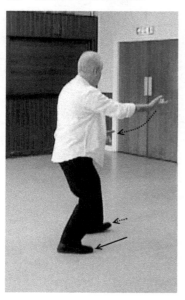

From the second Hsing-I technique (illustrated above) take a half-step back with your right foot and as you do so hold out the right palm; as though somebody is giving you something. Then step back a half-step with the left foot, extend Left Hand, palm-up….

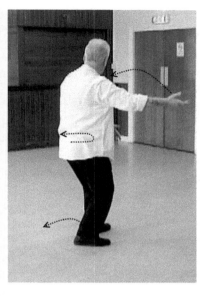

...then step forward bringing Right palm under Left; a bit like being in a tugging contest and you reach forward to get some more rope! Step back again taking the weight onto your right leg, the right hand is still forwards and the left hand near the right elbow.

...then take your left foot to the left (6 o'clock or North direction) using a diagonal step. Your left hand comes around towards the left hip and the right hand comes down in an arc (see white arrow on illustration above and right) to lower abdomen level. End up in Kneeling Stance (body facing toward 6 o'clock).

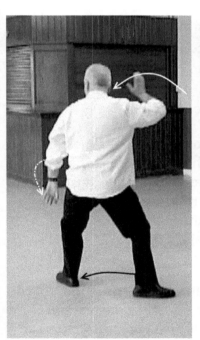

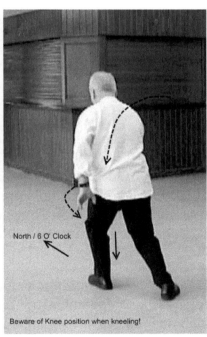

North / 6 O' Clock

Beware of Knee position when kneeling!

Shih-fu's Tip: Do not, under any circumstances, lean forwards as you execute the last part of this technique. Remain upright and balanced, calm and composed. It is also of paramount importance that you step back as far as possible so that when the left knee is bent it only comes forward over the centre of the left foot; otherwise knee strain and cartilage injury is possible.

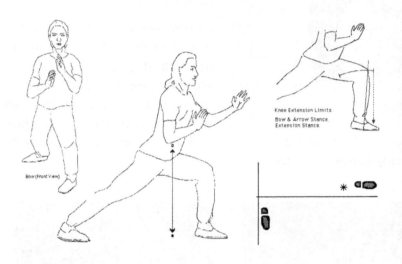

Maintaining good knee positioning is something that almost every Chinese Martial Art or Health Exercise has in common. Above you will see that 'Bow and Arrow' stance has been used to illustrate correct position and relationships. The relationship of the head, shoulders, elbows, hands, waist/hips, knees and feet are of paramount importance in the Art of T'ai Chi Ch'uan.

As stated earlier: **Do not** attempt to learn any exercise form from a book. You need a competent instructor whose experience and credentials need to be checked for credibility. Poor instructors can unwittingly cause injury, so the public need to be aware and wary.

Students may also cause self-injury by not listening to or following advice properly.

24 - Stand up and bring Left foot back to Bear, perform Open and 'Open and Close Hands'. Stand up and push back from your right foot to bring your weight back. Form Bear Stance and perform Open and Close Hands.

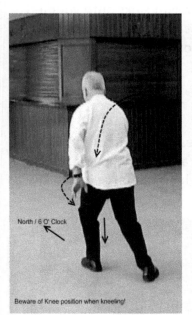

North / 6 O' Clock

Beware of Knee position when kneeling!

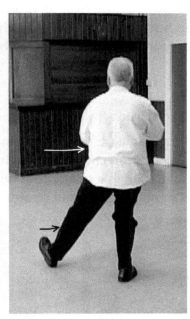

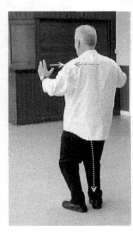

Weight is on the left foot, so use this to push backwards into Bear Stance. Perform Open and Close Hands. On closing, lower your weight onto your right leg and, for comfort and ease of movement, slightly turn out your left leg and allow your body to sink and twist anti-clockwise.

When beginning the next movement, the left hand will be in front of the right hand and the hands will perform a small arc outwards; like describing a rainbow.

Shih-fu's Advice:

When pushing back try not to go too quickly, do not raise your body height too much or straighten the leg, otherwise you may lose balance.

When finishing the Close Hands, shift most of your weight to your left foot (knee bent) and allow the torso to sink into the hips and the hips to turn slightly to the right as your weight sinks onto your left leg. (Pictured bottom right) Let your right hand come in front of the left as you prepare for the "paint a rainbow" movement in prelude to the kick.

25 - Perform Left Crane Kick (3 o'clock).

The more fit or supple you are determines the height of the kick. Technically the kick can come up as high as chest height as the hand "slaps" the shin. If unable to kick that high do not force it, just kick as high as you can manage without strain.

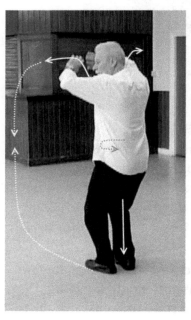 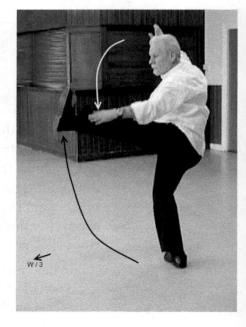

Shih-fu's Tip: It is within everyone's interest to remain as fit and as supple as you can possibly be. By regular stretching you will decrease risk of illness, injuries and stiffness of muscles and joints. Most people think about stretching the muscles but there are "hidden" benefits under the skin such as making the blood vessels more "elasticised" and stronger. Regular stretching helps blood flow and the nervous system, massages the internal organs and improves general mobility.

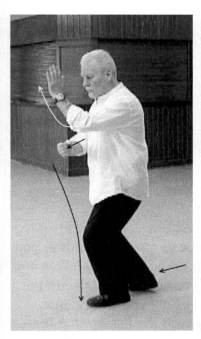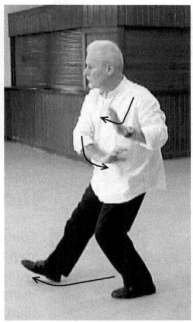

Place Left foot forward towards the 3 o'clock direction (West). Half-step forwards with Hidden Punch Under Left Elbow as you perform a half-step (picture above left).

26 - Follow through with 'Working the Shuttle', Right style.

From the previous position, continue to step forwards (pictured above right) and slightly out (leaving space between the feet both ways) to the right. Let your arms swing through, slowly, in an arc whilst turning the right palm outwards, as though covering your eyes from the sun.

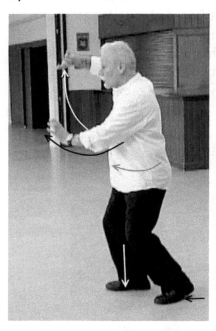

Continue the forward arc until your left hand rests at chest level and your right hand is at shoulder level. Do not raise or tense the shoulders. Relax the shoulders, waist and arms as much as possible.

27 - Execute Hsing-I Block & Punch.

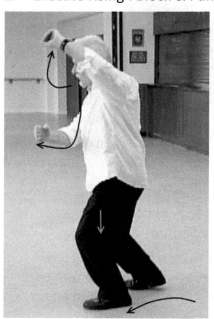

Continue to move forwards as you step through with the left foot and swing your arms through into the Hsing-I ("Xing-yee") technique. Lightly curls the fists so that there is no tension in the arms. Perform a half-step as you complete the technique.

Continue this same action but "mirrored" on the other side, stepping through with your right foot and follow step (half-step).

Keep the action at the same pace as all previous movements and do not speed up as you swing through or step!

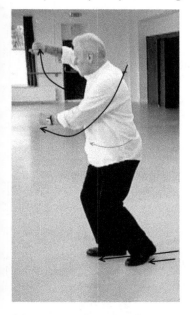 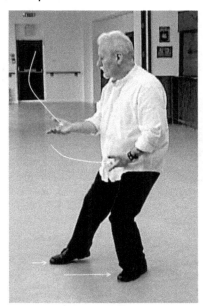

28 - Venomous Snake Darts Out (Picture above right).

Step back a half-step, extend Right Hand, palm-up (as shown top left) and the left hand withdraws to just in front of the Tan T'ien ("Dantian").

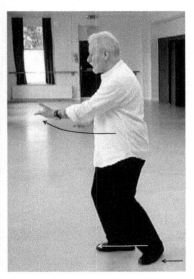

Then step forward bringing the Left palm under Right and forwards: as though you are pulling a rope and stepping forwards in order to get a better grip to pull back with.

Step back, being careful not to lean or trip, and hold the hands (next page) with the left hand forward most and the right hand level with the left elbow.

Take the weight onto your left leg, and then step right, to 6 o'clock (North) into Kneeling Stance as you bring your Left hand over in an arc to floor (6 o'clock).

Heed the previous advice about knee positions!

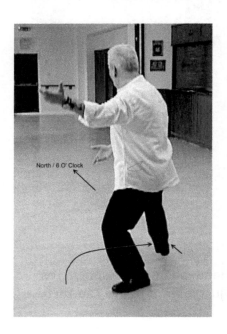
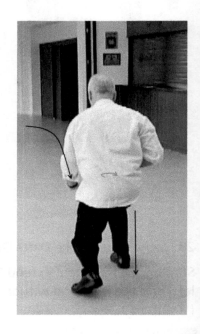

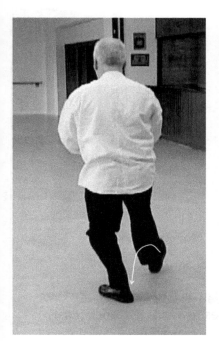
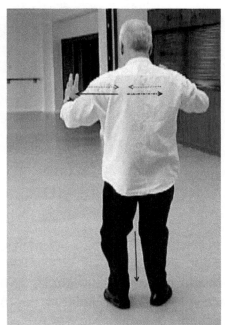

Step back by pushing with your lead foot and perform 'Open and Close Hands'.

30 - Right Crane Kick (9 o'clock) in 'Wu Style'.

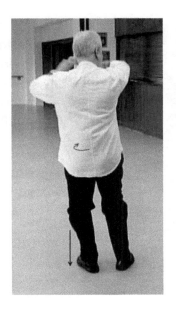

406

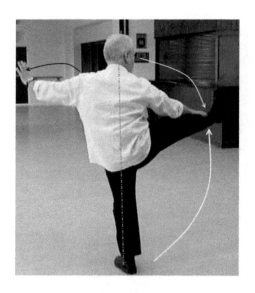
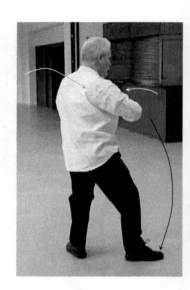

Turn and kick with your right leg as high as you can manage then place your foot down pointing the toes towards 3 o'clock (East) direction.

Note: follow the same advice as for the other side as well as your teacher's personal recommendations.

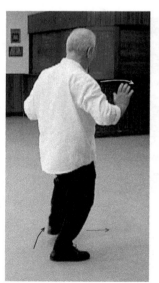

31 - Dive for Needle at Sea Bottom.

Perform Left Toe Kick towards 8 o'clock (below right), then place foot forwards toward 3 o'clock. Your hands are slightly apart and in front of your chest; as though holding a small ball.

Note: Make sure you step forwards as far as you comfortably can. This is to protect the knee when you "dip" down!

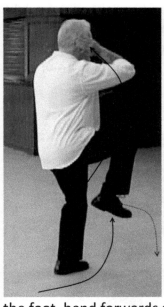 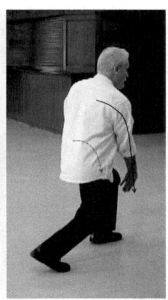

Kneel as though picking up something from just below your left knee. Do not over-extend the knee! Do not lean forwards either.

32 - Needle at Sea Bottom. Left foot is in the lead. Keeping the knee over the foot, bend forwards as though going to rub the inside of your right leg with your left hand; do not actually touch the leg and do not "lean" off-balance!

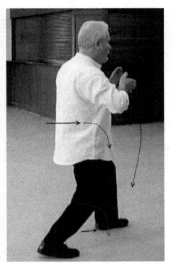

Push from your front foot to stand up straight (right knee remains crooked) and as you stand up raise your right hand covering your ear; do not actually touch the ear (see illustration on left).

This movement should be accompanied by the toes pointing downwards on the raised leg.

This technique was introduced to give more dynamic physical exercise values to the Form. Most people, especially as they get older, do not do as much physical work as they used to. This technique will help strengthen the knees, back and "open" the upper chest cavity.

As you return to the upright position you stand upright on your right leg to repeat the same technique on the other side. Stand firmly on your right leg and raise the left knee, toes pointing down, and the left hand beside the left ear. The right hand remains in front of your chest.

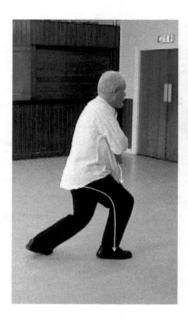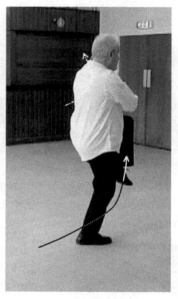

Perform "Needle at Sea Bottom" again, this time keeping your weight on your left leg as you "dip" to the "sea bottom". As you stand up, place your right foot down and transfer weight to it so that you are able to pivot the left foot on the heel bringing the toes around to point to 10 o'clock. When this is done, transfer weight to the left foot and pivot the right toes outwards.

33 - Turn to face 12 o'clock and perform Open and Close Hands, then continue to flow into the next movement.

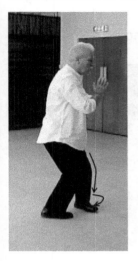 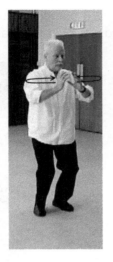 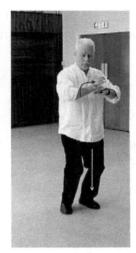

34 – As you finish, drop your weight onto your left leg. You may wish to turn the left toes inwards a little in preparation. Execute a Right Toe Kick towards 2 o'clock. At the end of Open and Close Hands, transfer the weight to your left foot and bring your left hand in front of your right. Perform "Paint the Rainbow" with your hands, only in a small arc, and then toe-kick to ankle height with the right foot. Place the Right foot forwards and right so as to turn towards 3 o'clock direction. (As shown in right picture)

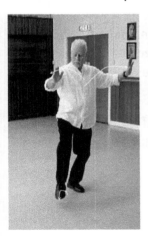 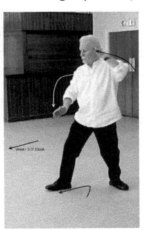

Note: Please be careful of twisting or pivoting, especially with older people or those with arthritis, etc. Instructors need to know how to guide a person through detailed pivoting techniques to avoid injuries caused by wrong weighting.

35 - Needle at Sea Bottom (Right style). Transfer the weight to the right leg. Keeping the knee over the foot, bend forwards as though going to rub the inside of your right leg with your left hand; do not actually touch the leg and do not "lean" off-balance!

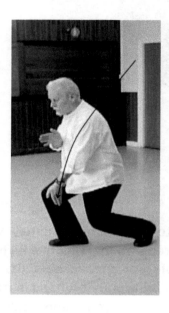 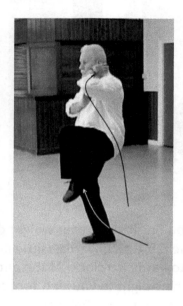

As you return to the upright position you stand upright on your right leg to repeat the same technique on the other side. Stand firmly on your right leg and raise the left knee, toes pointing down, and the left hand beside the left ear. The right hand remains in front of your chest. Perform "Needle at Sea Bottom" again, making sure that balance and control are all correct and the knees are "protected".

Then perform Golden Cock (Sun Style), as you stand up, placing your left hand near to your left ear as shown in the illustrations on the left. Repeat the other side.

36 -Opening and Closing Hands.

As you step the right foot down from "Needle at Sea Bottom", pivot on the right heel to bring your toes pointing to 2 o'clock. Then pivot the left toes to face 10 o'clock, so you end up facing the 12 o'clock or South direction in Eagle Stance. Perform Open and Close Hands as you conclude Part Three of the Form. On "close", drop weight to left leg, body turns slightly right.

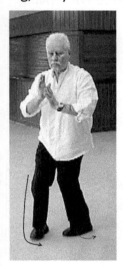

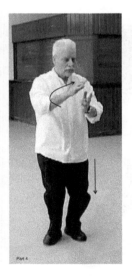

Note: The illustration left shows the blending of part three into part four opening as you convert Open and Close Hands to Brush Knee and Twist Step, sinking your weight to the left leg this time.

Part Four.

37 - Brush Knee Twist Step.
From Eagle Stance transfer weight to left leg as you rotate the hands and "offer the ball" with your left hand.

Step your right foot out to the 3 o'clock direction and perform "Brush Knee and Twist Step". This ends with the Follow Step and Push. This time, hold the weight on the right leg, instead of moving backwards as you did in Part One of the Form.

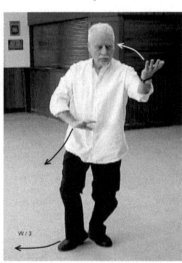
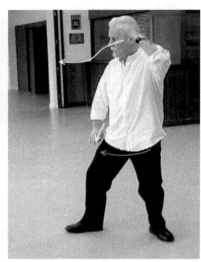
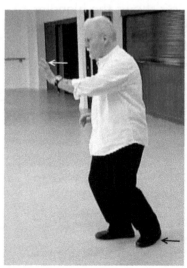
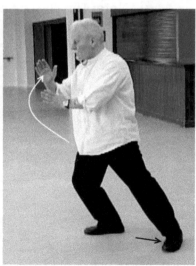

38 - Too Lazy to Tie Coat (Right side). Hold the Weight on the front leg. Step the left foot backwards (picture below left), at the same time bring your left hand backwards and down (as shown) and your right hand upwards and forwards.

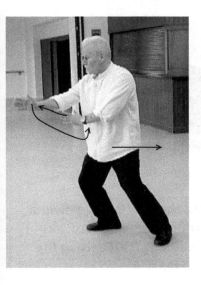 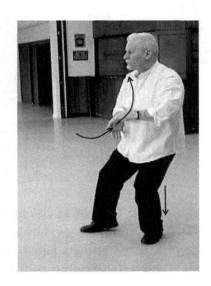

Take the weight back and place the left "sword Fingers" upon the right wrist - this part of the technique is known as "fixing the sleeves" - as you step back to Cat Stance. Bring the hands in towards the Tan T'ien as you do this.

Bring your right palm, with left Sword Fingers attached, up the centre line and up to chin level. Turn the fingers outwards as you take your weight back onto your right leg - the left leg and foot forms Monkey Stance - and look at your right palm as you turn; use only a slight waist movement and do not lean backwards or sideways! (See images above.)

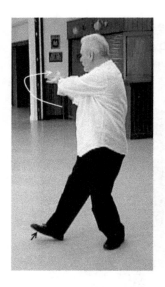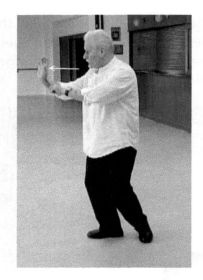

Bring your palm upright as you push from the rear leg to deliver a palm-strike at shoulder level by transferring your weight to your right leg (pictured above). Finish the movement "Lazily fixing the sleeves" with a Half-Step up with your left leg.

This whole movement must be done smoothly and without any loss of balance – do not lean - or concentration.

Learning the applications will greatly enhance anyone's understanding of the Form. The technique above known as "Too Lazy to Tie the Coat and Fix the Sleeves" contains at least two basic applications; I say "at least two" because you could fit in more than two! However, like most Taijiquan sets, the techniques blend together seamlessly, often disguising their true meaning.

39 - Opening and Closing Hands (Turn to 12 o'clock)

From the last position, transfer weight to left foot and pivot to face 12 o'clock. Perform Open and Close Hands as you have done before.

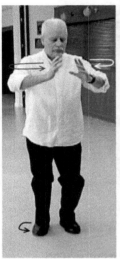 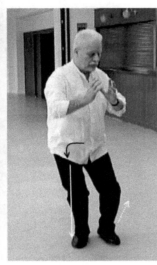

Shih-fu's notes:

The inclusion of this movement from simple Ch'i Kung (Qigong) by Sun Lu'tang was a master stroke. His original intention was said to be to create a suitable style of T'ai Chi Ch'uan for health as well as being practical for self-defence by women and men of all ages in China. This movement, although leaning towards the "health" side in obvious terms, has also got very practical applications in self-defence, so nothing is wasted and everything has more than one meaning; typical of a "classical" T'ai Chi Ch'uan Form!

As stated above, practising the Form with a mind to applications will help improve the quality of your Form. More importantly practising in that way will also develop "Ye" which in turn will develop qi and li energies. Some people may argue that they are only practising Taijiquan for health; therefore they need not be bothered about such things as the self-defence applications. This is a wrong way of looking at it and westerners get confused between health issues, like thinking that because they are moving (physical) they will be healthier. The Mind and the Qi/Ch'i also need to play a part in better health as they all work together in the body.

40 - Single Whip.

Step back to the Left - towards the 8 o'clock direction - with your left foot. Your hands are in front of your chest but not touching.

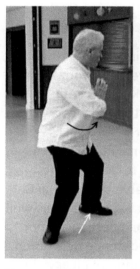 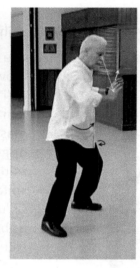 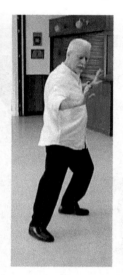

Next, push the hands forward gently as though swimming and parting the water. (The whole of Single Whip is shown above)

Separate your right palm whilst keeping your weight upon your left leg. The eyes are looking at your right palm in this instance (shown by dotted line and arrow) and you should allow your hips to "sink" naturally onto the left leg.

41 - Three Point Stance & Punch Under Elbow.

Turn your right foot and right hand in (as shown in image left) and transfer your weight to your right leg. Withdraw into Left Cat Stance. From this movement your weight should "corkscrew" onto your right leg and you use the left vertical palm to deflect a punch to your left side of head. This posture is "Three Point Stance" and your teacher will guide you as to what the proper angles and adjustments are.

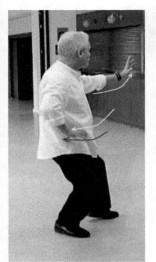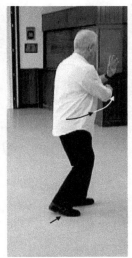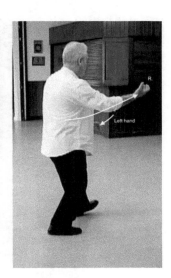

From the conclusion of Three Point Stance, step up with Hidden Punch Under Elbow (image above centre). This uses the classical Follow Step routine which was imported from Pa Kua Ch'uan (Eight Diagrams Boxing) and Hsing-I Ch'uan, a true beauty of Taoist Arts and speciality routines.

As a note of interest here, Hsing-I Ch'uan (a.k.a. Xingyiquan) uses a principle called "centre line". Many of the Sun Style Ch'uan use this method too.

The Romanised Chinese word Ch'uan (拳) can mean "fist", "hand" or "Form"; as in a Set of Chinese Boxing techniques strung together.

42 - Repulse The Monkey (6 o'clock).

Rock your weight back from left foot to right, at same time raise the right hand with palm-up in front of you (as shown left) as though holding a book in your open palm to read. The left hand begins to swing down- and-left as you prepare to step towards 6 o'clock with your left leg.

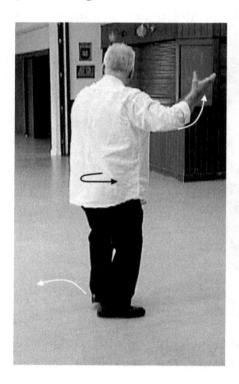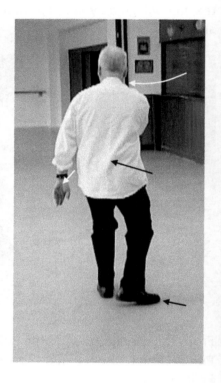

Step leftward towards 6 o'clock (as shown in picture on the left here) and complete the sweep with your left hand as you execute a push with the right hand and use Follow Step to complete the movement.

Note: Your Shih-fu will explain what the "push" is, but it is not a push! We just use that word to describe a technique which is too complicated to describe using text. Likewise the Follow Step has certain subtleties that cannot be explained on paper that well. This, like many other aspects of T'ai Chi Ch'uan, is why you really need a very good teacher; one who has himself or herself had these techniques and fine points explained to them and is able to demonstrate it as well as see and correct students who are doing it wrongly.

43 - Repulse Monkey (12 o'clock)

(Right Style)

Perform the Turning Step to turn to your right and back towards the

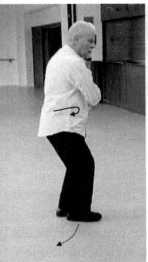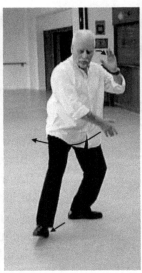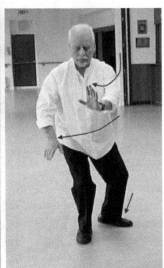

12 o'clock direction (image top left on this page).

With your weight on your left leg, step the right foot around and out diagonally (image immediate left) as you prepare to repeat the same technique, this time on the opposite side.

Continuing this flowing movement, half-step up as you deliver the "push" at chest height. The fingers of the right hand are slightly "raised", due to the nature of this technique's application, but there should be no unnatural tensions in the body or limbs at all.

Applications for this Form are varied and consequently you may see different practitioners performing this at variable heights, etcetera. One application conveys a rather wry Chinese sense of humour which reflects in the name of the technique.

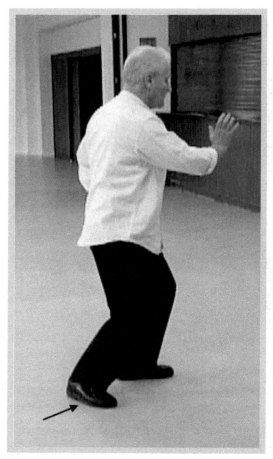

Tips: When extending your arm, in the push or strike modes, do not over-reach: this is illustrated below in the same technique but seen from the other side, so easier to understand arm positions and balance, etcetera.

Keep your weight vertical above your lead foot and stay relaxed. Allow your weight to sink and settle by relaxing into the stance. Because you are physically double-weighting to one side it is very important to counter this with the use of qi. Ask your Shih-fu to teach you how to avoid the pitfalls of double-weighting in this and similar techniques.

44 - Brush Knee Twist Step.

Stepping left towards 9 o'clock, perform "left style" Brush Knee and Twist Step as you have done before. When you have completed this technique, leave the weight on your left leg (as it is in the top right illustration) in readiness for the next part.

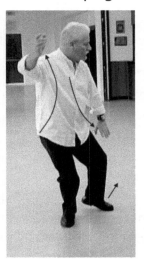 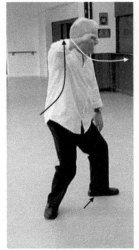 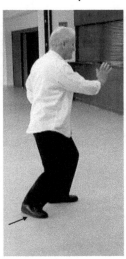

Safety Note:

The action of stepping off to the left, or right when done on opposite side, can have quite a strong torque effect on the ankles. For those with arthritis or other joint problems the effect can be felt on the ankles, knees or hip.

For the sake of safety and ease of movement generally, students should be taught how to pivot their foot slightly before stepping; e.g. in the illustration top left, pivot the right foot on the heel to turn the toes towards 11 o'clock or SSE direction before stepping out with the left foot.

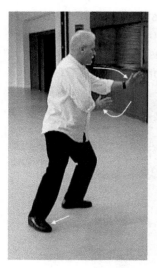 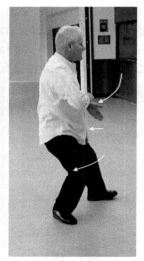

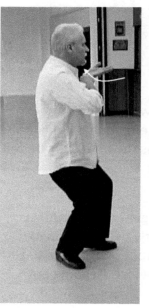

Step back with your right foot to give support without losing ground. Bring your right hand down and back towards the abdomen as the left hand circles forward-down-and-back to join the right hand images above).

Place your "sword fingers" on left wrist (image, left) and then transfer your weight to the rear leg as you bring both hands up the centre-line to just under the chin. Continue with a forwards thrust of the upright palm and a weight shift to the left leg.

(Continued on next page)

Then pivot the waist slightly as you take the palm to your left shoulder in Monkey Stance.

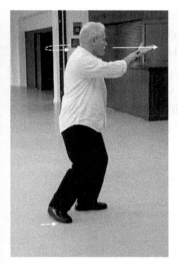 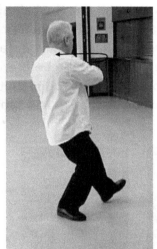

Finish by transferring weight forward again with the enhanced palm-push. In this instance you pivot on the left heel after changing most of the weight to the right leg.

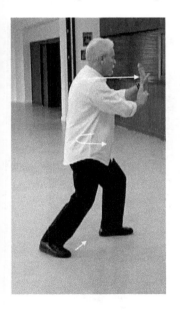

46 - Opening and Closing Hands.

Turn to face 12 o'clock directions you have done before, by shifting weight carefully and pivoting on the ball-of-foot or heel; depending on which way you are coming from, left or right. In Perform Open and Close Hands with the same relaxed state and focused consciousness that you have done before. Just because this is the end of the Form does not mean to say that you can allow yourself to "drift off" as this will be disruptive and spoil all the work you have done so far.

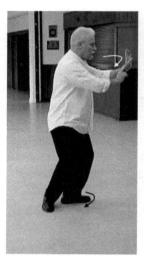
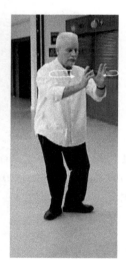

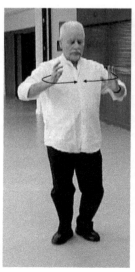
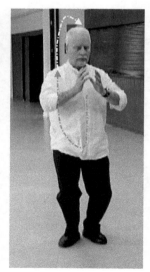

Closing Form.

Shih-fu's Advice: You have generated much new Ch'i whilst doing your Form. Now is the time to save that energy and store it at the Tan T'ien, but first you must use Open and Close Hands to link the last technique and the closing Form. Stay alert but calm.

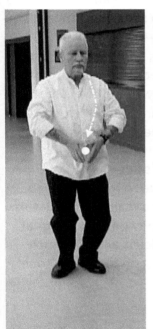

(Illustration left)
Bring your qi from the centre, up your spine and over your head as you bring both hands down, then up the centre-line.

Continue smoothly and without hesitation to bring your ch'i down the front of the body to the Tan T'ien (Dantian or Tanden) as you store the ch'i there (illustration on top right) - Tan T'ien indicated by a white circle.

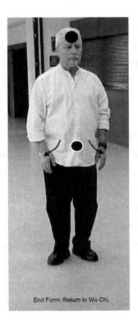

(Illustration right) When you have centred the ch'i you must return to your Wu Chi State (Wuji), from whence you started the Form. The black circles indicate Wu Chi; as described in the accompanying book to this series 'Practical Philosophy of Tao'. Remain there for a few moments or until you re-start the Form and do it another two times at least.

End Form: Return to Wu Chi.

End Notes:

This Form has been made more manageable for older people with balance problems, general weakness or those who suffer from arthritis or one of its many related diseases. Based on the variation of Competition Sun Style, that Dr Lam teaches under the title of "Tai Chi for Arthritis", which in itself is a variation of the Sun Style Competition Form that is a variant of the Sun Style Family Form, this 46 Form variation has been converted back to something more like the original "family style" of Sun ("Soon-g") Lu-t'ang; itself a compilation of Wu/Hao, Hsing-I and Ch'i Kung; with all respects to the Sun family for the changes; many older people in the western world cannot manage the twisting kicks and awkward turns of the original Form; this may be due to differences in skeletal structure between many Chinese and Westerners – a medical report publishes some years ago noted the differences between most Westerner's knees, for example, and most Chinese people's knees, the latter being bigger, thicker and stronger; perhaps due to more manual labour and squatting over the years. One of the main causes of this stronger knee would be Chinese toilets, whereby one has to squat and crouch over a hole in the floor. This practice is actually much better for evacuation of the bowels than sitting on a western toilet is.

Shih-fu Symonds has taught Tai Chi for Arthritis since 1998, having been qualified by Dr Paul Lam over a four year period of training, but in his experience he noticed that there were some extra beneficial "physical aspects" that could be added. Adding to the Form a part he inserted as "Part Three", made a noticeable difference to his class of mainly older students. The inserted part is "variable" in performance, according to the health and ability of the individual, and makes the whole Form more beneficial to the legs, back, chest and shoulders, also improving strength and balance. After much consideration the improvements were made in the same vein as Sun Style was developed in the first place; borrowing some movements from Hsing-I (which Shih-fu Symonds has also studied) in the main and also from the original Sun Style Form. Although these changes are made with no disrespect to Sun Style or Dr Lams TCA, they were made to benefit students with special needs, many of whom improve health and ability so much that they go on to learn more traditional Forms and/or much more active lives.

This teaching within T'ien Ti Tao is done in a completely traditional and non-commercial manner.

Apologies are offered to anyone who practices the traditional Sun Family Forms and who feels that they do not like the changes to the original Form, or feels that all people, even the sick, should do the full traditional Forms. Master Sun, Lu-tang, it is said, developed his original Form as much for health as self-defence, although he did include some spinning kicks which people with disabilities find difficult. In traditional China you would find that Doctors would send along people with heart conditions, high blood pressure and arthritis to a T'ai Chi Ch'uan class to help them gain strength. However, in old China and still in many places today, other more debilitating diseases like MS and Osteoporosis were either unheard of or sufferers were kept "hidden" from public view. In the western world we have people asking for T'ai Chi for *Health* specifically because their "dis-ease" prohibits them from some of the more difficult moves of the traditional Forms, like squatting low, stooping, high kicks and spinning turns. Any "modernisations" effected herein, alongside Dr Paul Lam's changes and any others, are considered to be essential and not just a whim.

The Future?

Through the efforts of Dr Paul Lam in creating a plan for those less able, this type of class has taken off. Many forward thinking medical practitioners around the world have studied and the benefits and found them to be positive. T'ai Chi Ch'uan was, it is said, originally developed as a health exercise through "Chinese Boxing" practice; giving a wider range of movement than most other methods of exercise. Therefore I see this as a natural progression in the constant development of T'ai Chi Ch'uan. There may be some people who do not like this and see it as an assault on their "traditional Forms", be they Yang, Chen or what have you? It is not. This is as natural a part of T'ai Chi Ch'uan as any other. Let us face facts, there are many, many styles and different systems of Taijiquan around the world, many hundreds if not thousands in China.

The fact that it is partaken of as a health enhancing and physical strengthening exercise is nothing new at all, either in the West or the East. For many centuries Chinese doctors have said to their patients with arthritis, high blood pressure and multitude of other ailments "Go do T'ai Chi Ch'uan"! Many older people in China have taken up this form of exercise specifically on their doctor's advice and for health reasons alone. Out of those many thousands not many have ventured too far into the "deeper aspects" and philosophical twists and turns that seem to cause much "snobbery" in the Western world and such silly comments as "That's not real T'ai Chi" whilst implying theirs is, of course; Utter nonsense.

T'ai Chi Ch'uan is like any other subject that has *depth* and you do not have to be a Theoretical Physicist like Stephen Hawking, CH, CBE, FRS, FRSA or Astronomer aficionado the likes of Patrick Moore or Mike Poxon to appreciate the innate and wonderful beauty of the stars and planets that we can see from earth. You do not have to be an expert engineer to appreciate driving a well-made car and nor do you have to be an expert to appreciate T'ai Chi Ch'uan if you just wish to enjoy the health benefits and how much it makes you feel good; and enhances life and longevity too.

As the modern saying goes "Get in there!" Given time you may find that your practice gets better, deeper and more profound. The more you do the more you gain. Experts who complain that people are not doing "real T'ai Chi" are just speaking without thinking it through. Everyone has to start somewhere, but not want to share the same depth of enthusiasm, at least at first. A good teacher should inspire, and then lead students gently into the next stage. Those who want to know more will ask, or absorb.

Personally I enjoy both aspects as much as I enjoy teaching those who want better health, and equally as much as teaching those who wish to learn the fuller aspects and philosophical arms of the deeper traditional systems. Having been studying T'ai Chi Ch'uan seriously since 1975 I can honestly say that I am still learning! Here I am reminded of an interview in a Hong Kong published Martial Arts magazine in the 80's: A Martial Arts Journalist asks an old T'ai Chi Ch'uan Master "How long do you think it takes to learn T'ai Chi Ch'uan roughly?" The old master said, "*Roughly*? Oh, about two life times!" This means that if you wish to learn it smoothly" it may take four or more lifetimes!

Such is the joy of T'ai Chi Ch'uan.

Footnotes:

There are many people teaching T'ai Chi exercises "for health" and the viewpoint of T'ien Ti Tao is that this is fine as long as (1) the person teaching has a good and well trained background in T'ai Chi Ch'uan and Ch'i Kung, (2) that medical conditions are taken into account because this is important, especially in the western world; you could be sued and you should understand individual's needs and abilities; you "lead" gently to improve health the same way as you would lead gently to improve abilities in traditional practice.

The Rights and Wrongs.
One problem which can be heard regularly is that "old apple" whereby one person declares publically that his/her Form or Style has this and the other person's does not, so therefore the other person could be doing something wrong. In one example I read where someone suggested that "in real T'ai Chi Ch'uan… the movements are designed to open the meridians in a specific order…" The answer to that is that in *some* styles they do, in other styles they do not. You cannot judge one style of T'ai Chi Ch'uan just by knowing another. Do you remember the reference earlier in the book about Mr Jou, Tsung Hwa? He suggests, after many years of studying all the Five Major Forms, that one should study Chen, Yang and Wu, just to get an idea what the concepts of T'ai Chi Ch'uan are. This implies that which we already know, each of these three styles has a vastly different appearance, and approach, to the others.

My advice?

Find the one you like and practice that until (a) you start to master it or (b) you decide it is time to change, but do not study one and debase another that you do not know.

Chapter Thirteen

T'AI CHI ASSOCIATED EXERCISES

Compatible exercise to deepen your understanding,
solo or partner practice.

WATER

The element which gives us life
Can also bring some grief and strife;
With flooding comes death and pain,
Caused by torrents of falling rain.

Snow-caps melting into mountain stream,
By which animals graze and walkers dream,
Serving all of life along its winding course,
From minuscule bugs to the noble horse.
Droplets of dew cling to grassy stem,
The sun makes it glitter like precious gem.
Surfers gybe atop ocean wave;
Dancing on many a sailor's grave.

The sun turns sea to misty clouds
That drifts over land like heavenly shrouds.
Cooling it falls over land as rain or snow,
Where children play and food will grow.

From sea to sky to earth then lake,
Finally water from the tap we take.
We brew our tea and drink our beer,
And sometimes we will shed a tear
Which drops to the ground, evaporates;
For a future eye that teardrop awaits.
Water so often taken for granted.
(©Shih-fu Myke Symonds - c.1986)

T'ai Chi Partner Exercises.

In this chapter we will take a look at some of the better known adjuncts to Taijiquan practice. These are used either as separate exercises systems, introductions, qi boosters or methods to concentrate particular effects and enhance practice, health and strength.

Taiji Ruler System

T'ai Chi Chih/Ruler (The nearest English pronunciation guide for Chih – ruler - is "Chr"). Another exercise of Taoist origin, the Chih has been used in T'ien Ti Tao's health classes as it has been shown to have a healing effect on diseases relating to the digestive system and other common ailments that we find in busy modern day living. There are different sets of Chih, set out according to needs of the developer. Generally the Ruler can be used for health or Health Qigong/Ch'i Kung but it can also be used in conjunction with the T'ai Chi Ch'uan Form, to develop stronger ch'i flow.

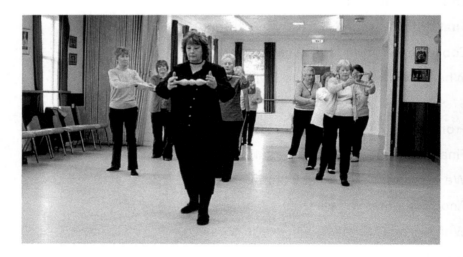

The history or origin of the Ruler system, a 7 stage system of qigong, is clouded in myth and legend, as are many of the stories concerning things Chinese. Suffice it to say that during the Sung Dynasty (960-1278c.e.), a famous Taoist hermit by the name of Chen Hsi Yi (also known as Fu Yao Tzu and Chen Tu Nan), was asked by his long-time friend, the Emperor Chao Kang Yan, to teach him esoteric methods to develop his inner powers, so that he could be a better and wiser ruler of his subjects. The exercises that were taught to the Emperor were passed down as a family treasure, a secret, for many centuries. One of the descendants of Emperor Chou was called Chao Chung Tao, and he brought the Ruler method into the public during the last years of his life.

Master Chao was born in 1844 and died when he was 122. He attributed his long life to the practice of the Ruler System.

In the 1860's, the grandmother of Chao began teaching him the Ruler system; she herself was well over 100 years of age at that time. How he came to study was an interesting tale in and of it. It seems that Chao came from a well to do family, and as a youth, he was very fond of all manner of Martial Arts. After studying various forms and styles from a young age, his Grandmother called in the teachers, and asked for any one of them to attack her. The teachers were incredulous at the offer, until the grandmother started to insult their methods and skill levels. One of them got up and dashed towards her, intent on giving her that which she requested. To the astonishment of young Chao, and the other teachers present, the old lady repelled the attacker, knocking him to the ground in one move. After seeing this, young Chao inquired of his grandmother as to what marvellous technique she had used. She replied that if he was to find out, that he must practice, and discover the secrets himself. After that experience Chao Chung Tao devoted himself to training under his grandmother's instruction.

Ch'ang Chuan or Zhang Zhuan.

This exercise literally translated as "Standing like a post", and named that way for good reason, is one of the kingpins of static qigong. It may be Yin on the outside but the Yang on the inside is as powerful as a large waterfall! Your instructor will tell you exactly what to do and why you are doing it, but below is the basic guidelines to help you recall the sequences in the correct order whilst you are learning.

There are five transitions to this preparation:

1. Stand in Eagle Stance (Wuji Zhang), hands by the sides. Eyes closed. Gather your thoughts and energies.

2. When you are ready, transfer your weight to your left leg. Move your right foot approximately twelve kun/inches to the right.

3. Transfer your weight to your right leg and then slowly glide the left foot up beside the right foot.

4. Keeping your weight on your right foot, take the left foot out to the left to a distance of approximate equal to the width of the shoulders. Bear Stance. Place the left foot down and distribute the weight to 50/50 proportions. The toes should be pointing slightly inwards. Bend your knees so that the patella comes out no further forward then the first joint of the toes.

5. With relaxed shoulders, raise both arms as though floating upwards whilst holding a large beach ball between your hands and chest. The elbows are bent and slightly downwards. Imagine that you are holding a small ball between the hands. Imagine also that there is a medium size ball between your knees, thus forcing or "springing" them outwards. Your jaw should be relaxed, teeth

slightly parted and mouth relaxed with the tip of the tongue on the upper palate. Gaze at the "ball of ch'i" between the hands.

Once in Three Circles Stance focus your thoughts on the Tan T'ien ("Dantian") breathing and remain in this posture for at least eight minutes. Let your mind clear of all thoughts. After eight minutes have elapsed concentrate on the Tan T'ien for approximately one minute.

6. When finishing: Slowly bring your hands in towards the body, without touching, and rub the palms together briskly. Close your eyes. Place the palms over your eyes and visualise absorbing the ch'i as you "dab" your palms over the eyes. Slowly open the eyes as you remove the palms for the last time.

7. Return slowly to Wuji Zhang Stance and then walk about briskly for a minute or two. Some variants in the walking warm up consist of opening and closing the hands, circling the arms or just concentrating on breathing.

8. Stand quietly for a few moments whilst the ch'i settles and you "return" gently to the outside world.

This exercise is not only beneficial before practice of T'ai Chi Ch'uan but can be practised every day as a healthy Ch'i Kung exercise. Try to increase the time in standing in Three Circles Stance by one minute each week for three weeks, then by week four to eight minutes. After six months you should find that you can maintain the Three Circles Stance for around thirty minutes. By this time you should be able to feel your ch'i moving around in your arms, legs and body, building up in intensity. At this stage you are likely to experience many involuntary actions, like trembles, spasms, twitches, itching or vibrations in the legs, arms or body. When this happens do not be alarmed or try to fight it. It is perfectly natural and harmless as it part of the transformational progression of your body's bio energy controlled processes. Relax and it will pass. This is a manifestation of the old adage, "In stillness movement will be created".

Advanced methods of Zhang Zhuan can include some variation to posture or how you perceive your posture. Martial versions also exist and are very powerful in developing Taijiquan even further. You will need a very good teacher to show you and guide you carefully through these exercises as doing them incorrectly can cause problems.

In T'ien Ti Tao Ch'uan-shu we usually commence Taiji Form practice with the New Standardised Pa Tuan Chin (Eight Strands of Silk Brocade): Book – 'Qigong & Baduanjin' ISBN: 9780954293222.

These exercises can help beginners become more gently attuned to the practice of T'ai Chi Ch'uan as they have similar qualities. Pa Tuan Chin can also strengthen the body as well as build the ch'i.

T'ai Chi Ball

We have big balls and small balls used in Chinese C'hi Kung/qigong, each used differently. The small balls come in pairs, are made of metal with Cloisonné enamel work motifs or designs on the surface. Inside a hollow brass case are some small bells, so that when the balls 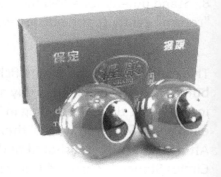 are turned in the hand a pleasant chiming sound can be heard; this should be heard instead of a "clunk" of the two balls banging together, they should not clunk. You should be able to buy some of these from most Chinese Gift Shops, or via mail order.

Many people who suffer from arthritis in the hands and fingers find that playing with the balls is very helpful and can bring some relief. The two balls are cupped in one hand and gently move the fingers to manipulate them, so swapping them from side to side, without banging them together. This is much harder than it sounds. Not only will this simple exercise help relieve the symptoms of arthritis in the hands but it will also strengthen the fingers. I would highly recommend this for anyone who does a lot of typing on computer keyboards, helping avoid or reduce risk of Repetitive Strain Injuries.

Big T'ai Chi Balls.

The larger T'ai Chi Balls were traditionally made from a round Gourd; dried out, hollowed and hardened. These would have "lucky coins" inside to make a jingling sound as they are rolled around. The large ball is passed from one hand to the other, may be rolled across the arms or upper back, and passed around the waist. The specific movements may be designed to meet each different style of T'ai Chi Ch'uan. The ball may weigh anything from just a few pounds/kilos to around 20 plus, so do not think that a football would do!

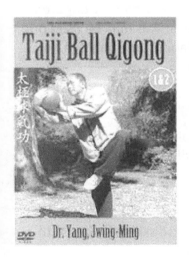

Taiji Ball Qigong

Dr. Yang, Jwing-Ming

If you would like to know more about this I would suggest visiting Dr. Yang Jwing Ming's website or obtaining his video or books on the subject. He is a man who has studied many styles and aspects of traditional Chinese Arts, one at a time, and has vast knowledge to share with the world on these.

This is Dr Yang's DVD entitled "Taiji Ball Qigong" which may be obtained either direct from his web-site or via mail order outlets.

The effects of T'ai Chi Ball are many, including building strong, flowing qi, a strong back legs, arms and shoulders, focus and concentration, practical skills in the application of Taijiquan and so on. Many of the "old school" practitioners use the Taiji Ball for enhancing their health and skills.

While it is not necessary for keen or advanced practitioners to play Taiji Ball it will enhance strength and skills. Most people in Europe or USA may be thwarted by the fact that trying to find a purchasable Taiji Ball is even worse than trying to find information about the practice! At the time of writing this – late 2014 – the sale of them in UK is non-existent, and even trying to find a shop in China is difficult. Alternatives that are more readily available, just to get you started, might include ten-pin bowling balls, medicine balls or even a carved wooden ball; if you can find someone to make one.

T'ai Ching Bang.
The Taiji Bang is a small stick, approximately the diameter of your grip and about 12" long. This simple implement is used with a set of exercises to strengthen the wrists and arms. Used on a regular training course it will increase flexibility of the wrists, strengthen and "elasticate" ligaments and arm muscles. This may be used prior to learning one of the heavier T'ai Chi weapons, the Taijidao, for example.

T'ai Chi Push Hands.
This is an integral part of any Taijiquan training. Depending on the style, this may be either Push Hands or Adhering Hands. Quite a profound difference exists between to two. Push Hands is more often associated with Yang Style, Adhering Hands with Wu or Li.

While the object of the exercise is to increase skills in relation to working with another person, the two styles may be said to be obviously different. The main difference is in stances and postures. In the former the stance may be higher and wider with more of a "face on" posture. In the latter the posture should be more natural and "slanted" with a smaller or more natural stance.

As T'ai Chi Ch'uan is a self-defence system it is highly recommended that all students are taught this and that they reach a proficient skill level. In Li/Lee Family style the proficiency of one's Adhering Hands was tested in Instructor Grading sessions. The application varies from person to person, but the requirements should be the same; e.g. to relax and react, not be tense or forceful! The finer points are not suitable for inclusion in a book as, like the main Form itself, it needs to be shown by a competent instructor with a watchful eye.

Partner Work.
In Jingquanshi we have exercise that can be performed with a partner other than I Fou Shou. These are also quintessential for the understanding of Taiji energies. For simplicity we use western terms, such as "Floating, sinking and drifting hands", then there is "Snake hands" (and yes, we know a snake does not have hands!) and Whirling Arms or Adhering Legs. All of these aspects help to improve skills and knowledge and to deepen the effects of applications. There is far too much to these exercises to put into one chapter and a book is not really the appropriate place; many descriptions defy words.

Chapter Fourteen

Teaching Supplements.

Including 'Flash Cards' to copy and use in class.

Flash Cards.

On the following pages you will see some "flash cards" as they are generally called these days. The author gives permission for these pages *only* to be photocopied onto separate sheets of A4 or Letter size paper and used in classes.

The first image is Wuchi. This describes the pre-universal state, before the "big bang" or creation of order from chaos. We use this image to reflect the mental and physical state that we attain before starting the Form.

The second image is T'ai Chi. This represents, among other things, creation, beginning and expansion.

The third image is one that we are all more familiar with, Tao. This symbol is often called Yin & Yang because this graphic illustrates perfectly the relationship of the two main forces. It also demonstrates power, advancement, harmony and change, plus many other aspects that we find in Universal Nature and of course T'ai Chi Ch'uan.

The other symbols are explained after that and are simple enough to draw or explain. Each has relevance in practice. If you are a student, ask your teacher to explain these things. If you are a teacher, then you should already know about them and their place in T'ai Chi Ch'uan.

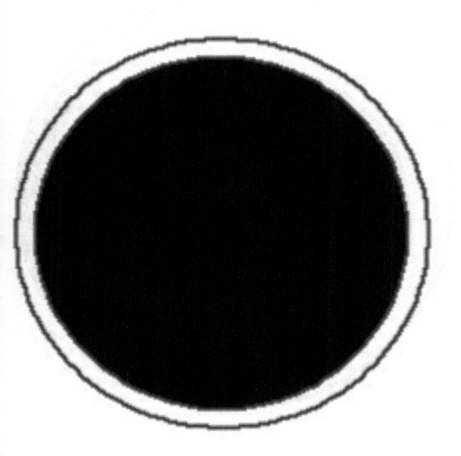

Wu Chi or Wuji.

A state of emptiness or inaction.

Related to the philosophical state of the Universe before the so-called "Big Bang"; sometimes referred to as "random chaos".

In Taijiquan we become motionless, as much as humanly possible, and empty the mind of all thoughts, feelings and actions, except awareness.

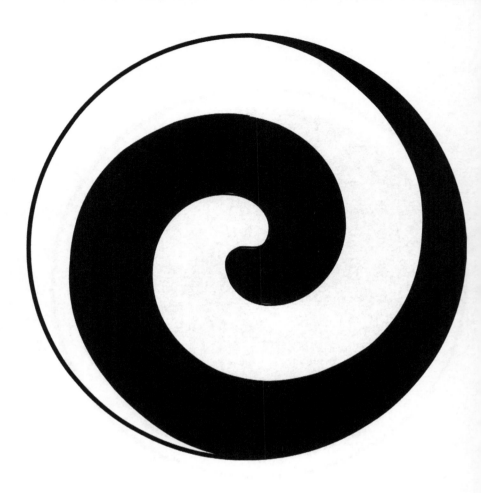

T'ai Chi; illustrated with spirals expanding outwards from the centre.
This represents "creation" from the "big bang".

In the Form we begin moving when stimulus demands. Stimulus
creates reaction, reaction creates action and action begins to spiral
or expand from the centre.

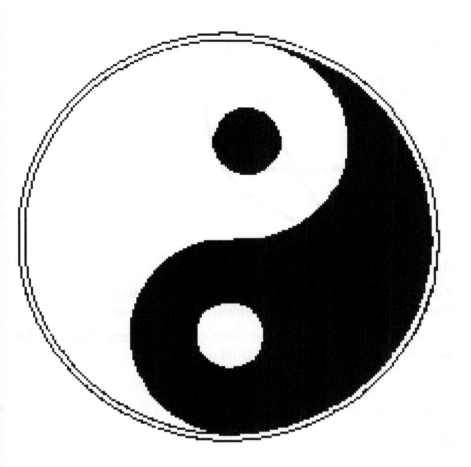

Tao: Yin and Yang (also called "T'ai Chi" sometimes).

This graphic illustrates clearly the result of "creation" at it continues to evolve, revolve or spiral. It is Yin and Yang, each following the other, each supporting the other.

Yin creates Yang and Yang creates Yin. Neither is more important than the other and neither could exist without the other. In all movements great attention should be paid to Yin and Yang at all times.

450

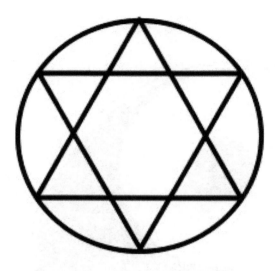

Dual Monism.

Yin – the triangle that points down wards- is a Monism.
Yang – the triangle that points upwards – is a Monism.

The two combined are Dual, so being called "dualism". Because the two are inseparable this forms Dual-monism.

Pa Kua/Bagua.

The natural actions of creation and expansion, contraction and change (dual-monism) form all things that we know within the Universe.

The sister Art of T'ai Chi Ch'uan is Pa Kua Ch'uan. This uses the Pa Kua in a very effective and innovative manner to guide the trainee through the various Boxing sequences that reflect the philosophical principles of the Pa Kua. Fascinating studies and another great "style"!

Taoist Philosophy uses images to describe each main factor and in the above illustration we see the Pa Kua or Bagua. These simple yet clever symbols use a Trigram made of three lines, either solid (Yang) or broken (Yin) to describe Universal features or actions. Here on the right we see a Hexagram, made up of two Trigrams, this one shows the Yin over the Yang, which examples "wise control" or passive control, exemplified in Taijiquan.

The symbols of the Pa Kua can be used to describe not only Nature's phenomena but also the basic movements of T'ai Chi Ch'uan; e.g. K'en = Shoulder press, Ch'ien = Ward-off, K'un = Roll Back, etcetera. Chapter 7 already deals with this and there is no need to elaborate further. Those who practice proper or "real" T'ai Chi Ch'uan will know about these principles. If someone has a Form which does not adhere to these basic principles then it is simply not Taijiquan at all but just soft, empty movements.

It matters not whether you teach the Chinese names with each technique but students should understand the philosophy of the technique. Each technique has a principle which should link and flow with the next one.

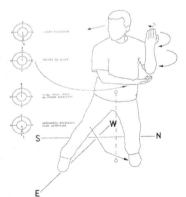

E.g. this is "Ward-off" followed by "Roll back" and then "Press"; "push" is an option. The teacher's job is to explain when and where each technique is used, or maybe used. Students must remain relaxed and in harmony with all the principles of T'ai Chi Ch'uan otherwise their practice will be almost futile.

In the western world where muscles and outward image seems more important than inward image and deeper understanding it may be easier to become blasé or confused about the Chinese principles. The Chinese are deep thinkers, generally, and do not take much for granted. Practice of this Fine Art is done internally, not externally; the mind leads the body and the spirit leads the mind, the mind then learns how to lead the qi and the body follows.

As I wrote this section one of my students diligently asked for more details of Ch'ang Chuan – "Standing as though holding a post" – ch'i kung. It was my pleasure to inform him of the finer details that will both enhance his health and his understanding and performance of the T'ai Chi Ch'uan.

Teachers have to learn too. My advice to teachers is to tell students that they must practice, practice and practice more. My Old Master, C. Chee Soo, used to say "Practice makes *almost* perfect". There should be a stage in everyone's training when they wonder "what?" or "why?" a certain technique is done this way, or what is happening inside the body, to the ch'i or what exactly is the purpose behind a specific action. Encourage students to ask questions. If you dear reader are a student, then ask your teacher questions about posture, ch'i or techniques at any time you have the inclination to wonder about it. A teacher should never tell you not to ask questions or to be quiet; that would be a probable sign that the teacher does not actually know the answer or does not genuinely know the Arts! Sometimes an answer may be verbal and other times a demonstration of the movement, or more precisely how the movement is created.

A student needs to be willing to learn, open to instruction. The teacher will demonstrate, or explain and demonstrate. The student tries to learn. After this comes the questions and "polishing up". You will always be polishing up!

You may be surprised at the complexity of the Art at first, but later you may be fascinated by the simplicity of it too. Like the practical philosophy of Tao that T'ai Chi Ch'uan is founded upon, the principles are at first as hard to grasp as a bar of soap in the shower! Do not try to read things into the practice that are not there, or be too intellectual about it. Tao is simple, uncluttered and natural. When Shih-fu Soo was asked "Just how can we attain Tao?" he paused, thought and then replied "It's like sitting in the bathtub and trying to grab the bar of wet soap. The harder you try to grip the soap the more it eludes you. Relax, open your hand, cup the soap and allow it to sit there. Finding Tao is like this. This same wonderful analogy I shall use for T'ai Chi Ch'uan also.

Relax, feel the movements and let it come naturally. We have to try at first, in order to learn the postures and principles, but after we have learned then we must relax and let them come to us. Just do not get lazy or sloppy! If you are lucky enough to have a genuine teacher of this wonderful Art then he or she will be able to explain the principles of the movements, the Mind, body and ch'i, as well as the levels of practice, the art of breathing, breathing without breathing, heel breathing or even back breathing. A teacher will be so familiar with the correct principles that s/he will spot the slightest postural tension, toe or knee in the wrong position or even mind in the wrong place. The Chinese say "It takes ten years to make a teacher, twenty years to make a good one!"

KUOSHU

National Arts. The Chinese traditional "Five Excellences".
These may include Ch'uan-shu (Boxing skills), Calligraphy, Art,
Cooking and/or herbs, plus Healing. These five skills are said to make
the perfect person.

How does this translate into modern society? This depends on your
point of view somewhat. Staunch Chinese traditionalists may say
that the original concepts are "it" and that should not be changed.
Others may say that as times change we adapt and that a certain
amount of change is inevitable. This is one argument that I shall not
try to settle; "Each to his own" as they say.

Ch'uan-shu is one requirement that I would not argue. I think that
anyone of a reasonable age should learn at least a basic style of
Chinese Boxing before approaching the more highly developed and
specialised T'ai Chi Ch'uan. This is simple foundation building.

A Picture Is Worth A Thousand Words.
Art may constitute the traditional Chinese Art, using calligraphy

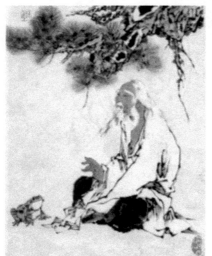

brushes and charcoal inks, to the
Chinese, but may be using Oils or
Watercolour in the west. It might
also include photography, the art of
seeing, framing and composing, or
even playing skilfully a musical
instrument. There are many aspects
to Art. Studying and practising
several Arts is said to make a
person whole.

You Are What You Eat.

Diet and cooking is another area which should be understood. The human body is designed to run on herbs, for the "design" is that of a herbivore system. Pedantic detail is not going to be argued here, suffice it to say that over a few thousand years some have had to adapt to a carnivore diet to survive, but that does not change the design. Full details can be found in this series' sister book, 'Tai Chi Diet: food for life'. However, if you want an inspiring example, there are Taoist living to between 120 and 140 years in Wudang that simply live on herbs (natural plant food from the jungle), water and Qigong.

Other aspects of lifestyle are important too. Where you live affects your health; traffic fumes and exhaust dust, diesel fumes, chemical spray and many other "unseen" elements. Try if you can to avoid anything unnatural things, and if you cannot then try at least to move to a cleaner area. Not so easy on this small island!

Clothing is all man-made. For better health avoid materials such as nylon. The Chinese traditional work and leisure attire is made of cotton, hard wearing and practical. Importantly cotton does not interfere with the flow of the ch'i. Personally, like many other people, I do not condone the making of silk in which millions of silk moths Pupae are boiled to death to obtain their cocoons. Many Chinese wear an artificial silk or "acetate" material for smarter clothes. Dress sense is also covered in the diet book and, I believe, mentioned in 'Qigong & Baduanjin' book too. High heels can be detrimental to balance, even on trainers; if you look at trainers most have a high heel of at least two inches. Flatter shoes offer better balance and foot control. Pay attention to detail.

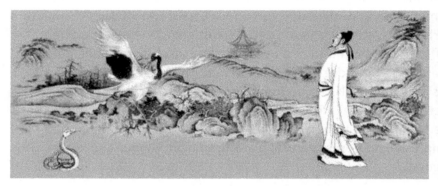

Chinese painting depicting Ch'eung Sam-feng witnessing the fight between a Crane and Snake that inspired him to create a "complete Taoist Boxing exercise.

Closing Notes.

Since my early childhood days of punching, throwing and "shadow boxing" practice in the house I was born in, it has always been my destiny. Spiritual Guidance has kept me on the long and often arduous path to learning, improving and seeking the truth. While most people wondered what I was doing, why I was being "different" and some even accused me of being a troublemaker or rebel, just because I did not agree with their way; these types are often bullies or in later life people who try to assert their opinions on others, become a bully hiding behind a uniform or similar, but just because the two personalities are Yin and Yang does not make it acceptable! Oft times I felt that I would rather be in another life, doing "easier" things or having a less stressful time of things. Yet still life finds me persisting with the task of communications, opening doors to the general public and trying to help more people become aware that *they* have the power to change things, *you* have the power and that power is rooted in Tao; the Natural Way.

To be a practitioner of T'ai Ch'i Ch'uan is a wonderful thing indeed. To be a teacher of T'ai Ch'i Ch'uan is a privilege and one that must never be abused; no "power or position" in society should ever be abused; abuse includes snobbery, the "I am better than..." syndrome (ego) and of course taking advantage of those in your care as well as abuse of powers in any society position. To be a teacher of Taoist Arts means that you are holding valuable tools, knowledge and personal empowerment, that can set many people free. The human form consists of flesh, organs, blood, bones and spirit. The body can be beaten, the bones broken, the blood spilled, but the spirit cannot be killed for it is pure energy and survives the body, but builds in strength and wisdom. Human energies, like the materials, are all part of the Universe. Tao is the Universe, we are part of Tao. Never forget that.

Those with serious mental health problems, dictators, forceful politicians, terrorists, despot rulers, violent attackers and murderers cannot alter Tao and cannot defeat energies, including the indomitable human spirit. Madness divides. Unity is Tao.

Practice should be maintained. At times it may be difficult or even tiring: e.g. when having to repeat a movement many times in order to get it right. One may flag mentally, for the Mind is not always in either a receptive or positive state, just like Tao and Yin/Yang, it has its fluctuations. Allow yourself a rest, but whatever you do, do not get bored or drift away! Your losses would be great and all that good that you have built up may come undone fairly quickly. Maintain the better health, the mental focus and the calmer persona that you have built up in practice.

When the initial movements have be learned, to a stage where you do not have to think too much about what you are doing or which way you are going, then look at its meaning. Look at the direction, relating to Pa Kua, or the action that it takes. Learn to relax, sink and be natural in all your movements. That alone will take several years to master! Then you can go on to develop even deeper skills, more mindful actions.

T'ai Chi Ch'uan is not a pool to dip toes into; it is an ocean, as deep and as wide as all the oceans on Earth and with unending secrets in its depths, wonders in the shallows.

Re-read this humble book from time to time, just one chapter at a time, so that you may digest it better. Even in this basic work there is much hidden in the depths, between the lines, or like a jigsaw puzzle, connections to be made. Diligence and observation are aided by perseverance.

Enjoy.

Shih-fu Symonds

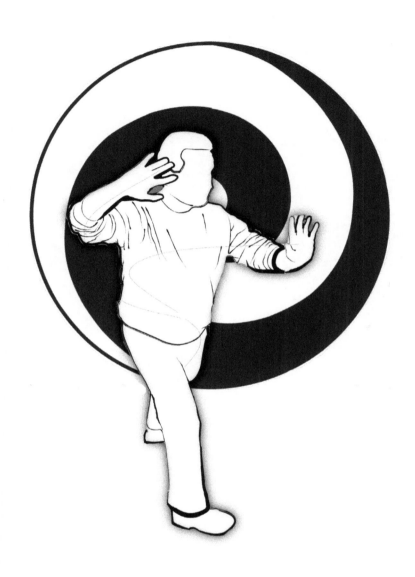